THE SWEETENER TRAP & HOW TO AVOID IT

BEATRICE TRUM HUNTER

Basic Health
PUBLICATIONS, INC.

The information contained in this book is based upon the research and personal and professional experiences of the author. It is not intended as a substitute for consulting with your physician or other healthcare provider. Any attempt to diagnose and treat an illness should be done under the direction of a healthcare professional.

The publisher does not advocate the use of any particular healthcare protocol but believes the information in this book should be available to the public. The publisher and author are not responsible for any adverse effects or consequences resulting from the use of the suggestions, preparations, or procedures discussed in this book. Should the reader have any questions concerning the appropriateness of any procedures or preparation mentioned, the author and the publisher strongly suggest consulting a professional healthcare advisor.

Basic Health Publications, Inc.

28812 Top of the World Drive • Laguna Beach, CA 92651

949-715-7327 • www.basichealthpub.com

Library of Congress Cataloging-in-Publication Data

Hunter, Beatrice Trum.
  The sweetener trap and how to avoid it / by Beatrice Trum Hunter.
    p. ; cm.
  Rev. and updated ed. of: The sugar trap and how to avoid It / Beatrice
Trum Hunter. Boston : Houghton Mifflin, 1982.
  Includes bibliographical references and index.
  ISBN 978-1-59120-179-3
  1. Sugars—Health aspects. 2. Sweeteners—Health aspects. I. Hunter,
Beatrice Trum. Sugar trap and how to avoid it. II. Title.
  [DNLM: 1. Sweetening Agents—adverse effects. 2. Diet. 3. Dietary
Sucrose—adverse effects. 4. Food Habits. WA 712 H945s 2008]

  QP702.S85H86   2008
  613.2'83—dc22

                                          2008026120

This book was published originally as *The Sugar Trap, and How to Avoid It* by Houghton Mifflin in 1982. The present edition is revised and updated.

Editor: Cheryl Hirsch
Typesetting/Book design: Gary A. Rosenberg
Cover design: Mike Stromberg

Printed in the United States of America

10 9 8 7 6 5 4 3 2 1

Contents

To H. J. Roberts, M.D.,
with homage.

THE SWEETENER TRAP: HOW DID WE GET CAUGHT?

It is important to remember that refined and processed sugars have been added to a wide range of products. Although labeling regulations do not currently require the content of the different sugars to be described, if some kind of sugar (corn syrup, fructose sugar, dextrose, honey, etc.) is listed as one of the first two or three ingredients, then one can reasonably assume that there is a lot of sugar added to the product.

—"DIETARY GOALS FOR THE UNITED STATES," PREPARED BY THE STAFF OF THE SELECT COMMITTEE ON NUTRITION AND HUMAN NEEDS, U.S. SENATE, 2ND ED. REV. DECEMBER 1977

Although we are toothless at birth, already we have acquired a sweet tooth. We have developed taste buds in our fourth month in the womb. Almost immediately after birth we respond to sweet tastes with smiles, and to bitter tastes with grimaces. As newborns, we display the same positive responses to sweet tastes as we do later as adults. With surprising precision, as infants, we are able to distinguish different levels of sweetness; like adults, we prefer high concentrations.

An inborn preference for sweets is believed to be an evolutionary adaptive mechanism that guides us to choose nutritious fruits and vegetables that are high in energy-rich carbohydrates. Many other animal species also have learned the survival value of selecting sweet plants. Our aversion to bitterness in infancy is thought to be another survival mechanism: steering us away from toxic alkaloids present in many bitter plants.

In recent times, however, our taste for sweetness has become maladaptive. As we learned to extract and concentrate the sweet components from plants, we succeeded in separating sweetness from nutrition. Our greatly increased consumption of concentrated sugars, divorced from their nutrients, is incriminated as an important factor in a wide range of health problems. The problems are compounded by the extensive use of non-caloric sweeteners.

The sweetener trap is baited early. At birth, we are offered sweetness, either with lactose, the breastmilk sugar, or with cane, beet, or corn sugars in infant feeding formulas. Sugars and sweetened foods continue to be offered in commercially prepared solid baby foods and toddler foods. Our sugar consumption is greatest between our twelfth and fourteenth years. As we mature, generally we continue to enjoy sweet tastes, and culturally acquire tastes for bitterness and for subtle mixtures of sweetness, bitterness, saltiness, and sourness.

EARLY IMPRINTING

"A company called Munchkin Bottling arranged to have soft drink logos like Mountain Dew and Pepsi placed on baby bottles. Babies are four times more likely to consume soft drinks from these as from standard bottles."

—Kelly Brownell, Ph.D., director of the Yale Center for Eating and Weight Disorders, *Food Fight: The Inside Story of the Food Industry* (McGraw-Hill, 2004)

Indisputably, we humans enjoy sweetness. In some circumstances, it is believed that our enjoyment of the food's taste may affect how well we utilize the food. In this respect, sweetness may play an important role.

In our cultural traditions, sweetness has been associated with goodness. More than sixty English phrases include sugar, and as many include honey and other syrups, all conveying positive ideas about taste, smell, appearance, acts, and characteristics. Terms of endearment include "you're my sugar," "sweetie pie," "sweetheart," and "honey."

SUGAR—A CHEAP AND PLENTIFUL ENERGY SOURCE

Sugars and starches are classified as carbohydrates, and along with proteins, fats, minerals, vitamins, and water, constitute our total nutrient content of foods and beverages consumed. Nutritionists are in general agreement that a diet comprised of about 50 percent carbohydrates is normal and healthy. However, the carbohydrates should be from fruits, vegetables, whole grains, and legumes. Instead, many of our carbohydrates are from refined sugars and flours. Because sugar is the cheapest and most plentiful food energy source available, proponents suggest that we could consume even higher levels than those being used without overstepping the bounds of moderation. They argue that in a well-balanced diet, having enough calories provided by carbohydrates and fats keep us from having to burn our protein for energy. Furthermore, they claim that sugar is eaten with foods and beverages, many of which contain specific nutrients, so the total dietary intake is not "empty calories."

This argument is specious. Sugars are simple carbohydrates; starches are complex. We utilize them differently. We metabolize sugars rapidly, and starches slowly. The candy bar is noted for its "quick energy"; a baked potato provides slow, sustained energy. Total blood fat levels of triglycerides and cholesterol are increased significantly by high-sugar diets, but not by high-starch diets.

Is sugar a cheap calorie source, as sugar proponents would have us believe? Although growing plants from which sugar is derived may require low-energy use, its refining process is energy-intensive. According to the Census of Manufacturers' standard industrial classifications, the processing of sugar beets and the refining of sugarcane, along with the milling of wet corn and the processing of malt beverages—all sources of "empty" calories—account for 20 percent of the total energy used to process food in the United States. The production of one pound of refined beet sugar requires 4,360 kilocalories, and cane sugar, 2,610 kilocalories. Yet each returns only 1,746 empty nutritional kilocalories. In Brazil, it was found that less energy was needed to ferment and distill sugar into alcohol than to refine it.

HOW MUCH SUGAR DID OUR ANCESTORS EAT?

According to historical studies, 200 years ago, Americans consumed only about four pounds of sweeteners from all sources, according to "Working Papers," *Commonwealth Research Publication*, Vol. 1, No. 3, Bolinas, California. A similar amount is quoted, also, in *Nutrition Reviews*, Vol. 32, 1974. By 1894, consumption of processed sugar in the United States reached 40 pounds, as recorded in *Historical Statistics of the United States, Colonial Times to 1959* (U.S. Bureau of Census, 1960).

Can we really view our present sugar consumption as moderate? Not by standards of human experience through many centuries, nor by those who still live elsewhere on traditional diets. Prehistoric humans consumed carbohydrates mainly from wild fruits, berries, starchy tubers, and other plants. Infrequently, they found concentrated sugars from other sources such as wild honey or licorice root, but such findings were so rare that they were recorded as special events in Stone-Age drawings and other artifacts. Currently, in a few areas of the world where people still eat their traditional foods, simple carbohydrate consumption is exceedingly low and infrequent.

HOW SUGAR BECAME A MAJOR PART
OF THE AMERICAN DIET

In the human experience, carbohydrates have been consumed commonly as complex carbohydrates. Two major events reshaped this traditional pattern. The first event was the technological development of sugarcane refining by means of centrifugal machines introduced in the mid-nineteenth century. The second event, at the end of the eighteenth century and the beginning of the nineteenth century, was the development of the sugar beet during the Napoleonic Wars, as a solution to the British blockade of continental ports, which cut off sugar supplies. The outcome of these two events was a shift away from predominantly complex carbohydrates, and a move toward simple, refined carbohydrates.

Sugar proponents insist that our sugar consumption has not increased over the last hundred years but has remained at a level of more or less 100 pounds per person annually, except during World War II when rationing forced less consumption. Our sugar consumption has *not* remained stationary over the last hundred years. This canard is founded on figures drawn from a base period of U.S. sugar consumption from 1910 to 1913, the time when collection of sugar statistics began. *Prior to that period, consumption was significantly lower.* As consumption began to increase dramatically, the need to gather such information became apparent.

A study by scientists from the Agricultural Research Service (ARS), U.S. Department of Agriculture (USDA), released in 1974, showed that per capita use of refined sugars rose 33 percent from the beginning of the twentieth century. By the early 1970s, Americans were consuming about 102 pounds of refined sugars per person annually. By 1977, the total of all sugars and other caloric sweeteners, exclusive of non-nutritive ones, reached 137.8 pounds per person annually. The annual consumption fluctuated somewhat, due to the introduction of low- and non-caloric sweeteners, but currently, the total consumption remains undesirably high, at 141.5 pounds per person.

According to another USDA study, the increased use of sucrose (sugar) is largely traceable "to the desire of food manufacturers to create unique food products with a competitive edge." Among examples cited was the practice, begun in 1948, of adding sugar to breakfast cereals in order to boost slumping cereal sales. The effort was successful, and ever since, "the profusion of varieties of cereals, soft drink, and other products represent efforts to protect market shares." Currently, more than 90 percent of cereals marketed to children are sugar coated (*Sugars in Nutrition*, Academic Press, 1974).

Not only are traditionally unsweetened foods now sweetened, but also sweetness levels are much higher. For instance, formerly bread recipes did not have sweeteners among their ingredients, and early cake recipes had far lower levels of sweetening than current ones.

Statistics for sugar consumption are divided between its industrial use to manufacture processed foods and beverages, and its home use. In 1925, almost two-thirds of all sugar was used by consumers directly within the home, and only one-third was used by industry. Gradually, there was a shift, and industrial use accounts for the major portion of all sugars used. Correspondingly, direct household use has declined.

SUGAR AND CALORIES

". . . The leading source of calories in the United States is sugared beverages, which accounts for about 7 percent of all calories consumed. This is a big part of our problem since it is so easy to consume calories in liquid form. The No. 2 source is cake and sweet rolls . . ."

—Meir J. Stamfer, M.D., Ph.D., chairman of the Department of Epidemiology, Harvard University School of Public Health, quoted in *Newsweek*, January 16, 2006

What caused this shift? Home decline was not due to lower sugar consumption, but rather from increased purchases of convenience food products. The manufacture of pre-sugared items and ready-to-eat products proliferated, especially since the 1960s. The soft drink industry uses a large part of the industrial sugar supplies, and the remainder is used mainly by bakers, canners, confectioners, and processors of ice cream and dairy products. We purchase less sugar for home use, and *we have less control over the levels of our sugar consumption than people did at the turn of the last century.*

The USDA study also showed that higher incomes result in increased purchases of convenience foods. Additional factors contribute to increased refined-sugar consumption. One is the higher proportion of teenagers and young children in our population, groups likely to consume above-average quantities of sugar by as much as 20 percent. Other factors include the development of new uses for sugar. The 1970 cyclamates ban temporarily led to the greater use of sugar to partially replace cyclamates.

Even using the 1910 to 1913 base period cited by the sugar proponents, the radical transformation of our total carbohydrate consumption is apparent. During this period, the average American ate 498 grams of total carbohydrates daily, consisting of 342 grams from starches, and only 156 grams from sugars. By 1974, the average American ate more fats and protein at the expense of somewhat fewer total carbohydrates. But the decline of total carbohydrates to 397 grams is less significant than the composition of the carbohy-drates. Starch consumption declined to 197 grams; sugar consumption rose to 200 grams. This meant that we were eating fewer complex carbohydrates such as potatoes and bread, and more simple carbohydrate such as sugar. Sugar's percentage of our total carbohydrate consumption in the 1910 to 1913 period was 31.5 percent; by 1974, it had risen to 52.6 percent. Thus, even using the sugar proponent's statistical base period, the rise in sugar consumption is well defined. A release by the Society for Nutrition Education in 1975 reported that sugar and high-sugar products had reached a stage that "the average Ameri-can now consumes his or her own weight in sugar yearly" (*Nutrition News*, Jul 1975).

THE COST OF SUGAR AS A CONTROLLED COMMODITY

The U.S. government has controlled the price of sugar for more then 200 years. At first, the goal was to raise revenue; later, to protect domestic producers' economic interests. What evolved is an elaborate system of price-support programs, import tariffs and quo-tas, developed during the Depression era and into the early years of World War II. As a result, Americans are fleeced by paying artificially high prices for sugar. Since 1985, the price of raw sugar has been from 8 to 14 cents a pound higher in U.S. markets than in world markets. By the time that sugar is sold at retail prices in the United States, the dif-ference doubles.

The decline in starch consumption due to the increased sugar consump-tion was well recognized by nutritionists. In devising the Dietary Guidelines in 1977 and the first Food Guide Pyramid in 1992, repeated recommendations urge Americans to increase consumption of complex carbohydrates and to limit consumption of added sugars and refined flours.

Another unjustified claim of the sugar defenders is that sugar is eaten with foods and beverages, many of which contain specific nutrients and make a contribution to the diet. Yet the very types of foods and beverages that have the highest levels of sugar are those that lack other nutrients, too. Soft drinks, candies, and chewing gums account for a sizable amount of sugar use. Other products, such as frozen desserts, pies, puddings, and cakes, not only have high sugar levels, but also contain objectionably high levels of undesirable types of fats and/or refined flours, and have insignificant levels of desirable nutrients such as proteins, beneficial fats, minerals, and vitamins. A high intake of sugar depletes the body of nutrients. In metabolizing the sugar, the body is forced to draw on its own supply of nutrients that have been present in the raw sugar cane but stripped from refined sugar.

Sugar consumption is likely to increase, due to our dietary patterns, which in turn, are altering radically some of our traditional cultural patterns. Home food preparation from basic commodities has continued to decline as more women work away from home. Advertising has convinced many individuals that convenience foods save time and money, although these claims are not necessarily true. With more discretionary income, many people have turned to built-in convenience, and the food industry has complied. At present, the major portion of the foods we eat is processed outside the home and the majority of these foods contain added sugars. According to predictions, increased consumption of such foods will continue, and may become nearly total. Also, Americans are eating away from home more frequently. This trend, too, may accelerate. Cultural patterns are disrupted, as many Americans no longer sit down together as a family to share meals in common, but snack individually and erratically throughout the day, in a pattern that has been termed "grazing." Snacks *can* consist of nutritious foods, but many of the ones commonly consumed are high in sugars.

SOME SYNERGISMS WITH SUCROSE

Sucrose exerts synergist effects with other ingredients, such as refined flours and salt, both of which are commonly found, along with sucrose, at high levels in the Western diet, especially in processed foods. A strong correlation exists between the increased consumption of sweetened starch-type snack foods and dental caries, and has occurred even when the per capita sugar consumption has remained constant (Dr. Abraham Nizel, *Edible TV*, Select Committee on Nutrition and Human Needs, U.S. Senate, Sept 1977). When sucrose and sodium chloride (table salt) were combined in the diet of experimental animals, sucrose had a synergistic effect and produced more hypertension than did salt alone (*American Journal of Clinical Nutrition*, Mar 1980).

SUGAR'S UBIQUITOUS PRESENCE

Sugars are well recognized in certain types of foods, where they are expected, such as in cakes, candies, puddings, jellies, and frozen desserts. But sugars are not apt to be recognized readily in foods that traditionally were not sweetened. Today, hidden sugars may be present in a wide variety of convenience foods purchased for home use or used in restaurant preparations, including cured ham, luncheon meats and frankfurters; bouillon cubes, soups and gravies; peanut butter, potato chips; dry roasted nuts; coatings for fried or baked poultry; restructured poultry; mixes intended to stretch the protein content of chopped beef; some canned and frozen vegetables, frozen and canned entrées; plain cottage cheese; instant coffee, both regular and decaffeinated, and instant tea mixes; and roasted coffee. Even iodized salt contains some sugar (to stabilize the iodide). In tests, some catsups contained a greater percentage of sugars than ice cream; some salad dressings had three times more sugar than cola drinks; and at least one non-dairy creamer contained a greater percentage of sugar then a typical chocolate candy bar.

SOFT DRINKS ARE LIQUID CANDY

"Doctors say having one regular soda is like enjoying liquid candy" intones Dina Bair, Medical Watch reporter for Chicago's WGN-TV. "In fact, it's the same as a bag of M&Ms. The problem is on average most people have three sodas a day. That's three bags of candy. At 250 calories a bag, that meant 750 calories . . . " But that's just the tip of the iceberg, Bair says, the perils of pop approach the level of a national health scandal, and she says she has sound bites from experts to prove it."

–Pierce Hollingsworth, Contributing Editor, "Artificial Sweeteners Face Sweet 'n Sour Consumer Market." *Food Technology*, July 2002

Sugar's presence need not be listed on all food labels. Even when added sugar is listed, consumers are unable to judge the amount present, because percentages of sugars are not required to be listed. Nor do present nutrition labeling regulations require that the sugar portion be stated in a listing of carbohydrates. For example, a fruit-flavored yogurt may list carbohydrates as 49 grams, compared to 17 grams for plain yogurt. Consumers cannot know how many of the 49 grams are derived from fruit and how many are from the sugar in the fruit jam that flavors the yogurt.

When consumers learned that ingredients are listed on labels in a descending order of predominance, many were surprised to learn that some presweetened breakfast cereals contained more sugars than grains. The discovery was made by noting that sugar was listed first, even before the grain. The cereal processors responded with a ruse. By reformulating and using a number of different sweeteners, they could retain the same high sweetening level in the products, but the label information made it appear that grain, listed first, predominated. In reality, it did not. For example, the original label of one hypothetical product might read: "Contains sugar, wheat, vegetable oil" (followed by other ingredients). After reformulation, the label might read: "Contains wheat, sucrose, vegetable oil, brown sugar, corn syrup solids, malt powder," (followed by other ingredients). No longer is it apparent that the total sugar content is greater than the total grain content.

PROMOTING SUGAR

According to Marion Nestle, professor and chair of the Department of Nutrition and Food Studies at New York University, supermarkets have a rule to sell as much sugar as possible. They devote 25 percent of shelf space to high-sugar products.

Consumers who read food and beverage labels assiduously may still fail to recognize the presence of sugars and sweeteners that appear under many guises. All the following are sugars and sweeteners: sucrose, dextrose, corn syrups, high-fructose corn syrup (HFCS), crystalline fructose, sorbitol, xylitol, mannitol, turbinado, raw sugar, brown sugar, molasses, sorghum, honey, maple syrup, malt syrup, maltol, and more. Some terms, such as maltodextrin and polydextrose are unfamiliar, yet they contain sugars. At times, misleading phrases are used, such as "fruit sugar" or "natural carbohydrates." While the -ose ending of words indicates that the substance is a sugar, not all sugars end in these letters.

CANDY TOOTHBRUSH

"I've seen a lot of bad sugar-delivery methods, including the liquid candy-filled baby bottle, but somehow the 'candy toothbrush' I just saw at the store seems particularly outrageous. The plastic hollow 'toothbrush' has holes in the brush . . . where, judging from the cartoonish picture on the side, foamy candy bubbles out. So you can just coat your teeth directly with sugar foam . . ."

—Jill Nienhiser, *Wise Traditions*, Fall 2005

Consumers remain ignorant about sources of hidden sugars that are used in certain industrial practices before foods reach the home or restaurant. Sugar may be added to hog feed prior to slaughter of the animals. This practice is reported to improve meat flavor and color in cured pork products. A dehydrated molasses blended with corn syrup may be added to hamburgers and other ground meats used in restaurants to help reduce shrinkage and improve the meat's flavor, juiciness, and texture. Breading, intended to coat seafood before it is deep fried, may contain sugar. Raw potato slices may be dipped in sugar solution before they are deep fried. Whole salmon may be glazed with a sugar solution before it is vacuum-packed and frozen. Honey solutions may be injected into pieces of chicken before they are fried.

HIGH-SUGAR CONSUMPTION AND HEALTH

Perhaps the first observations of human health problems related to high-sugar consumption were reported in the first century A.D. by three Hindu physicians, Caraka, Susruta, and Vaghbata. They had observed a disease that was fatal at the time (and is recognized by modern physicians as *diabetes mellitus*) and suggested that large amounts of sugar were bad for people suffering from this disease. Such warnings were not recorded again until the early nineteenth century, when refined sugar was affordable to the prosperous classes on continental Europe, in England, and in America. For the first time, quantities of sugar were consumed by the wealthy. Between 1850 and 1900, worldwide sugar consumption increased tenfold; between 1900 and 1940, it tripled. In time, its use would escalate dramatically.

In the sixteenth century, a German traveler in England, after seeing Queen Elizabeth, suggested that the good queen's blackened teeth might be due to sugar indulgence. Perhaps this was the first recorded observation that high sugar consumption may lead to dental problems. As sugar consumption increased in the developed countries in more recent times, the relationship to dental problems became apparent. Although the sugar interests vehemently reject most suspected relationships between high sugar consumption and many human health problems, they grudgingly acknowledge its role in tooth decay.

By far, the most significant human study of sugar's dental effects was conducted in Sweden, known as the Vipeholm Dental Caries Study, and reported in 1954. More than 400 mental patients were given controlled diets, and observed for five years. The adults were divided into various groups. Some ate complex and simple carbohydrates at mealtimes only, while others supplemented mealtime foods with between-meal snacks, sweetened with sucrose, chocolate, caramel, or toffee. Among the conclusions drawn from the completed study was that sucrose consumption could increase caries activity. The risk increased if the sucrose was consumed in a sticky form that adhered to the tooth's surfaces. The greatest damage was inflicted by foods with high concentrations of sucrose in sticky form, eaten between meals, even if contact with the tooth's surfaces was brief. Caries, due to the intake of foods with high sucrose levels, could be decreased if such foods were eliminated from the diet. Individual differences existed. In some individuals, despite avoidance of refined sugar or maximal restriction of natural sugars and total dietary carbohydrates, caries still developed, due to other factors.

SUGAR AFFECTS MORE THAN THE TEETH

In 1977, Dr. Herman Kraybill at the National Cancer Institute noted some of the adverse effects from high levels of sugar consumption. In humans, high-sugar intake replaces nutrient-rich foods. It contributes to the formation of dental caries. It may affect the processes of growth and maturation. If the metabolism of an individual is faulty, high-sugar intake contributes to overweight, can cause and aggravate diabetes, and may result in low blood sugar and allergies. High-sugar intake increases the risk of pancreatic cancer. It is implicated in high fat levels in the blood (both cholesterol and triglycerides). It is a suspected contributing factor in the development of atherosclerosis. In addition, Kraybill cited possible adverse health effects in humans, based on laboratory experiments. In test animals, high levels of sugar consumption increase the demands on enzyme systems of the liver and kidney, impair glucose tolerance, speed up kidney disease, and shorten the life span of the animals. Since Kraybill's litany of adverse effects from high levels of sugar consumption, many other research findings link sugar consumption with additional health problems, including an impairment of the immune system.

ENLISTING THE GOVERNMENT FOR GUIDANCE

By the 1970s, increasing numbers of nutritionists, physicians, dentists, researchers, and public health officials were voicing concerns about the public health effects from high levels of sugar consumption. A growing body of incriminating evidence associated high-sugar intake with dental caries and obesity. Additional data suggested links between high sugar consumption and a wide range of other health problems not previously linked to sugar.

In 1973, the Select Committee on Nutrition and Human Needs of the Senate (commonly called the McGovern Hearings after its chairman, Senator George McGovern, D-SD) held hearings on sugar in the diet. Professionals from here and abroad attested to the various health problems created by high sugar consumption, including conditions such as diabetes, coronary heart disease, hypoglycemia, and behavioral problems.

Information collected from these hearings, as well as in hearings held by the committee concerned with other aspects of the American diet, led to the issuance in February 1977 of the Dietary Goals for the United States. Among the recommendations, Americans were urged to increase total carbohydrate consumption so that it would comprise 55 to 60 percent of the total caloric intake, but *to reduce sugar consumption by about 40 percent so that it would account for only about 15 percent of the total caloric intake.* In order to achieve these changes, the committee recommended that Americans increase consumption of fruits, vegetables, and whole grains, and decrease consumption of sugars and food products high in added sugar.

The recommendations were reasonable and similar to dietary goals previously officially recommended by other countries. Nonetheless, publication of the Dietary Goals sparked a sensational controversy that raged for months and continues to flare up spasmodically. Affected interests, such as the sugar industry and food and beverage processors entered the fray. Some nutritionists also joined battle for various reasons, but mainly in objection to recommendations concerning fats and salt, rather than sugar. As a result, ten months later, the committee was forced to issue a revised version of the Dietary Goals. Although certain recommendations, notably concerning salt, were weakened, sugar reduction recommendations were strengthened. The committee urged Americans to increase consumption of complex carbohydrates and naturally occurring sugars from about 28 to 48 percent of total caloric intake, but *to reduce consumption of refined and other processed sugars by about 45 percent to account for about 10 percent of total caloric intake.*

SUGAR AND OBESITY

"Compared with individuals who consume small amounts of foods and beverages that are high in added sugars, those who consume large amounts tend to consume more calories but smaller amounts of micronutrients. Although more research is needed, available prospective studies suggest a positive association between the consumption of sugar-sweetened beverages and weight gain. A reduced intake of added sugars (especially sugar-sweetened beverages) may he helpful in achieving recommended intake of nutrients and in weight control."

–Dietary Guideline Advisory Committee Report, 2005

GOVERNMENT REEVALUATES HEALTH IMPACT OF SUCROSE

As part of a review of all food additives identified by the term Generally Recognized as Safe (GRAS), the Food and Drug Administration (FDA) organized a task force to evaluate the health aspects of sucrose as a food ingredient. The report, prepared by the GRAS Review Committee of the Federation of American Societies for Experimental Biology (FASEB) consisted of a four-year review of scientific literature. In 1976, the committee concluded that "reasonable evidence exists that sucrose is a contributor to the formation of dental caries" at the then current use level, and especially with sticky sweets consumed between meals. Also, the committee noted that undesirably high total-caloric intake of sugar may lead to obesity. However, the committee expressed the view that any link between sucrose and diabetes was circumstantial, and that there was no clear evidence in the available information on sucrose that demonstrated a hazard to the public when used at the then current levels and in the manner practiced. However, it was not possible to determine without additional data whether an increase in sugar consumption—that would result if there were a significant increase in the total amount of sucrose, corn sugar, corn syrup, and invert sugar added to foods—would constitute a dietary hazard.

SUCROSE AND "QUICK ENERGY"

"All carbohydrates stimulate insulin release; the more refined they are, the more dramatic is the release. Sugar (sucrose) is the most dramatic. This is because the bond in sucrose (consisting of a molecule of glucose and a molecule of fructose, two simple sugars) is very easily broken. Sucrose is rapidly absorbed by the body, releasing a surge of glucose into the bloodstream, which then stimulates the release of insulin to lower the blood sugar again. This is what lies behind the advertising pitch of 'quick energy.' Most college students have learned that a candy bar before an exam gives them a quick pick-up (a swift rise in their blood sugar) only to be followed a few hours later with the fatigue symptoms of lowered blood sugar."

—Carl C. Pfeiffer, Ph.D., M.D., *Mental and Elemental Nutrients* (Keats Publishing, 1975)

Four years later, at the end of 1980, at the completion of the first comprehensive GRAS list review, FASEB placed sucrose in Class 2, an indication that although the present levels of use were presumably safe, further data were needed.

Two researchers at the Carbohydrate Nutrition Laboratory of the Nutrition Institute, U.S. Department of Agriculture (USDA), Drs. Sheldon Reiser and Bela Szepesi, criticized FASEB's conclusions. The men charged that abundant evidence demonstrated that sucrose is an important dietary factor in diabetes, obesity, heart disease, and other health problems. They reported that ample data demonstrate the dramatic rise in diabetes incidence that occurs about one generation after a culture begins to consume high sucrose levels. Reiser and Szepesi cited the clear cause-and-effect case of Yemenite Jews who, after relocation in Israel for thirty years, experienced a "dramatic and tragic" diabetes increase from high sucrose consumption. Reiser and Szepezi's discussion of the Yemenite Jews was based on the testimony of Aharon M. Cohen, M.D., before the Hearings of the Select Committee on Nutrition and Human Needs, U.S. Senate, on April 30, 1973.

Reiser and Szepesi noted that high-sucrose intake in laboratory animals induces diabetes, but high-starch intake does not. Virtually all the clinical diabetes symptoms can be induced by feeding the animals with high-sucrose levels, but are not induced by high-fat or high-cholesterol intake.

The FASEB report did acknowledge that a segment of the population appears to have a genetic predisposition to experience large and permanent increases in blood triglycerides (fats) if they consume sucrose-containing diets. In sensitive individuals, these effects have been observed with sucrose levels as low as 20 to 25 percent of the total caloric intake of humans. *These percentages are well within the average sucrose intake range of Americans.* This type of elevated blood fats (hyperlipidemia) has been associated with health problems such as abnormal glucose tolerance, diabetes, and heart disease. Reiser and Szepesi charged that FASEB should not have concluded that sucrose intake at present levels represent no health hazard. There are millions of carbohydrate-sensitive adults in the United States. Sucrose, by itself, may be a very important cause of heart disease and diabetes in 10 percent of the population. For the remaining 90 percent, sucrose by itself may not be a *primary* risk factor. However, by virtue of its synergistic interaction with dietary fat, triglycerides, and cholesterol, sucrose must be considered as an important risk factor in vascular diseases and diabetes development. Reiser and Szepesi strongly recommended that sucrose from all sources (except fresh or processed fruits without added sugars) be decreased by a minimum of 60 percent and be replaced by complex carbohydrates from vegetables and whole-grain cereals. These recommendations reaffirmed those made earlier in the Dietary Guidelines for Americans.

In order to implement necessary reform, Reiser and Szepesi made several suggestions. There should be a concerted national effort to identify carbohydrate-sensitive individuals. These individuals should have sugar intake exclusively from fresh and processed fruits without added sugar. To protect the remaining population, food and beverage processors should be required to identify the amount of added sucrose on the labels of their products. Further, a national campaign should inform the public about the health hazards associated with high sugar consumption. We still await official actions on these worthy suggestions made by Reiser and Szepesi more than three decades ago.

DOWNPLAYING SUGAR'S HEALTH EFFECTS

In early 2003, the Sugar Association attacked a report issued jointly by the World Health Organization (WHO) and the Food and Agriculture Organization (FAO) on diet, nutrition, and health. The commonsense recommendations in the report were that people should increase consumption of fruits and vegetables, and cut down on fat and sugar consumption. According to Chris Mooney in his book, *The Republican War on Science*, the Sugar Association, an organization composed of members of the sugar industry, was enraged by the report's suggestion that people limit their intake of so-called free sugars to 10 percent of daily calories. (Free sugars, as defined by WHO, are sugars added to food products by manufacturers, cooks, or consumers. The free sugars include concentrated sugars present in honey, syrups, and fruit juices, as well as commonly used table sugars.)

In a letter dated April 14, 2003, the Sugar Association warned WHO that the association would "exercise every avenue available" to challenge the report. The association announced that it would urge members of the U.S. Congress to cut off WHO/FAO funding.

This action was followed by sugar processors and other affected industry groups such as the Corn Refiners Association (HFCS producers) requesting Tommy Thompson, Secretary of HHS, to remove a draft version of the objectionable report from WHO's website. Members of what is known as the "U.S. Senate Sweetener Caucus"—political allies of the sugar interests—including Larry Craig (R–ID) and John Breaux (D–LA) requested Thompson to instruct WHO to "cease further promotion" of the report.

On April 23, 2003, the Sugar Association, in a press conference, challenged the scientific basis of WHO's recommendation. The association cited an earlier report issued by the Institute of Medicine (IOM, an organization of the National Academics), but distorted IOM's findings. IOM had concluded that a sugar intake up to 25 percent of calories in the diet was a maximum intake level beyond which nutrient losses would occur. This statement was twisted to mean that a 25 percent sugar intake was acceptable. The statement by IOM was *not a recommendation,* but rather was *a cautionary warning.* The association's distorted interpretation was seized promptly and reported widely by segments of the media.

THE SUGAR INTERESTS AND POLITICS

". . . The Bush administration's food industries ties are, of course, extensive. As George W. Bush ran for reelection in 2004, his campaign listed among its 'Rangers'—fundraisers who raise at least $200,000 in donations—the sugar magnate Pepe Fanjul. Meanwhile, in the campaign's class of 'Pioneers' raisers of a minimum of $100,000—was Robert E. Coker, a United States Sugar Corporation senior vice president. Other Rangers and Pioneers included executives from Coca Cola . . . "

—Chris Mooney, *The Republican War on Science* (Basic Books, 2005)

Ironically, these recommendations had a wry twist. Between 1970 and 1980, Americans became weight-conscious. Although they succeeded in reducing total caloric intake by about 10 percent, they achieved it by consuming a greater proportion of calories from sugar. The increased use of sweeteners, chiefly in soft drinks, actually increased per capita sugar consumption. This increase, combined with a lower total food intake, resulted in a substantial rise in the proportion of calories from sweeteners. Despite the drop in caloric intake, the incidence of obesity increased in our population. By the end of the twentieth century, obesity was recognized as an epidemic in the United States. It also became pandemic as obesity became a problem in most developed countries, and was dubbed "globesity." Since then, official recommendations in subsequently issued Dietary Guidelines and revised Food Guide Pyramids merely offer the vague advice to "moderate use of added sugar." There is *no* advice to use highly processed foods and beverages sparingly, and *no* mention at all of the high-intensity synthetic sweeteners that are adding to the obesity problem. There is *no* mention of the linkage of high-fructose corn syrup with obesity. These unmentioned factors are ignored, but remain as the unnoticed 800-pound gorilla in the room.

Part One

TRADITIONAL SWEETENERS AND EARLY NONTRADITIONAL NEWCOMERS

Chapter 1

REFINED SWEETENERS: DESIRED, BUT UNDESIRABLE

The refining of sugar may yet prove to have been a greater tragedy for civilized man than the discovery of tobacco.
—J.A.S. DICKSON. M.D., *THE LANCET*, AUGUST 15, 1964

If only a small fraction of what is already known about the effects of sugar were to be revealed about any other material used as a food additive that material would be promptly banned.
—JOHN YUDKIN M.D., *SWEET AND DANGEROUS* (WYDEN, 1972)

Plants contain many types of sugar. For example, arabinose, raffinose, stachyose, and xylose are all plant sugars. Sucrose, however, is the most widely used sugar in our food supply. Sugarcane, the most abundant source of sucrose, is nature's most efficient solar energy trap. Like all green plants, the sugarcane collects solar energy, and by photosynthesis, converts it into sucrose. This process occurs deep inside the leaves, in cell parts called chloroplasts. With favorable conditions of temperature and moisture, the chloroplasts absorb carbon dioxide from the atmosphere, sunlight forces the release of oxygen, thereby making it possible to manufacture sucrose, which is stored in the plant's stem. Each sugarcane stalk contains about 15 percent sucrose.

When we eat sucrose, we reverse the photosynthesis process by converting the sucrose back into energy. Consumed sucrose is digested, converted into dextrose in the small intestine, and stored in the liver as glycogen. Oxygen ignites the energy cycle. Glucose, as needed, is released from glycogen into the bloodstream and metabolized by the body to create energy. The body releases carbon dioxide and water, which can be used by plants to create more sucrose. Thus, the completed cycle begins anew.

THE FIRST COMMERCIAL SUGAR

It is thought that at least 8,000 years ago sugarcane originally grew in the South Pacific. From there it was transported to India where, for the first time, juice was extracted from the cane and evaporated to a solid state called *khanda* (candy) in Sanskrit. Perhaps this product was the first processed food.

Sugarcane was known in China, where the juice was used medicinally by herbalists. By the tenth century, the Persians and Egyptians found a simple method to produce crystallized sugar from the cane. During the Crusades, samples of "honey from reeds" were taken back to Western Europe as a curiosity. Sugar remained as an expensive rarity. One of the earliest records of sugar use in Western Europe dates back to the thirteenth century when Henry III requested 3 pounds of sugar "if so much is to be had" for a notable feast. By the sixteenth century, due to brisk trade, sugar become more affordable and was used as a sweetener in British confectionery. By the seventeenth century, the growing of sugarcane and the manufacture of sugar, as well as molasses and rum, were well-established industries in tropical countries, and formed an important link in the slave trade.

The year 1800 added a new dimension. The British blockade of French ports cut off West Indian cane-sugar supplies to France. Napoleon requested French scientists to find a suitable substitute. Many plants were examined. Benjamin Delassert produced a crystallized sugar from beets and won Napoleon's Cross of Honor. Napoleon acted swiftly and energetically to establish several hundred sugar-beet refineries in order to free France from further importation of "English" sugar. The development of beet sugar challenged cane sugar's pre-eminence and enabled areas with temperate climates to compete with tropical countries for sugar markets. As rivalry rose, production increased, sugar prices declined, and the product became accessible to more people.

Both cane and beet sugars have many versatile characteristics, and both are particularly attractive to food and beverage processors. Sugar acts as a preservative with fruits, jellies, jams, and preserves, and enhances fruit flavors. In products such as canned cherries, sugar makes them plumper, less acidic, and more palatable. Sugar is useful as a curing agent for processed meats. Sugar contributes bulk and texture to ice creams, baked goods, and confections. Sugar supplies "body" to the liquid in soft drinks and makes them more appealing in the mouth than if the liquid were thinner. Sugar serves several functions in baked goods. It acts as a medium for fermentation, contributes to crust color and flavor, and retains moisture in products, which extends their shelf life.

Both cane and beet sugars are sucrose. Chemically, their structures are identical, and they are used interchangeably. Both are 99.9 percent pure, and chemists affirm that they cannot be distinguished from one another. Nonetheless, individuals highly sensitive to beets may suffer adverse reactions to beet sugar, but not to sugar derived from cane. Similarly, those who are sensitive to sugar from cane may tolerate sugar from beet.

HOW DO WE PERCEIVE SWEETNESS?

Some individuals perceive sweetness intensity at lower levels than others. Little is known about the biophysical and chemical mechanisms involved. Why are such diverse molecules as saccharin, maltol, glycine, chloroform, lead acetate, and some beryllium salts sweet? Only a few single sugars (monosaccharides) and multiple sugars (polysaccharides) are sweet. Why is cotton, a polysaccharide, tasteless, yet corn, another polysaccharide, sweet? Nor is the basis of our sweetness perception well understood. How does the sweet molecule act positively with our tongue's taste receptors? Our tongues have more then a half million taste cells, clustered in groups of about fifty cells to form taste buds. The ends of the buds are composed of tiny fingerlike projections called microvilli. Tastes occur at the microvilli that are constantly bathed in saliva. Strangely, taste can be perceived with some substances by intravenous stimulation, not in direct villi contact. Formerly, it was thought that specific taste nerves existed capable of responding only to one type of stimulus, thus giving rise to the idea of primary tastes of sweet, bitter, salt, and sour. Now, it is believed that differences exist among taste-receptor cells, but most are not specialized but respond to several tastes.

Cane sugar sensitivity was reported to the medical community as early as 1925; and beet sugar sensitivity, the following year. The possibility of cane sugar as an allergen has received scant attention, although it is part of a botanical family of cereals, with various members as common allergens. In addition, cane sugar, consumed frequently in the typical American diet, fulfills another requirement as a suspicious food allergen. Documented case studies reported in medical journals have demonstrated chronic allergic symptoms from cane-sugar consumption, as well as from intravenous injections of invert sugar derived from cane. (Invert sugar is a mixture of sucrose and dextrose in special form; see Glossary.)

An extreme example of cane sugar sensitivity was reported in a fifty-five-year-old man, who suffered from allergic rhinitis, fatigue, headache, and depression. Within a few minutes after an allergy test injection of a common concentration of an extract of cane sugar, he reported a heavy sensation in his head. He yawned several times, and developed facial flushing. These symptoms were followed rapidly by a state of extreme apprehension, crying, and other signs of acute depression, as well as physical symptoms, including chills. Although this case may appear extreme, it demonstrates the allergenicity of cane sugar experienced by an individual who was sensitive to it.

Sensitivity to beets as a vegetable has long been recognized, but the recognition of sensitivity to beet sugar was not discerned. For a long time, beet sugar was the main source of granulated sugar consumed in a certain well-defined geographic area of the United States, especially where beet sugar mills were located. They were in regions somewhat distant from cane sugar refineries. The beet sugar refineries included the entire western half of the country, and to some extent the north central states, notably Michigan, Minnesota, and Wisconsin. More recently, sugar-refining areas are not so well defined. Processors now make their sugar selections based on wholesale prices of beet or cane. Due to this changed practice, beet sugar use in food and beverage processing no longer is confined to certain regions, and products containing beet sugar are in national distribution, along with products with cane sugar.

As with cane sensitivity, there are documented case studies of beet sugar sensitivity, observed by physicians. One reported case of beet and beet sugar sensitivity was of a thirty-two-year-old women who, in being tested with beet sugar, developed an acute psychotic condition characterized by disorientation, regression, and depression. The condition persisted for three days, followed by residual amnesia and other symptoms. Her reactions were recorded on film and shown at the American College of Allergists in February 1951. The case was reported by her physician, a pioneer in food allergy, Theron G. Randolph, M.D., in "The Role of Specific Sugars," in *Clinical Ecology* (Charles Thomas, 1976).

Federal labeling regulations fail to differentiate among the types of sugars used in processed foods and beverages. Obviously, this arrangement is convenient for processors but may be health threatening for a segment of the population. The word "sugar" on a food or beverage label offers no clue about its derivation. Yet, for health reasons, it may be a critical piece of information to know whether the sugar is derived from cane or beet. This is an illustration of the inadequacy of food label information for consumer protection.

SWEET, CHEAP SWEETENER GAINS FOOTHOLD
IN AMERICAN FOOD SUPPLY

More then half of all cornstarch milled in the United States is converted into corn sugar or corn syrups by means of hydrolysis with heat and acid or enzymes. The resulting products include dextrose (glucose), maltose, liquid and spray-dried corn syrups, liquid corn sugar, lump sugar, and crystalline dextrose.

A SUCROSE SPINOFF

A proposed spinoff of sucrose is waiting in the wings. Neosugar is a nondigestible sweetener being investigated as a potential sugar substitute. Neosugar is a combination of three fructooligosaccharides, similar to those found in plants such as onions, asparagus root, tubers of Jerusalem artichoke, wheat, and triticale. However, commercial neosugar is manufacturered from sucrose by means of a fungal enzyme. Neosugar is being researched by Meiji Sika from Japan, Beghin-Say from France, and Coors, the beer manufacturer in the United States. Neosugar is not hydrolyzed by digestive enzymes in the intestinal mucosa, pancreas, or internal organs. The researchers concluded that neosugar had the benefits of a low-energy sweetener, with effects similar to those of dietary fiber.

Corn sweeteners have extensive use throughout the food industry. Their low costs make them especially attractive. Also, they possess special characteristics that favor their use, to supplement rather than to replace sucrose. At a 2 percent concentration, dextrose is only about two-thirds as sweet as sucrose, but as more dextrose is used, the difference in sweetness between dextrose and sucrose decreases. (For the relative sweetness of sugar and sweeteners, see Appendix C.) At a 40 percent dextrose concentration, it is difficult to distinguish between the sweetness of dextrose and sucrose. Similarly, corn syrups have this characteristic. Thus, dextrose or corn syrups, combined with sucrose, yield a sweeter mix than would be expected. For this reason, processors can replace some sucrose with cheaper corn sweeteners in such products as syrups used in canned fruits, without loss of sweetness.

Glucose is the term for blood sugar in the body. Unfortunately, the same term is applied to the commercially processed sugar that is derived from cornstarch. Confusion has resulted. The blood sugar, glucose, needs to be maintained at a steady level within the body, and the human organism has mechanisms to sustain equilibrium. Large amounts of processed glucose, or other sugars consumed, unbalance this equilibrium.

Food processors began to use glucose in the late nineteenth century as a cheap sweetener and filler. Frequently, they substituted glucose for sucrose with canned fruits, candies, and other products. Also, commercial glucose was used to adulterate honey and molasses.

Harvey Washington Wiley, M.D., working with the Indiana State Board of Health in the late 1800s, became interested in examining food products, especially sugars and syrups, for their role as adulterants. He quickly discovered that "glucose and its near relations have been, are, and will continue to be the champion adulterants," as he described these sweeteners at a later date in his book *An Autobiography* (Bobbs Merrill, 1930).

Wiley considered glucose to be a dangerous sweetener due to its low level of sweetness. Large quantities could be consumed in foods, but with little recognition of its presence by consumers. Glucose could replace nutritious dietary components to an even greater degree than sucrose. For corn-sensitive individuals, substitution of glucose for sucrose, with incorrect label information, was deceptive and an economic cheat. Also, it was hazardous. Yet, even currently, from time to time, the FDA seizes products containing glucose as an adulterant.

In 1902, glucose was introduced in the retail market. Erroneously, the public thought that the product was made from glue. To overcome this prejudice, the product was renamed "corn syrup." Wiley, who by this time headed the federal agency that was the forerunner of the Food and Drug Administration, charged that the term corn syrup made the product misbranded and subject to seizure. A food was considered misbranded if it bore the name of another substance. An earlier product had existed that was a true corn syrup, made from pressed concentrated cornstalk juice.

Hearings were held before the Board of Food and Drug Inspectors. In support of Wiley's contention, the board decided that corn syrup was an inappropriate term for the new product. However, the corn refiners brought heavy political pressures on the federal regulatory agency, on congressmen, and on President Theodore Roosevelt. The refiners launched an organized campaign that, in retrospect, appears like a harbinger of actions that would be taken several decades later with other sweeteners. Individuals and trade groups organized massive campaigns of resolutions and protest letters flooded into Washington, D.C.

A new hearing was held. The refiners filed an impressive compilation of opinions from prominent chemists who endorsed the sweetener. Wiley charged that college and university scientists were paid to sign testimonials favoring the term corn syrup, with no comprehension of the larger issues of food adulteration and misrepresentation. The refiners' campaign was successful. The government reversed its earlier decision, and accepted the term. By February 1908 the issue was closed. Wiley had lost his long, hard struggle to keep glucose, as well as other dangerous substances, out of the American food supply.

Corn-derived sugars are allergenic for many corn-sensitive individuals, and had been reported as such as early as 1936 in the *Journal of the Kansas Medical Society* (vol. 27). At that time, corn ranked fourth among various foods listed in the order of incidence of sensitivity. In recent years, the greatly increased use of corn-derived sweeteners has made corn allergies more common than ever. Physicians working with food-allergic patients note that the incidence of diagnosed allergy to major foods is approximately as follows: corn and corn sugar are among the first three; beet and beet sugar, among the first six; and cane sugar, among the first twelve. Although some cases are identified, many more cases probably go undetected.

IS SUGAR ADDICTIVE?

"Laboratory rats given a high-sugar diet and then withdrawn from sugar experience changes in both behavior and brain chemistry similar to those seen during withdrawal from morphine or nicotine."

—Carlos Colantuoni et al., *Neuronal Report,* vol. 12, 2001

Symptoms of corn sensitivity may include chronic fatigue, gastrointestinal upsets, irritability, depression, rapid heart beat, intermittent chills, generalized muscle aches, chronic sore throat, postnasal discharge, intense itching of the eyelids and ear canals, and other health problems.

Theron G. Randolph, M.D., the pioneering food allergist mentioned earlier, noted that for many corn-sensitive individuals, chronic symptoms fail to subside until *all* corn sugars are eliminated *totally* from the diet. Randolph suspected that the practice of feeding dextrose intravenously frequently induced reactions in hospitalized patients who were corn-sensitive.

Not only is corn sugar particularly effective in maintaining corn allergenicity, but certain corn-sensitive individuals tend to react in tests with corn sugar more quickly than with other fractions of corn. Randolph noted in "The Role of Specific Sugars," mentioned earlier, that reactions to corn sugars such as dextrose (glucose) and dextrin have been observed within ten to twelve minutes; to cornstarch, within twenty minutes; and to corn oil, from two to three hours.

Corn-sensitive individuals need to avoid saccharin sweeteners that are mixed with dextrose; newer sugar substitutes that are mixed with dextrose and/or maltodextrins; granulated sugars labeled "superfine, pure cane granulated sugar with dextrose," talc-coated rice, to which glucose is added to make the rice look shiny; sorbitol and mannitol, sweeteners generally made from dextrose; and confectioner's sugar that may have cornstarch added to prevent the product from caking.

Chapter 2

TRADITIONAL SWEETENERS: OVERRATED?

No one form of sugar—whether honey, granulated white sugar, brown sugar, or molasses—is any better than another, according to Kay Munsen, Iowa State University extension nutritionist. When food experts talk about eating more "naturally occurring" sugars, she explained, they are not talking about less processed forms of sugar like honey. They mean sugar already present in fruits and vegetables.
—*CHICAGO TRIBUNE*, FEBRUARY 15, 1979

When the word "sweeteners" is used, most people think of raw, brown, and white sugar, or syrups such as molasses, honey, maple syrup, or sorghum. These common sweeteners are familiar; some have had a long tradition of use. Erroneously, many people regard these sugars as "natural." They are natural only in the sense that they are derived from plants. But all have been extracted and concentrated, and they should be regarded as processed sugars. The term "natural sugars" should be limited to those sugars present in fruits, vegetables, and milk, which have not been extracted and concentrated. How desirable are the traditional but processed sweeteners?

RAW SUGAR

At a sugar central (large-scale sugar mill), the juice is squeezed from sugarcane by means of heavy rollers, then filtered and boiled in a huge vacuum pan to make the crude sugar crystallize. The newly formed crystals are centrifuged to separate them from the molasses, which is the remaining liquid that did not crystallize.

At this stage, the crystals are "raw sugar." Being coated with molasses, they are brownish and sticky. These crystals are shipped to a refinery for further processing. The film clinging to the crystals is removed and the resulting product is refined white cane sugar, also known commonly as table sugar. Technically, it is sucrose.

26

Meanwhile, back at the sugar central, the molasses is further processed and the crystals formed range from yellow to brown. They have a distinctive taste. These are the so-called yellow sugar and brown sugar. Viewed microscopically, these sugars are still white inside, with molasses coating. Due to the sticky molasses, these sugars clump. As consumers know, the molasses coating dries out, and these sugars harden after prolonged storage.

The remaining molasses is processed still further, as many as seven or eight times, to extract as much crystallized sugar as is practical. With each processing, the molasses becomes progressively darker. The process ends after as much crystallization as possible is obtained. The remaining syrup is blackstrap molasses.

Reputable writers who discuss natural foods generally warn about raw sugar's shortcomings. Many stores refuse to stock raw sugar or products made with it. Nevertheless, a persistent myth continues that somehow raw sugar is superior to refined white sugar. In part, this myth has been perpetuated by processors and sellers of raw sugar. Restaurateurs are urged by advertisements in their trade journals to make packets of raw sugar available on dining tables. The product "says you're aware of natural food trends among today's health-conscious consumers," and offers "new texture, new and more natural color," announce raw-sugar sellers in *Restaurant Business, Restaurants & Institutions,* and other trade journals. The raw sugar packets are labeled "unrefined, natural sugar." Fact or fiction?

POLICY OF ORGANIC MERCHANTS, INC., REGARDING SUGARS

In a flyer distributed to a group called Organic Merchants, Inc., natural food store personnel were informed that:

> No Organic Merchant sells white sugar or any product containing white sugar because it is a foodless food . . . Organic Merchants do not sell brown sugar or "raw" sugar or any products containing brown sugar either, because the plain fact is that brown sugar is a shuck (for those not familiar with the term, let's call brown sugar phony). It does not seem to me to be good judgment to ban white sugar because it is refined . . . and then turn around and sell a product which is made from . . . the very same white sugar.

—Fred Rohe, *The Sugar Story,* undated, distributed by Organic Merchants, Inc.

So-called raw sugar offered at retail markets as well as at restaurants is not the raw sugar consisting of newly formed crystals centrifuged and separated from molasses. This type of sugar is sold in some countries, but not in the United States. The Food and Drug Administration (FDA) considers such sugar unfit "for direct use as a food or ingredient because of the impurities it contains." The FDA forbids its sale, and rightly so. At this stage, raw sugar may be contaminated by particles of sand, earth, molds, bacteria, yeasts, sugar lice, fibers, lints, and waxes. Some samples of such sugars have been found to contain up to 3 percent of such undesirable extraneous substances.

If raw sugar is washed once by centrifuge under careful sanitary conditions, some but not all of the dirt will be removed, along with some solid matter and bacteria. If the resulting product meets the minimal sanitary level established by the FDA under its Filth Tolerance Allowances, the sugar is cleared for sale. This sanitized product is known as turbinado sugar. According to the Sugar Association, Inc., contaminants may be present in turbinado sugar.

Raw sugar, as produced in this country, actually is white sugar with traces of cane or beet pulp added back to approximate the appearance and taste of genuine raw sugar. Or, depending on the degree of color desired, molasses may be added back to refined white sugar, ranging from 5 to 13 percent molasses. A special crystallization process is used for some light-colored sugars, designed to create an illusion of rawness. Whatever iron content is claimed for the sugar comes mainly from the tiny particles of the metal worn off the machinery in which the sugar is prepared from the cane.

In 1972, the Federal Trade Commission (FTC) took action against a company producing a raw sugar product, charging that the company engaged in false advertising. The agency charged that the product was not an organically grown, but rather a processed food. It did not have unique qualities unavailable in other types of sugars. It was not a significant source of vitamins and minerals, nor was it a significantly greater source of these nutrients than refined sugar; neither type of sugar contains nutritionally significant amounts. The absence of chemicals and preservatives did not make the product substantially different from, or superior to, other sugars.

In addition to FTC's litany of false statements, there is no justification for the claim of "unrefined, natural sugar" on raw sugar labels. Such products have undergone several refining processes, including use of various substances such as lime, phosphoric acid, charred bones, diatomaceous earth, and carbon, for purposes of clarification, adsorption, and whitening.

SUGARCANE JUICE

In recent years, there have been attempts to upgrade the nutritional quality of sweeteners from sugarcane. Sugarcane juice and evaporated sugarcane juice (crystallized) are available.

In tropical areas where sugarcane is grown, it is a common sight to see people chewing on sections of cut cane to extract the juice. Cane juice, with its accompanying nutrients intact, has a modicum of sweetness. Refined sugars, stripped of their original nutrients, are concentrated in their sweetness. Unlike refined sugars, cane juice consumption does not lead to dental decay.

In southern Florida, Cuban snack bars serve "guarapo," the juice of freshly squeezed sugarcane. This greenish juice, served chilled, is only mildly sweet. In the same areas, vendors in open-air markets and street fairs may offer chunks of sugarcane. The sellers peel off the fibrous exterior of the cane and cut the interior flesh into bite-size pieces. In chewing the chunks, one extracts the cane juice.

Cut sections of sugarcane, called "batons," are found in Hispanic, Caribbean, and southeast Asian markets, as well as in specialty food shops and supermarkets in large cities. The ends of the batons may be waxed to seal in the cane juice. The stores also may stock canned cane juice.

If you have a piston-type citrus press, you can extract cane juice at home. Peel the baton, and with a sharp knife, cut it into small pieces that will fit into the press.

Evaporated sugarcane juice, in crystallized form, has become available. In tropical areas, granulated sugars from cane have had a long history of production as a cottage industry, and these sweeteners have been staple sweeteners for thousands of years. Produced in homes, under primitive conditions, the qualities and flavors of such sugars vary. They have a high moisture content, ferment readily, and are difficult to store or transport. However, such sugars retain their original nutrients.

In the twentieth century, Swiss pediatrician and health advocate Max-Henri Beguin was convinced that by applying modern techniques, he could produce a sugar that retained its nutrients, was uniform in quality, and had stability. The product that evolved from his efforts was registered first as Sucanat (a composite of *sugar cane natural*), and later as *Organic Sucanat*.

Strict rules guide the production of this organic evaporated sugar-cane juice product. The rules were formulated even prior to the federal certification requirements established by the U.S. Department of Agriculture (USDA) for organic crops. Before fields are certified to grow organic sugarcane to Sucanat specifications, there is a three-year waiting period. During this time, no pesticides, herbicides, chemical fertilizers, or any other chemical can be used on the land. After initial certification, the fields are audited annually by independent organic agencies.

Sucanat production begins with hand-harvesting of the sugarcane, and processing it within twenty-four hours at a certified organic facility. The juice is extracted through a series of roller mills, and then clarified and filtered to remove bagasse pulp and any other soluble matter. The cleaned cane juice is concentrated by evaporation, followed by a crystallization process to remove any residual water, and to yield a dry, free-flowing granulated sugar with the original nutrients intact. The process differs from the traditional one for making table sugar, in which the nutrients present in the cane juice are removed during centrifuging and crystallization, and the resulting refined sugar consists solely of sucrose. Also, Sucanat differs from table sugar in its structure, appearance, and flavor, as well as its composition. Sucanat has less bulk density than table sugar, but it can replace table sugar, cup for cup.

After Sucanat was introduced in the late 1980s, it was promoted as the "organic 100 percent whole food sweetener." One advertising statement declared that "Sucanat has more calcium than broccoli; more vitamin A than Brussels sprouts; more iron than raisins; more potassium than potatoes; and about the same vitamin C as fresh tangerines," in the National Foods Merchandiser (Sept 1990). Sucanat's producer felt that the claim was valid, based on nutritional comparisons for equal quantities of the mentioned foods, as they were evaluated in the USDA's Handbook No. 8: *Nutrient Composition of Foods*, as well as by independent-certified laboratory testing.

THE COMPOSITION OF SUCANAT

An independent laboratory analysis of Sucanat supplied by its producer, showed the following composition of the sweetener:

Fructose: 3–10 percent   Glucose: 2–9 percent   Sucrose: 75–80 percent

Because the only element removed in processing Sucanat is water, the laboratory analysis showed that one cup* of the sweetener contained an average of:

Basic Nutrients	Carbohydrates	141.0 g
	Protein	1.05 g
Minerals	Calcium	165.0 mg
	Magnesium	127.0 mg
	Phosphorus	48.0 mg
	Iron	6.5 mg
	Sodium	5.0 mg
	Zinc	2.3 mg
	Potassium	1.125 mg
	Copper	0.3 mg
	Chromium	40.0 mcg

Vitamins	Vitamin A	1,600 IU
	Vitamin C	49.5 mg
	Riboflavin	21.0 mg
	Thiamin	21.0 mg
	Pyridoxine	6.0 mg
	Niacin	2.0 mg
	Pantothenic acid	1.8 mg

Key: Grams = g; milligrams = mg; micrograms = mcg; international units = IU

* Generally, sweeteners are added to foods and beverages in amounts of teaspoons or tablespoons. However, the cup measurement is used commonly in baked goods. The cup is the commonly used unit of measurement for comparison of caloric sweeteners such as table sugar, brown sugar, dried maple syrups, dried malt, or liquid honey. Compared with these other sweeteners, listed in the USDA's *Handbook No. 8,* Sucanat contains higher levels of nutrients. However, if used as a flavoring, Sucanat contributes only a minor amount of nutrients to the total diet.

The Center for Science in the Public Interest (CSPI), a Washington, D.C.-based independent consumer watchdog organization, challenged Sucanat's nutritional claim, and lodged a complaint with the FDA's Center for Food Safety and Applied Nutrition, and also with the National Advertising Division of the Better Business Bureau. In a press release in March 1991, Dr. Michael Jacobson, executive director of CSPI, charged that Sucanat's advertisements and labels were deceiving customers by comparing the nutritive content of the sweetener with the same size serving of fruits and vegetables. Jacobson noted that "Sucanat has miniscule amounts of vitamins and minerals. It is not rich in the vitamins and minerals like its label says." Jacobson added, "The label indicates that the products are almost pure sugar."

The Sucanat producers rebutted CSPI's accusations of false and deceptive labeling. Bruce Kirk, president of Pronatec, producer of Sucanat, retorted that "our label shows that Sucanat is 75 to 78 percent sucrose, while white sugar is 99.9 percent sucrose. In any scientific investigation, this would not be classified as 'almost [pure sugar],' as quoted in *Health Food Business* (May 1991). Kirk continued, "he [Jacobson] didn't even have Sucanat analyzed by an independent lab to show his accusations were correct." Kirk added that the FDA did not allow Sucanat to be labeled as a sugar "because our sucrose level is not high enough." Instead, the product is labeled as evaporated cane juice.

Kirk reported that the advertisement for Sucanat that CSPI deemed deceptive "ran at the beginning of what most people consider the baking season. Our ad shows a theme of baked goods. Most people who bake utilize more than one teaspoon of sweetener in their baking."

SPECIALTY SUGARS

"Nigel Willerton, CEO of Wholesome Sweeteners, based in Sugar Land, Texas, attributes the rising popularity of specialty sugars to consumers who are more concerned about the source of their food, the environment, and the use of pesticides and herbicides. Wholesome Sweeteners' sales of these sugars, which the company imports from five countries, have quadrupled in four years, reaching $26 million this year [2005]. Despite their growing market share, organic and unrefined sugar sales still account for a tiny share—about $39 million of the $10 billion-a-year U.S. sugar market . . ."

—"Ain't That Sweet!" by Stacie Stukin, *Time Bonus Section,* November 2005

Pronatec sought a public retraction by CSPI of all its statements concerning Sucanat. Also, Pronatec countered with its own advertisement in the May 1991 issue of *Health Food Business.* The company urged the public to "demonstrate your distain for this emotional reportage on the part of CSPI and cancel your subscription to their publication. They guarantee a full refund, even if you are in the last month of your subscription."

The skirmish ended. Neither side apologized. Organic Sucanat is available in natural food stores and in some specialty sections of supermarkets. The processor, Pronatec was renamed NutraCane, Inc. The sugar is distributed by Wholesome Sweeteners, a subsidiary of Imperial Sugar Company, both located in Savannah, Georgia.

Another attempt to upgrade the quality of sweeteners from sugarcane occurred in the mid-1990s, with the introduction of unbleached cane sugar for use by bakers and confectioners. According to the trade journal *Food Engineering* (May 1994), this product also was being sold to "processors of seemingly unhealthy foods seeking a better image." This group included, among others, processors of candies, chocolates, jellies, and soft drinks. According to *Food Engineering,* "market research indicated that unbleached cane sugar has a very strong appeal with health-conscious consumers and those who like foods made with unusual ingredients." Later, unbleached cane-sugar distribution extended to natural food stores and supermarkets with specialty foods. The retail product became available in large plastic bags and jugs.

The producer of this sugar claims that its sugarcane is grown pesticide- and herbicide-free, and that the sugarcane is processed minimally to remove impurities, but to retain the golden color and fine flavor of the juice. Unlike the processing of white sugar, this product is not stripped of nutrients, nor deionized, nor heated at high temperature, nor fractionated.

The producer reported that the product has a very fine granulation, which allows it to dissolve quickly. The sugar remains in the solution in hot or cold beverages.

This product is named Florida Crystals. The Natural Source Company in Indian Harbour Beach, Florida grows, harvests, mills, and markets the product, and is its sole distributor.

BROWN SUGAR

In countries where cane is grown, some brown sugars are made simply by cutting short the refining process so that the sugar retains some of the molasses that otherwise is washed out or removed in the final refining treatment. At times, brown sugar is made fraudulently by adding brown caramel coloring to white sugar.

The technique for brown sugar production in this country makes the product *more* refined than white sugar, and the additional process may offer health hazards. The raw sugar is washed to remove the molasses coating, and is centrifuged to separate the crystals. Then, it is heated to a melting point, filtered, and decolorized with animal-bone charcoal. With repeated boilings, the decolorized liquid becomes crystallized and concentrated. The "brown" color in this sugar results from the bone-charcoal treatment rather than from molasses residue.

Regarding this decolorizing process, long ago cancer expert Wilhelm C. Hueper, M.D., reported:

> In themselves, sugars may not be carcinogenic—but carcinogenic impurities may be introduced into sugars when concentrated sugar solutions are filtered for decolorizing purposes through improperly prepared charcoal containing polycyclic hydrocarbons. Chemicals of the dibenzanthracene type are eluted (washed out) from charcoal by concentrated sugar solutions . . . Traces may be introduced in this manner and remain in apparently chemically pure sugar (*Cancer Research*, May 1965).

In a baking trade journal, *Baking Industry* (May 1976), bakers were advised that:

> Substantial dollar savings are now available to bakers using brown sugar by "making their own." The concept involves simply mixing granulated [white] sugar with a special brown sugar-molasses product. Brown sugar use is increasing sharply because of the consumer trend toward natural foods.

Commercial bakers may use imitation brown sugar in liquid form. The product is intended to 'fortify' regular sugar or to replace up to 100 percent of brown-sugar flavoring.

A granulated brown-sugar product, introduced in retail markets, was described as a "low-calorie sugar substitute" that "looks, tastes, and smells like old-fashioned brown sugar." The product consisted of brown sugar and saccharin. How accurate was the description? "Sugar substitute" identified the saccharin portion correctly, but this noncaloric sweetener would hardly succeed in converting brown sugar into a low-calorie sugar. One cup of packed brown sugar has 821 calories; table sugar, 770. In the FDA's quest for greater accuracy in food labeling, in 1978 the agency announced that products could be labeled low-calorie only if they contain no more then 40 calories per serving.

No brown sugars contain any worthwhile amounts of nutrients. Nor do they contribute any significant amounts of vitamins or minerals to meet the body's needs.

MOLASSES

Molasses played a significant role in American history and caused John Adams, one of the Founding Fathers of the United States, to call it "an essential ingredient in American independence." Columbus had introduced sugarcane and its resulting molasses into Santa Domingo in 1493. By the eighteenth century, molasses—the instrument that balanced accounts with the Mother country—was regarded as the life blood of colonial commerce. Exports from the colonies of lumber, fish, cotton, and other agricultural staples failed to equal the value of manufactured goods imported from England, until the molasses trade tipped the scale.

Molasses was intertwined with the slave trade. Sailing vessels shipped colonist products to the West Indies and returned with molasses, which the colonists fermented and converted into rum. Part of the rum was consumed locally, but much of it went to Africa in exchange for slaves. Ships returned to America via the West Indies, where some slaves were debarked and promptly bartered for more molasses. The remaining slaves were shipped, along with the molasses, to the southern colonies.

England attempted to discourage this arrangement by passage of the Molasses Act of 1733, which levied heavy import duties. By 1764, England proposed even more stringent provisions. Molasses, as well as tea, became a precipitating factor in the American Revolution.

In colonial days, molasses imports were substantial in areas along the Atlantic seaboard. Even today, the customary molasses use still prevails. Maine and North Carolina continue a tradition of molasses consumption.

The quality of the molasses depends on the sugarcane's maturity, the amount of sugar extracted, and the extraction method. Quality also depends on whether the processor intends to produce molasses or sugar as the primary product. The three major types of molasses are unsulfured, sulfured, and blackstrap products. Unsulfured is made from the juice of twelve- to fifteen-month, sun-ripened West Indian cane. The harvested cane is crushed and heated in clarifying kettles. Then, the juice flows through a series of copper kettles, becoming more concentrated until it reaches the desired density. It is transferred to tanks where the molasses ages. This process has been used for more than two centuries. Modern machinery insures uniformity and sanitation in the product. The molasses is shipped by barrel or puncheon to warehouses in this country and then is blended. Because the character and flavor differ from each location, blending produces a uniform product. Some molasses may be kept in the warehouse for a year or two for further aging and mellowing.

Sulfured molasses is a byproduct of sugar refining. The efficient modern sugar plants, by extracting a high sugar level from the original cane juice, yield molasses of lower quality. Most sulfured molasses is made from cane grown outside of the West Indies, in areas where the ripening season is not long enough to allow cane to mature. The 'green' sugarcane is treated with sulfur fumes during the sugar-extraction process. As a result, sulfur residue remains in the molasses. Sulfur compounds are undesirable in the food supply. The FDA allows six sulfiting compounds as approved food additives. Health-conscious consumers avoid all foods treated with them. For individuals who are sensitive to these sulfiting compounds, reactions can be severe, including anaphylactic shock, and even death.

"First centrifugal" and "second centrifugal" are two types of sulfured molasses. The former is sugarcane juice boiled to the proper density in vacuum pans and then centrifuged to extract sugar crystals. A yellow-colored molasses remains, and is subjected to a second boiling and centrifuging. Additional sugar crystals are extracted. The remaining blackstrap molasses is darker and contains a larger percentage of natural gums and ash, and has a less agreeable flavor.

Blackstrap molasses is the waste product of sugar processing. Usually, it is sold to produce industrial alcohol for rum and yeast, and for use in animal feed. This molasses results from a third boiling, with more sugar crystals having been extracted. The remaining product, from which it is no longer profitable to remove any more sugar, is blackish in color, with a burnt, bitter taste. If the sugar refinery is imagined as a laundry facility where crude sugar is washed as clothes, blackstrap molasses would be equivalent to the wash water that carries most of the mineral matter and all of the gum, ash, dirt, and indigestible matter present in the unprocessed crude sugar.

Food processors use molasses because of its special characteristics. As well as having sweetness, molasses has the ability to mask certain unpleasant flavors such as the bitter taste of bran in bread. Molasses can mimic related flavors, such as chocolate, butterscotch, coffee, and maple. At times, molasses is added to foods and beverages with those flavors, to intensify them and reduce costs. Molasses is effective in controlling the water activity of foods, and appears to have a natural antioxidant component that helps retard food spoilage.

A CHEMIST'S VIEW OF SUGAR

Alsoph Corwin, a distinguished chemist emeritus from Johns Hopkins University, wrote "The Most Common Source of Chemical Contaminants" (an undated paper), in which he described what happens to sugar when it is subjected to heat. Hydroxymethyl furfural, a highly reactive and allergenic group of compounds, form by cooking foods that contain sugars. Using gas chromatography, Corwin demonstrated that the ones formed in acid solution usually are derived from furane or pyrane, and they include a wide variety of complex chemicals. The ones formed in alkaline media are even more complex, including carbon-ring compounds with a variety of functional groups attached. The conditions for these compounds to form are especially favorable in processing sugarcane juice to form blackstrap molasses. According to Corwin, chemists view its coloring matter as water-soluble tar. He reported,

> Blackstrap molasses is widely recommended as a 'health food' because it contains residual minerals which are removed from cane juice in the purification of cane sugar. Due consideration for food stresses, however, would dictate that the necessary minerals be obtained from a less risky source. So-called raw sugar, turbinado sugar, and brown sugar all contain varying amounts of molasses and all should be considered as rich sources of chemical contaminants formed by the cooking process. While some of the colored materials present in cooked sugar solutions have been identified, many of them are so complex that their structures are still unknown. All of them are artificial chemical contaminants.

Many food processors use liquid and dry molasses blends. Such products are not 100 percent molasses. One light-brown blend consists of molasses, wheat starch, and soy flour. The total sugar content is 60 percent, consisting of 30 percent sucrose and 30 percent other sugars. One medium-brown blend has a total sugar content of 53 percent, consisting of 37 percent sucrose and 16 percent other sugars.

One free-flowing granulated molasses blend consists of 75 percent molasses and 25 percent corn syrup solids; another has 75 percent molasses and 25 percent soy bran and cornstarch. Such blends are used for many processed foods, including breads, cookies, pies, health foods, mixes, cereals, and sausages. The strong molasses flavor acts as a masking agent with some of these products. Although the ingredients in such blends may be acceptable as food components, the word "molasses" on food labels is misleading. Consumers are unaware of the presence of corn, wheat, or soy constituents, any of which may be hidden allergens.

One molasses producer stated that "the natural sugar in molasses is taken up by the body without any undue strain and can be used in practically any quantity" (*All About Molasses*, American Molasses Co., 1952). This statement may sell molasses, but even today is poor advice. The text continued, "only liver compares favorably with molasses as a source of iron, and molasses rates even in this comparison as a less expensive source." Untrue. One 3-ounce serving of calves' liver provides 12.1 milligrams (mg) of iron; less expensive pigs' liver, 24.7 mg. One would need to consume a 12-ounce bottle of light molasses, which contains 21.2 mg of iron, to approximate the amount in pigs' liver; a 12-ounce bottle of medium-colored molasses supplies 29.6 mg. In addition to iron, the liver supplies many other nutrients at high levels. To depend on molasses as an iron source, one is forced to consume an undesirably high-sugar level.

TRACE ELEMENTS IN MOLASSES

Trace elements, small in amounts, but important in biological systems, including humans, animals, and plants, were studied extensively by Henry A. Schroeder, M.D. In his book *The Trace Elements & Man* (Devin Adair, 1973), Schroeder reported that the refining process resulted in severe losses of certain trace elements when sugarcane was converted to molasses. The loss of trace elements in one part per million (ppm) were as follows:

Zinc loss	8.28 ppm	Cobalt loss	1.26 ppm
Copper loss	2.21 ppm	Chromium loss	1.20 ppm

The remaining trace elements in molasses were:

Magnesium	250.0 ppm	Chromium	1.21 ppm
Zinc	8.3 ppm	Cobalt	0.25 ppm
Copper	6.83 ppm	Molybdenum	0.19 ppm
Manganese	4.24 ppm		

Carl C. Pfeiffer, M.D., Ph.D., was also interested in the effects of trace elements on biological systems. He examined the differences between the levels of trace elements in molasses derived from cane and molasses derived from beet. Pfeiffer analyzed molasses samples by atomic absorption spectrography, and reported his results in his book *Mental & Elemental Nutrients* (Keats Publishing, 1975). The trace elements in one ppm were as follows:

Trace minerals	Cane-derived molasses in ppm	Beet-derived molasses in ppm
Iron	20.4	30.2
Manganese	4.14	5.83
Zinc	1.08	3.02
Copper	0.55	1.75
Chromium	0.08	0.30

Pfeiffer noted that although beet molasses was higher than cane molasses in all trace elements measured, the use of beet molasses is limited to cattle feed.

Is blackstrap molasses better? A mystique has evolved and has been per-petuated about blackstrap's benefits and nutrients. Sulfur and blackstrap molasses, used as a spring tonic and as a lotion for pimples, are well-estab-lished rites. Folklore provides the notion that blackstrap molasses, mixed with cinders, enriches the blood; with goose grease, cures croup; and in the North Carolina hills, a mixture of blackstrap molasses with whiskey and linseed oil allegedly relieves whooping cough. Blackstrap molasses enthusiasts have termed it a "miracle" food.

Due to the concentration of blackstrap, it contains similar nutrients found in other molasses, but at higher levels. According to Dr. Roy E. Morse of the Food Science Department at Rutgers University:

There's a lot of iron in [blackstrap molasses] just as the health-food people claim, but there may also be arsenic and some other unpleasant things, which have become more concentrated with each run. The possible dan-gers from these components have caused the FDA to forbid the sale of true blackstrap as human food (*Food Facts from Rutgers*, Jul/Sept 1973).

The bitter unpalatable flavor of blackstrap molasses makes it self-limiting. For food preparation, blackstrap molasses is more palatable if it is blended with a sweeter molasses. Due to the stickiness of all types of molasses, they cling to the teeth. If not removed promptly, residues can lead to dental decay.

Is Blackstrap Molasses a Superior Molasses?

The following is a comparison of nutrients of average light molasses and blackstrap molasses.

	Average light molasses (1 tablespoon)	Blackstrap molasses (1 tablespoon)
Food energy	50.0 calories	43.0 calories
Carbohydrates	13.0 grams	11.0 grams
Potassium	183.0 mg	585.0 mg
Calcium	33.0 mg	137.0 mg
Phosphorus	9.0 mg	17.0 mg
Sodium	3.0 mg	19.0 mg
Iron	0.9 mg	3.2 mg
Riboflavin	0.01 mg	0.04 mg
Thiamin	0.01 mg	0.02 mg
Niacin	trace	.04 mg
Vitamin A	none	none
Ascorbic acid	none	none

—*Nutritive Value of American Foods in Common Units*, Agricultural Handbook No. 456 (ARS, USDA, Nov 1965)

Prudence dictates that molasses should be used sparingly as a flavoring agent, rather than depend on it for its nutritional content. Because molasses is mainly sugars and is highly concentrated, its use should be limited.

HONEY

Numerous books and articles have been written in praise of honey. Among the earliest of sweeteners, through many centuries, legends and folktales about honey have evolved in mythology, religious ritual, medical practice, and social custom. The high esteem for honey is reflected in expressions such as "the nectar of the gods," "youth elixir," or "molten gold." Numerous expressions in language incorporate the word honey to express pleasant tastes, personal qualities, and other attributes.

Honey has been found to have antibacterial and anti-inflammatory properties on bruises and cuts, and to stimulate tissue growth, according to the Honey Research Unit at Waikato University in New Zealand. Also, the National Honey Board in the United States reported that honey enhances the growth, activity, and viability of the beneficial probiotic bifidobacteria present in fermented dairy products such as yogurt.

Honey's current popularity is understandable. The term "natural" is positive; "synthetic," negative. Similarly, "unprocessed" is preferable to "refined"; "raw" favored over "heated." Synthetic sweetener safety and usefulness are questioned, and refined sugars are implicated in dental decay and other health problems. Honey symbolizes natural and unprocessed, with implied attributes to healthfulness and safety.

Nectar gathered by bees consists of more than 80 percent sucrose, which bees are able to metabolize by means of the digestive enzyme, invertase. In the time elapsing between gathering the nectar and returning to the hive, the bees have split the sucrose of the nectar into two simple sugars: glucose (dextrose) and fructose (levulose). This mixture, invert sugar, is sweeter than the original nectar from which it is derived. (Invert sugar, processed for food and beverage use, is made from sucrose treated with acid or enzymes to split the disaccharide into its separate components. This process, termed inversion, results in the commercial "invert sugar" on food labels. Its special properties of interest to processors are its resistance to crystallization and its moisture-holding capacity. Both qualities are useful in certain food formulations.)

Invert sugar, when eaten by human beings, provides a direct energy source because it requires no digestion. Fructose, highly soluble, does not crystallize readily, but glucose does. The proportions of fructose to glucose vary in different honey varieties. For example, tupelo honey from the flower's nectar of the gum tree has a high-fructose content and resists crystallization.

ANTIOXIDANTS IN HONEY

Recent studies identified antioxidants in honey. Although honey, by itself, may not serve as a major source of dietary antioxidants, it can provide a supplementary source of them. Researchers at the University of Illinois in Champaign-Urbana examined the water-soluble antioxidant capacity of nineteen samples of honey from fourteen different floral sources. Depending on the floral source and crop year, the antioxidant levels varied. The darker honeys provided the highest antioxidant levels. Antioxidants in buckwheat honey compared favorably with the ascorbic acid-related antioxidant content of tomatoes.

Other research, at Clemson University in South Carolina, found that honey plays a role in the prevention of oxidation in processed meat products. Meats prepared with 15 percent dried honey have greater yields, less oxidation, and remain free of bacterial growth for more than eleven weeks of refrigerated storage (based on information in *Food Technology,* Jan 1996).

Differences in honey color result from the compositions of plants. For example, samples of tested honey showed variation in their development of antioxidants, mainly flavonoids, traces of vitamins C and E, and beta-carotene. Honey produced from the pollen of Illinois buckwheat, a strong flavored honey, was found to have twenty times more antioxidants than light-colored, mild-flavored sage honey from California.

Honey is prized, not so much as a source of ready energy, but for its flavor. Dissolved aromatics give each honey its own distinctive flavor and appearance. The remaining components in the mixture are mainly water, a small amount of sucrose, dextrin, gums, and a modicum of minerals, vitamins, enzymes, and bee pollen with its own components. The presence of these substances, albeit in small amounts, is the prime reason for honey being as highly valued by persons interested in what are considered as natural or health foods.

Compared with other caloric sweeteners, honey consumption in the United States is minor, and remains at a fairly stable level. In 1963, the average American ate more than 107 pounds of cane, beet, and corn sugars annually, compared to only 1.1 pounds of honey. By 1980, cane, beet, and corn sweetener consumption had risen to 127.3 pounds; honey declined slightly to 1.0. Currently, honey remains as a minor sweetener. The Economic Research Service of the USDA, in 2005, estimated that the U.S. per capita annual deliveries for domestic food and beverage use in 2004 for honey was 0.9 pounds. Thus, consumption figures remain quite stable. Actually, honey production can be regarded as a byproduct. The main enterprise is to provide bees for their vital work in crop pollination.

As honey progresses from beehive to table, can it be considered truly as an "unrefined" product? First, honey needs to be extracted from the hive. Cottage-industry beekeepers may use a simple bee-escape device to remove bees and gently brush off any stray ones with a soft brush. To save time, large-scale packers may resort to toxic materials such as carbolic acid, nitrous oxide, propionic anhydride, or benzaldehyde. Allegedly, these substances dissipate quickly and leave no residues. However, repeated exposures to these substances may shorten the bees' lifespan.

Honey labels that state "unheated," "no heat used," or "unpasteurized" may be misleading. Generally, home-packers do apply heat to thin honey for easier extraction, to retard crystallization, and to destroy honey yeasts that cause fermentation and spoilage. The conscientious apiarist will extract with mild heat (only up to 120°F) and such honey retains its small amounts of nutrients. Studies showed that filtered honey heated to 150°F lost 27 to 30 percent of its thiamin; 22 to 45 percent, riboflavin; 8 to 22 percent, pantothenic acid; 15 to 27 percent, niacin; and 9 to 20 percent of ascorbic acid as reported in the *American Bee Journal* (vol. 95, 1955). Prolonged exposure to heat causes enzyme and protein breakdown, as well as impaired color and flavor. Large-scale honey packers may flush-heat honey briefly through heated pipes to temperatures above boiling.

"Buttered" or "creamed" honey is finely granulated, but this appearance is no guarantee that the honey has not been heated. The honey may have been heated, then recrystallized by seeding it with honey crystals to produce granulation.

Extracted honey is strained or filtered to remove impurities and to clarify the product. Some people seek label terms of "unfiltered" or "unstrained" honey. A small amount of pollen may be present in such honey. Along with the pollen, present in insignificant amounts, may be other particulates such as bees' wings and legs. These extraneous substances may not be aesthetic, but they are not harmful.

Filtration is used to grade honey; the greater the clarity, the higher the grade. "Fancy" U.S. Grade A, the top rating, is given to honey strained through a fine screen or cloth. "Choice" Grade B is strained through a coarser screen; and both "Standard" Grade C and "Substandard" Grade D, through even coarser screens. This USDA grading, used by most states, has *no significance* other than as a measurement of particle size of the extraneous matter filtered out of honey, and is *unrelated to quality.*

Actually, the USDA uses a rarely publicized quality rating with three factors on a 100-point scale. A maximum of 50, 40, and 10 points is given respectively for flavor, absence of particles, and clarity. Obviously, flavor should be more important than clarity. Neither the official grades nor quality ratings carry any marketing constraints, and legally all four grades are saleable.

The cottage-industry apiarist merely may strain the honey through a filter, or just allow it to settle overnight. Large-scale honey packers may mix honey with inert diatomaceous earth to remove particulates as the honey is pumped through a series of filtration discs. The diatomaceous earth does not remain in the honey.

As honey ripens in the hive, bees reduce its moisture content to less than 17 percent, which results in honey with a smooth, mellow flavor. The glucose in the honey releases hydrogen peroxide, which retards fermentation. At times, however, beekeepers who are eager to market honey early, extract unripe honey prematurely. Such 'green' honey with moisture frequently above 20 percent, has a disagreeable biting taste. Its low glucose concentration reduces its resistance to bacterial contamination, and such honey can ferment and spoil readily; mature honey does not.

Legally, honey is defined as "the nectar of the floral exudations of plants gathered and stored in the comb of honeybees" (*Beekeeping Bulletin*, No. 5, Department of Agriculture, Florida, Jan 1958). Writers Anstice Carroll and

Embree de Persiis Vona gave false assurance that "the surest way to get untreated, unheated honey is to buy it in the comb" (*The Health Food Dictionary*, Prentice-Hall, 1973). Commercial comb honey is not necessarily unheated and unfiltered. Such products may consist of processed honey that, along with clean empty honeycombs, is placed in containers.

One food trade journal described honey labeling as a neglected problem by the natural food industry, whose honey sales constitute a significant segment of the honey market. Terms on honey labels such as "natural," "old-fashioned," "country-style," "organic," or "undiluted" are meaningless. The term "organic" on honey labels has been justified by citing a dictionary definition of organic as meaning free from foreign particles. "Undiluted" has been justified because no water has been added to the honey. If it were added, the product would he considered adulterated and subject to seizure.

Domestic honey is derived from more than 300 varieties of plants. Label information about the honey's source may be imprecise. Honey, labeled as the product of a single source, such as sage, clover, orange blossom, or buckwheat, in fact may be blends of different sources. Some states, notably California, require that only 51 percent of the product be derived from one source in order to name a specific source on the label.

Honey blending is practiced to alter moisture content, improve flavor, or retard granulation. For example, the bitterness of orange blossom honey may be mellowed by blending it with a milder, lighter honey. Buckwheat honey is so strongly flavored that in many states it may comprise only 10 to 15 percent of a product labeled "buckwheat honey."

The Florida Department of Agriculture has established more stringent controls. Identifiable types or varieties of honey must be made entirely from the stated origin. Florida issues official tags or labels to mark containers "certified tupelo honey," "certified orange blossom honey," or others. Regarding honey blends, the agency cautioned Floridian apiarists in *Beekeeping Bulletin* No. 5, (Jan 1958) that:

Blending honey has reference only to the very best honey and not to any of inferior quality. A poor grade should never be in a blend, or it will ruin all. It is better to put the cheap honey up separately and sell [it] as such. This applies to both the color and flavor of honey. Some poor honey has a fine color, and some very fine honey has a poor color. It is seldom, if ever, advisable to blend dark honey with light, or honey of poor flavor with that of good flavor, but a blend should always be with honey of similar color and quality of flavor.

Blended honey is not necessarily inferior to single-source honey, but the label is inadequately informative to meet the needs of individuals who are sensitive to constituents of certain plants that may be present as hidden allergens.

The United States imports honey mainly from Canada, Mexico, Argentina, Brazil, and China. When China began to flood the global marketplace with its numerous exports, its honey exports to the United States in the late 1990s were especially worrisome. The honey from China, priced below actual production costs, causes losses of income by American apiarists. The U.S. Department of Commerce responded, by instituting tariffs from 34 to 184 percent. Some Chinese companies attempted to circumvent these stiff tariffs by devising elaborate honey-laundering operations and smuggling schemes. 'Middlemen' countries, such as Vietnam, Malaysia, Thailand, Mexico, India, and Turkey blended Chinese honey with their own or simply relabeled honey from China and then exported it to the United States and elsewhere.

Chemist Fredrick Accum, in his book exposing food adulteration *A Treatise on Adulterations of Food, and Culinary Poisons* (Longman, 1820), wrote, "Honey is frequently adulterated with starch, sand, flour, etc., for the purpose of improving its colour, or increasing its weight." Accum described his technique for detecting sand in honey. He dissolved the honey in water, and allowed any sand that might be present to sink to the bottom.

Accum was a pioneering muckraker from Germany. His exposés about food adulteration outraged the unethical processors who threatened his life. He fled to England and continued to expose the deceptive practices. His work influenced food reform.

Currently, honey adulteration continues, not with sand but with cheap sugars or syrups. Frequently, the FDA announces seizures. Since the development of the industrial sweetener, high-fructose corn syrups (HFCSs, discussed in Chapter 4), honey adulteration from this source has become commonplace and difficult to detect. Until 1978 the available testing techniques were inadequate. The adulteration grew to such proportions that the practice was an economic threat both to consumers and honey producers. Honey is in limited supply and is costly; HFCS is plentiful and inexpensive. In 1978, the Eastern Regional Research Center, a branch of the USDA, perfected testing techniques that were capable of detecting HFCS adulteration in honey and in bee feed. Such products are subject to seizure.

In contrast, another USDA branch's efforts are expended in the opposite direction. Researchers at the Bioenvironmental Bee Laboratory succeeded in simulating the aroma and flavor of bee pollen with a mixture of whey, yeast, soybean flour, dry skim milk, cottonseed meal, and corn gluten. The mixture, encapsulated in starch, was intended as feed for honeybees. The colonies fed this ersatz feed were found to yield as much honey and reproduced as readily as nectar-fed colonies (*Publications and Patents. Eastern Regional Research*

Center, USDA, Jul/Aug 1979). This type of research should be discouraged. Among other undesirable outcomes would be lack of crop pollination, and potential allergic food reactions to components in the bee feed induced in individuals who normally tolerate honey derived from flower nectar. Also, the image of honey as a natural food would become sullied.

Serious honey adulteration was discovered in 2000. Food inspectors in the European Union discovered banned chloramphenicol (an antimicrobial drug) present in honey from China. By 2002 and 2003, the FDA conducted numerous seizures of honey imported from China, containing this drug; Canada conducted similar widespread recalls of honey imported from China due to the same contaminant. Additional seizures were made of honey-containing prepared meals and snacks—all from China, and all containing illegal chloramphenicol. Mexico detained Chinese honey contaminated with illegal residues of the same drug as well as with streptomycin, tetracycline, and other antibiotics.

Food processors use honey in liquid and dry forms. As with molasses, such products are not 100 percent honey, but rather honey blends with other ingredients. One product contains only 60 percent honey, with added wheat starch and soy flour as drying aids, and calcium stearate to keep the dry form of honey from caking. Another is a blend of 60 percent honey and invert sugar, as well as other ingredients. An advertisement in a food trade journal promised food processors cost savings up to 30 percent with such blends. These products are used in many baked goods, breakfast foods, snacks, soups, sauces, sugar substitutes, and in a variety of canned, frozen, and tableted foods. Food processors were advised in *Health Food Retailing* (Feb 1980) that "use of the product in most cases requires no change in labeling statement." This indicates that consumers are misled. When the term "honey" appears as an ingredient on food labels, buyers do not expect that invert sugar is mixed with honey, or that 40 percent of the honey consists of other ingredients. In some cases, natural food outlets have sold products in good faith that were labeled in this manner, and later were found to contain sucrose in the carrier base.

In addition, imitation honey flavors, available to food processors, are described as looking, tasting, and performing like honey. Some of these flavors are created by adding beta-phenylalanine to a sugar such as glucose, and allowing it to react at high temperatures. Such products are designed as honey replacers in meat and dairy products, jellies, jams, cereals, baked goods, toppings, glazes, ice creams, candies, and other products in which honey sometimes is used as a sweetener or flavoring. These replacers are low in cost, do not crystallize, and store indefinitely. Some are a hundredfold sweeter than honey in their intensity, and processors can dilute them with invert sugar syrup, and thus save money.

How safe is honey? Generally honey is a safe food. However, there are a few practices worth noting. Sulfa drugs and other antibiotics may be used to control bee diseases in the hive. These medications are fed in sugar syrup before or after a honey flow. Empty combs may be fumigated with paradichlorobenzene (moth balls) or methyl bromide. Either substance may contaminate honey. Many apiarists, concerned about their bees as well as their own safety, and the quality of the honey, avoid using these adjuncts.

Pesticides may contaminate honey, but the problem is of a lesser order than with most foods. Worker bees probe deeply into blossoms, where pesticide concentrations are lower than on the exterior. Pesticide-exposed bees are apt to perish before they can return to the hive. Those who do return exhibit such radical behavioral changes, that they are refused admittance by the colony.

The pesticides most lethal to bees are among some that have been banned from use in the United States: DDT, lindane, chlordane, DNC (4, 4'-Dinitrocarbanilide), and dieldrin. DNOC (4.6-Dinitro-o-cresol) is less toxic. Although carbaryl (Sevin) is considered to be one of the less toxic pesticides, it is highly lethal to bees. One pesticide, octamethyl pyrophosphoramide (Schradan) appears not to be toxic to bees. This systemic insecticide is applied to plants before they flower. It appears in the nectar, and may be carried back to the hive. Schradan does not decompose and may be stored in honey. Up to 44.5 ppm of Schradan was found in some honey samples. Franklin Bicknell, M.D., in *Chemicals in Food and in Farm Produce: Their Harmful Effects* (Faber & Faber, 1960), estimated that this amount is equivalent to about 20 micrograms of this insecticide in a pound of honey.

Honey poisoning has long been known, having been described in 400 B.C. by the Greek writer Xenophon. Near Trabzon (formerly known as Trebizond) Turkey, Xenophon recorded that the troops found beehives, and . . .

> . . . all those who ate the honey went out of their senses and vomited and purged and not a man of them could stand on his feet. If they ate only a little they seemed like drunken men. If they ate much, like madmen; some even died of it. So they lay in heaps as if there had been a route, and they were very unhappy about it. Next day no one died, but about the same time of day they came back to their senses; in another day or two they got up dazed as if they had been drugged.

In modern times, honey poisoning in Turkey is recognized and still is experienced. Elsewhere, less common, the slight effects experienced by eating a small quantity of toxic honey probably are not well identified. Several outbreaks were reported in New Zealand, attributed to a toxin in the nectar from the tutu plant (*Coriaria ruscifolia*). Toxins have been detected in honey produced in the United States, and exported to Great Britain.

Honey from certain plants can be toxic. Nectar from rhododendron, azalea, oleander, and mountain laurel contain highly cardioactive glycosides. Honey from palmetto and black locust also may he toxic. Some honeys contain substances capable of inducing liver cancer and birth defects. Some 3 percent of all flowering plants produce pyrrolizidine alkaloids. These toxins are present in herbal garden favorites such as borage and comfrey. Tansy ragwort, a common western weed, contains alkaloids known to inflict liver damage in animals. Bees forage on ragwort during dry summer months. Researchers from Oregon State University found significant quantities (up to 3.9 ppm) of ragweed alkaloids in four samples of Oregon honey, as reported in *Science* (Feb 4, 1977). Heavily contaminated honey, being bitter, is unlikely to be sold uncut. However, frequently bitter honey is blended with milder ones. Even trace contamination of toxic ragweed alkaloids is cause for concern.

Fortunately, poisonous honey is not widespread. But it should be recognized as a problem. Bees gather nectar within a limited radius of approximately two miles. Generally, beekeepers are familiar with the flowers in their vicinity, and marketed honey is likely to be produced from safe flower sources.

Raw honey poses a distinctly different problem. Many people choose raw honey for its fine flavor, presence of enzymes, and lack of processing. For most of the population, raw honey is safe. However, it can be hazardous to very young infants.

Raw honey may contain *Clostridium botulinum*. The spores of this bacterium are responsible for botulism. In 1976, infant botulism was viewed by the Centers for Disease Control and Prevention (CDC), as an important problem that had gone unrecognized for too long. Infant botulism differs from the botulism that poisons adults following the consumption of toxins created in improperly canned or processed foods. *C. botulinum* spores are widespread in soils, dust, and raw agricultural commodities. The spores can be swallowed by infants, multiply in the gut, and produce toxins that cause botulism. Infant botulism became one more factor, among possible causes, of sudden crib death syndrome (also known as sudden infant death syndrome, or SIDS).

In July 1976, the Sioux Honey Association of Sioux City, Iowa, issued a press release, stating that honey and other raw agricultural products fed to infants less than twenty-six weeks old could produce botulism poisoning. This statement was prompted by epidemiological and laboratory findings at the California Department of Health Services. A two-year study showed that by 1978, of all foods tested that had been fed to infants who developed botu-

lism, honey alone was found to contain *C. botulinum* spores. Of more than sixty honey specimens tested in California, about 13 percent were contaminated.
These findings were confirmed independently by four laboratories in other
sections of the country, and were not unique for California honey. Although it
was believed that honey might account for less than a third of all California
infant botulism cases, the condition involved other risk factors. Also, any raw
agricultural produce, including all fruits and vegetables, can be sources of *C.
botulinum*.

Why is raw honey not safe for infants? The botulinum spores, ingested
by the infant, can grow in the intestine and produce enough toxins to make
the infant quite ill or die. Although all young infants are exposed to botulinum spores from various sources, not all infants become infected. Susceptibility may depend on the composition of the bacterial population in the
infant's intestine.

Is honey a superior sweetener? Many qualities are attributed to honey,
among which are its easy digestibility, antiseptic and laxative qualities, and
medicinal uses. These virtues may exist but they need to be separated from
any discussion of honey's nutritional value.

Tomb reliefs dating from the third millennium B.C. depict Egyptians collecting wild honey by smoking bees from their nest. Probably honey was
used far earlier. Wild honey was found infrequently, and therefore was eaten
infrequently. Therein lies the lesson. Honey, used infrequently and in small
amounts is an acceptable sweetener. If it is regarded as a flavoring rather
than as a sweetening agent, so much the better. Most basic foods do not
require sweetening; most food concoctions that do require sweetening are
items that should be consumed infrequently. Unfortunately, some people
reason that because honey is a natural sweetener, it can be used in any
amount without creating health problems, and in addition, it will provide
significant amounts of nourishment. The nutrients present in honey are supplied at exceedingly low levels. For example, one would need to consume
about 230 tablespoons of honey a day to meet the minimum requirements for
riboflavin. Similarly, honey's content of vitamin C is miniscule and far below
one's daily requirements.

Used sparingly as a flavoring agent, honey may be marginally superior to
other sweeteners. Honey contains more monosaccharides, which are sweeter
than disaccharides. Honey is about 1.3 times sweeter than sucrose, so less can
be used. Honey is utilized quickly. Both glucose and fructose have been predi-
gested in honey, so it goes directly into the bloodstream for quick energy. This
feature of easy digestibility is unfavorable, however, for hypoglycemics and
diabetics. But, if a person is allergic to corn, cane, or beet sugars, honey may
be a nonallergenic alternative.

THE NUTRIENTS IN HONEY

The following nutrient values are listed for one tablespoon of average honey in *Nutritive Value of American Foods in Common Units,* Agricultural Handbook No. 456, ARS, USDA, November 1965:

Food energy	64.0 calories	Iron	0.1 mg
Carbohydrates	17.3 grams (g)	Riboflavin	0.01 mg
Potassium	11.0 milligrams (mg)	Ascorbic acid	trace
Calcium	1.0 mg	Thiamin	trace
Phosphorus	1.0 mg	Vitamin A	none
Sodium	1.0 mg		

Honey samples analyzed by atomic absorption spectrograph for parts per million (ppm) of trace elements in honey were cited by Carl C. Pfeiffer, M.D. in *Mental & Elemental Nutrients:*

Trace element	Orange blossom honey (in ppm)	Clover honey (in ppm)
Chromium	0.02	0.05
Copper	0.05	0.08
Iron	0.59	1.81
Manganese	0.17	0.29
Zinc	0.98	0.82

Due to honey's stickiness, it clings to the teeth, and unless the mouth is cleansed promptly, honey can contribute to dental decay. This problem extends to all sweet syrups, as well as to dried fruits.

The conclusions are that honey, used sparingly, is an acceptable flavoring or sweetening agent, but, honey is overrated as a good source of nutrients.

MAPLE SYRUP

Maple syrup, like honey, is perceived as a natural, pure, unrefined, and nutrient-rich sweetener. Does reality match these perceptions?

We are indebted to Native North Americans for their introduction of maple syrup into our diet. They used a hatchet technique called "boxing" to tap sugar maple trees, either with a diamond or Y-shaped incision into the tree. At the bottom of the cut they drove the hatchet deeply into the base of the "box" and inserted a flat splinter to guide the dripping sap into a wooden trough. They concentrated the sap either by boiling it in earthenware pots or by freezing it repeatedly and discarding the sap ice. Early settlers followed similar practices, which were recorded in family Bibles. Maple syrup and maple sugar were valued because sugarcane was scarce and costly.

The maple products varied greatly. Some iron-boiling kettles produced syrups of light color and mild flavor; others, dark and strong. If the syrup was allowed to boil at length, a dark mass of burnt crystallized sugar would form. In 1794, one Vermonter described maple syrup production as one made under so many unfavorable circumstances that "it appears for the most part rough, coarse, dirty, and frequently burnt, smoky, or greasy" quoted by Helen and Scott Nearing in *The Maple Sugar Book* (John Day, 1950).

By the 1850s, maple syrup processing equipment was transformed radically. Stave buckets replaced hollowed-log troughs. Horse- or ox-drawn sleighs replaced sap yokes, and sap gathering in the sugar bush became easier. Syrup quality was controlled better when sheet-iron boilers with wooden sidepieces replaced iron kettles. The boiling equipment was suitable for indoor housing and the sugarhouse evolved.

As the population increased and land availability decreased, maple syrup producers tapped the same trees yearly. They learned conservation and used drill bits only large enough for reed spouts, called spiles, to be inserted in the trees. The newer spiles inflicted less damage to the trees than the spiles used earlier.

Even after cane sugar became more accessible and relatively inexpensive, maple syrup continued to be popular due to its distinctive flavor, and value as a home-produced crop. Maple syrup reached markets farther and farther away from its origin. In 1898, Vermont syrup products were exhibited at the Philadelphia Exposition. The demand for maple sugar exceeded the demand for sugar. By 1890, Vermont maple production had peaked at about 14 million pounds yearly, but by the turn of the century, had declined. To bolster the market, the University of Vermont and the State Agricultural Experiment Station jointly conducted research on maple sugar production, which resulted in many improvements.

Current maple syrup production still consists basically of tapping trees, gathering, concentrating, and filtering the sap, and marketing the products. While modest cottage-industry efforts remain simple, large-scale producers use sophisticated equipment and techniques.

In 1962, the FDA sanctioned use of paraformaldehyde pellets as sanitizers for maple tree tapholes. The pellets kill harmless bacteria normally found in maple trees that retard sap flow. The long-lasting and slow-dissolving pellets keep tapholes open longer and thus increase sap flow and profits. With pellet use it became possible to begin tree tapping in the Northeast as early as January. Experiments showed that trees could be tapped even as early as November, and then, by using pellets, tapholes still were productive the following April. The pellets, having a lower boiling point than syrup, presumably evaporate during the processing. For safety, some producers discarded the first sap run.

The pellet, sanctioned by federal and state regulatory agencies, was denounced by some maple syrup producers. They felt that maple syrup symbolized purity as a food and this image would be lost. With a sizable maple sugar industry involved, the Canadian Food and Drug Directorate (renamed the Health Protection Branch, Health and Welfare Canada) resisted pressure to sanction pellet use. Some American producers, having used the pellet, reported unfavorable results, including tree damage below the tap holes and early runs yielding syrup with a leafy taste.

Pellet use may lower syrup quality. If the sap is collected when the tree chemistry changes from "sweet water" to substances used for tree growth, the sap is described as tasting "buddy" and useless for producing a table-grade syrup. Even one or two buddy-stage trees can contaminate and downgrade an entire pooled sap from a sugar bush. When this occurs, a bacterial culture (*Pseudomonas geniculata*) may be added and allowed to ferment, to mask buddy syrup and convert it into an acceptable commercial product.

Maple syrup producers were not required to state on labels that their products were from sap from pelletized trees. Some producers did add label statements that their products were untreated; others, if questioned, supplied the information.

In 1982, the state of Vermont banned the use of paraformaldehyde pellets, in order to maintain the public's high regard for maple syrup as "pure" and "natural." In 1991, the Environmental Protection Agency (EPA) made paraformaldehyde use for this purpose illegal nationwide. In 1993, Canada also banned its use in maple syrup production.

It was thought that the galvanized buckets and tin evaporators used in the past might leach minute quantities of lead into the sap. However, the sap did not remain in the collecting buckets very long and the evaporators quickly "limed" over with mineral deposits from the sap. In 1995, Vermont set a goal for a maximal amount of lead in maple syrup at 500 parts per billion (ppb).

The traditional techniques for producing maple syrup continue, but newer equipment used by most syrup producers differs significantly. Stainless-steel evaporators have blind-soldered seams, so that the boiling sap does not touch the soldered part. In large-scale operations, plastic bags replace the metal collecting pails. Plastic pipe systems, permanently installed in the sugar bush, facilitate work in sap collecting. The pipes are cleaned by chemical flushing before the first sap run. Although migration of substances leached from the plastics and sanitizing chemicals may occur, after long boiling, it is thought that such contaminants are not apt to remain.

Maple syrup grading is confusing for consumers. As with many agricultural commodities, it is based on appearance rather than on taste. Color is the prime factor in grading, provided that the syrup meets requirements for density, flavor, and clarity. "Fancy" is the highest quality syrup by state standards in Vermont, followed by Grades A, B, and C. But federal USDA grades are U.S. Grade AA for light amber; A, medium amber; B, dark amber; and Unclassified. For many people the highest federal Grade AA is the wrong color. It comes from the first sap flow and lacks a strong maple flavor. Grade A, made from late season run, is darker with a more distinctive maplelike flavor. Generally, food stores stock Grade A. Grades A, B, and Unclassified account for most of the maple syrup market.

Many Vermonters prefer their Grade B and rarely is this grade exported outside of the state. Grade B is less refined than Grade A, and maple syrup aficionados claim that it has a superior flavor.

As early as the 1880s, one of the well-known blends was introduced into the American marketplace as an economical substitute for costly pure maple syrup. In the beginning, the product contained 45 percent maple syrup. As maple syrup became more expensive, over the years, gradually the percentage of maple syrup in the blend was reduced. Another well-known blend, introduced in 1966, contained only 15 percent maple syrup. Over time, the percentage of maple syrup was reduced in this blend, too. Ultimately, the level was so low that the company officials felt that the amount scarcely flavored the product, and decided to eliminate it entirely. As quoted in the *New York Times* (May 4,1975) a company representative observed:

> Americans have come to like—even prefer—the taste and consistency of imitation syrup. Our consumer tests showed that many people like the artificial stuff better than the real thing. . . Over the years, they've gotten used to it.

This conclusion was reinforced by another survey, sponsored by the International Maple Syrup Institute. Of more than 2,000 consumers interviewed, fewer than 200 could distinguish between pure maple syrup and the imitations.

Maple syrup production, labor intensive and seasonal, is an expensive sweetener to produce. Gradually, through the years, maple sugar production dwindled. Around 1900, more than 5 million gallons were produced annually;

by 1972, production had declined to only 1 million. At the same time, demand increased. In 1971, market studies showed that some 18 million American households occasionally used pure maple products, mainly syrup and some maple sugar. Unfortunately, the studies also revealed that half of the consumers who *thought* that they were buying pure maple syrup actually had chosen blends with less expensive ingredients such as corn syrup, water, sugar, and artificial colors and flavors. Such blends are known as pancake or waffle syrups.

One product labeled Canadian Brand Imitation Maple Butter had a prominent logo of a maple leaf. The product, made in Massachusetts, consisted of glucose, cane sugar, milk, cornstarch, salt, and imitation maple flavoring. Another product labeled Vermont Maple Orchards Creamy Sugar and Butter Spread, contained neither maple syrup nor butter, and consisted of 85 percent cane sugar syrup.

Such practices became so widespread that, belatedly, countermeasures were instituted jointly in a two-nation campaign by the International Maple Syrup Institute in Quebec, Canada, and the United States Maple Syrup Information Bureau in New York City. The effort was to protect consumers from misrepresentations by means of an industry-wide use of a distinctive logo showing sap dripping into a bucket, combined with a maple leaf. Display of the logo would guarantee the purity and grade of the maple syrup. A representative of the Institute was quoted in *Food Product Development* (Jul 1979) as saying, "We are advocating legislation which will assure the public that they are getting the food they are paying for."

From time to time, the FDA seizes maple syrup products that are adulterated and misbranded. Generally, less costly cane or corn syrups have been substituted in whole, or in part, for more costly maple syrup.

In addition to the maple syrup blends, imitation maple flavors are available to food and beverage processors, in powder and liquid forms. These replacers are used in many processed foods including canned hams, processed meats, cereals, baked goods, candies, ice creams, and syrups. One prominent flavoring company in its advertisement in *Food Processing* (Feb 1978) stated that its artificial maple flavor "tastes as authentic as a cold morning in Vermont."

Is pure maple syrup a superior sweetener? *Consumer Reports* (May 1979) reported on its analysis of pure maple-syrup products. They contained about 70 grams of total sugars per five tablespoons of syrup. This quantity, estimated as an average amount poured over a stack of three pancakes, served as a measure. In contrast, the total sugars in syrup blends ranged from about 30 to 50 grams of total sugars per serving.

In the same analysis, the predominant sugar in maple syrup products was sucrose; in syrup blends, dextrose; and in one low-calorie syrup blend, fructose. Small amounts of fructose, maltose, and lactose were present in all the syrups tested. None of these sugars are more—or less—"natural" than any of the others.

Calories ranged from 272 to 313 per serving in all of the tested syrups except the low-calorie one. That product contained about three times as much water as the other syrup blends, and had 82 calories per serving.

Consumers Union, the testing organization that conducted this analysis, suggested that in many cases, choosing syrup blends would serve just as well as pure maple syrup, and with a far lower cost.

This poor advice encourages consumers to select poor-quality food products. Also, persons with allergies usually tolerate maple syrup, but may react unfavorably to blends that contain cane, corn, or beet sugars, especially if they appear as hidden ingredients in blends.

A headline in the *Brattleboro* [Vermont] *Daily Reformer* (Dec 6, 1975) proclaimed, MANY NUTRIENTS ARE IN PURE MAPLE SYRUP. This statement was based on information supplied by Dr. Mariafranca Morselli, from the botany department of the University of Vermont. She reported that maple syrup retains nutrients even though the sap is boiled, concentrated, and filtered. She claimed that pure, filtered maple syrup contained "significant amounts" of calcium, potassium, manganese, magnesium, phosphorus, and iron, and trace amounts of riboflavin, pantothenic acid, pyridoxine, niacin, biotin, folic acid, and amino acids.

The nutrients Morselli listed so impressively may be found in pure maple syrup, but they are not present in sufficient amounts to make any significant contribution to the diet unless the syrup is consumed at undesirably high levels. As with molasses and honey, maple syrup needs to be viewed as a pleasant flavoring agent, rather than as a food that offers an important contribution of nutrients. As with other sticky syrups, maple syrup should be removed from the mouth quickly, in order to avoid dental decay.

SORGHUM

Sorghum, one of the oldest cultivated grains, and consumed by humans and animals, also yields sugar, syrup, and starch. Sorghum yields about 180 to 230 pounds of raw sugar per ton of stalk. Although sweet sorghum was recognized as a potential sugar source for more than a century, its full development awaited more recent research. The major sugar production methods used with cane and beet were ineffective in removing the large amounts of starch present in sweet sorghum. Although it was possible to produce sorghum syrup, it was not possible to produce it as a crystallized sugar. Conventional processes to recover sugar from cane or beet require temperatures near 200°F.

At such heat, the sorghum starch granules gelatinize and thicken the syrup to reduce or even totally prevent sugar crystallization.

In the early 1970s, researchers at the Agricultural Research Service (ARS), USDA, developed a technique to remove the sorghum starch by modifying the refining procedures used with sugarcane. But the method was inapplicable to sugar beet facilities, and crystallized sorghum was not perfected for commercialization. By the mid-1970s, ARS announced that sweet sorghum soon might join the ranks of cane and beet as a source of crystalline sugar. In a factory production test, researchers were able to produce 22 tons of raw sugar from sweet sorghum equal to cane sugar's purity. This production was the culmination of a long, intensive effort involving the development of new sorghum varieties; improved growing, harvesting, and processing techniques; and innovative research. At last, it became possible to mill sweet sorghum in conventional mills, and free the raw juice from starch by standard clarifiers. Sorghum syrup looks and tastes like light-colored molasses derived from sugarcane. The FDA has seized some sorghum syrups adulterated with less costly corn syrups. In contrast to other sweeteners, sorghum consumption is minor.

By the early 1990s, a sorghum syrup was developed for processed food applications. Named *Sorgo,* the syrup was made available by Crompton and Knowles.

This syrup is composed of 68 to 72 percent sucrose and invert sugars. Its sweet flavor is more intense in the darker grades from compounds extracted from the sorghum plant, and the flavor intensity develops further during the processing.

The distributor reports that the sorghum syrup is a nutritional source of calcium, iron, potassium, and phosphorus. Sorghum syrup somewhat resembles cane sugar molasses. However, it is lighter in color and milder in flavor. Sorghum syrup is suitable for baked goods, chewy confections, sauces, glazes, and as a table syrup.

COMPOSITION OF TRADITIONAL SWEETENERS

Comparing the traditional sweeteners reveals that they do not differ very much in composition from one another. Following is a list of each of their values for one cup of sweetener.

Type of sweetener	Grams	Calories	Carbohydrates*
Brown sugar, packed	220	821	212.1
Molasses, 1st extraction, light	328	827	213.2
Molasses, 2nd extraction, medium	328	761	196.8

Type of sweetener	Grams	Calories	Carbohydrates*
Molasses, 3rd extraction, blackstrap	328	699	180.4
Molasses, Barbados	328	889	229.6
Maple syrup	315	794	204.8
Sorghum	330	848	224.4
Table blend, mainly corn	328	951	246.0
Table blend, cane and maple	315	794	204.8
Table sugar, white	200	770	199.0

*in grams

–*Nutritive Value of American Foods in Common Units,* Agricultural Handbook No. 456 (ARS, USDA, Nov 1965)

MALT

To the general public, the word malt may be associated with malt beer or malted milk; to food and beverage processors, malt serves additional functions. Bakers use diastatic malt, which is from sprouted grain, usually barley. The grain is roasted with low heat to retain enzymes, then ground, and made either into syrup or powder. Added to bakery dough, the enzymes in diastatic malt split the starches present in the flour into maltose and dextrin. These sugars, known as yeast foods in baking, assist fermentation and production of soluble proteins used by the yeast. These enzymes play comparable roles in the fermentation of beer and other malt beverages.

Several nutritional benefits result from sprouting grain. The sprouting process reduces the undesirable phytic acid, and increases the vitamin content. Germination produces other beneficial changes, too, that result in improved digestibility of the food, and increased bioavailability of nutrients from the food.

Bakers use malt extract, too. It imparts a good flavor and color to baked goods. The extract is not very sweet. It has about the same sweetness level as corn syrup, and only about a third the sweetness of invert syrup. Dehydrated malt extract is available in a readily handled crystalline form.

Bakers also use malt syrup, which is dark in color and strong in flavor. It is made entirely from malted barley. For lighter, sweeter syrups, malt extract is blended with corn syrup in various proportions and used by bakers as yeast foods. Higher percentages of corn syrup and lower percentages of malted barley are blended for use in certain types of baked goods, confections, ice creams, breakfast cereals, pretzels, vinegars, and pet foods.

Traditionally, dextrins (polysaccharides made from cornstarch) were used as carriers of water-insoluble flavoring oils and other substances. After various processing steps, the dextrins help to convert liquid flavors into dry powder, which can be used to formulate many dry foods and beverage mixes, without suffering flavor loss.

By legal definition, a food additive is any substance, other than a basic foodstuff, that is present in food as a result of any aspect of production. Thus, dextrins used for this purpose are regarded as a food additive. In 1958, dextrins were granted Generally Recognized as Safe (GRAS) status. With a greatly expanded use in processed foods, in 1979 the FDA curbed dextrins' use. If processors use dextrins above the established upper limit, dextrins lose their GRAS status, and are regulated.

Maltodextrins were developed as replacers for dextrins as well as for gums and starches used in food and beverage processing. Maltodextrins are hydrolyzed carbohydrates. Some products are made from dent (field) corn, and the more expensive maltodextrins are made from the more costly waxy maize corn. The sweetness level of maltodextrins is lower than that of dextrose. Maltodextrins serve many functions as processing aids. They permit processors to spray dry even the most difficult, highly hygroscopic (moisture absorbing) food ingredients without clogging the equipment. Dry mixes remain free flowing, without lumping or caking. Maltodextrins, unlike sucrose, have excellent suspension in solution, and inhibit crystallization. Being bland, maltodextrins do not overpower delicate flavors present from other ingredients. Because of their low reducing sugar content, maltodextrins can be used in baked products in which corn syrup solids are undesirable. Maltodextrins are favored especially for creme fillings, glazes, snack food coatings, pie crusts, and cracker fillings.

Now commonly used, maltodextrins have replaced dextrins in converting liquid flavors into dry powders. They are found in many dehydrated products, such as soup and gravy mixes; doughnut, cake, cookie, and icing mixes; in powdered citrus drinks; instant coffee and tea; and cocktail mixes; spice blends, seasoning, and salad dressing mixes; and coffee whiteners. Additional uses are in candies such as marshmallows and jelly beans; frozen eggs; frozen desserts; infant foods; peanut butters; whipped toppings; and sausages.

Malted ingredients are marketed in a number of forms and degrees of sweetness. They include malted whole grains, malt flours, malt extracts, and malt blends with other sweeteners.

One traditional method of producing malted-grain products is by sprouting. Customized kilning of wheat meets a desired flavor and/or function, such as dark, or light-colored malt, or the presence or absence of enzymatic activity. Because each type of grain requires different conditions for optimal sprouting, more and more malted grains are being produced by different proprietary processes.

The wheat products include flakes, nuggets, kibbles, meal, and flours, intended for use by bakers and cereal manufacturers. Use of these malted products permit a reduction in the quantity of sweeteners added to product formulations, as well as cost savings. Grainulose is a blend of wheat, rye, and rice syrups. Sunspire is from malted barley.

A syrup based on tapioca is available from Ciranda, in Hudson, Wisconsin.

GRAIN SYRUPS

As an outgrowth of advanced malting techniques, wheat, rye, and rice syrups can be produced. They serve as alternatives to malted barley syrups and blends. They offer sweetness, enhance flavor and color, and add body and sheen to cereal-based products such as breakfast cereals, baked goods, snacks, confections, beverages, and pet foods. These syrups tolerate high baking temperatures, and each one has its distinctive characteristic of flavor, color, and sweetness level. Use of these syrups can allow a reduction of other sugars and colors used in formulations.

Rising sugar prices created interest in low-cost alternative sweeteners, especially when sweetening is not the ingredient's main function. Among products that can replace sugar is a byproduct of beer brewing. Spent barley malt and rice grain—wastes from beer processing—contain soluble sugars that can be dried and milled to produce a sweet-flavored and colored sugar replacer. The inexpensive products can replace up to 20 percent of more costly sugar in many food products such as breakfast cereals, breads, crackers, corn chips, and flavored snacks; up to 25 percent in cookies, and up to 35 percent in pancake and waffle mixes.

Rice Syrup

Numerous rice syrup products have been developed. They are more costly to produce than corn syrup, but they may have a healthier image. Corn syrups, made from highly purified starch, suffer mineral losses from the original plant. In contrast, rice-based syrup is minimally processed, and retains a small amount of fat, which helps retain vitamin B.

Some syrups are promoted as rice syrups, but rice is merely a small constituent of the syrup. Such syrups may contain numerous other sweeteners such as liquid glucose, sorbitol, high-fructose corn syrup, dextrose, monohydrate, and high maltose syrup, along with the rice.

Other rice syrups do consist mainly of rice, without added colors or preservatives. They are produced from rice, water, barley, and an enzyme starter that converts the rice starch into complex sugars. By using the enzyme, use of the harsh process of acid hydrolysis is avoided. The complex sugars are absorbed into the bloodstream slowly, compared to more rapid absorption of simple sugars. Rice syrup, processed in this manner, is composed mostly of maltose, an oligosaccharide that requires more time for digestion than do the simple sugars such as sucrose, fructose, or glucose.

To produce such rice syrup, the grain is cooked for a long time at a low temperature. This allows the enzyme from the malted grain to ferment in the liquid mash. The liquid is cooked again at a low temperature until the rice syrup attains a good consistency and with the maximal conversion of starches into complex sugars.

Other rice syrup products combine rice with fruit juices. One type combines rice maltodextrin from partially milled brown rice with pear juice concentrate. This sweetener, available to food and beverage processors, has applications in beverages, baked goods, confections, and other food products. Another type combines rice syrup with grape juice, and is offered to processors as a fat replacement in food products and sports drinks.

Some processors promote the fact that their rice products are made from brown rice. As a whole grain, it is the least processed form of rice, and is more nutritious than white rice. The brown rice provides more proteins, calcium, phosphorus, potassium, niacin, fiber, and vitamin E than does white rice. The syrup made from brown rice is a source of complex carbohydrates as well as being a sweetener. Briess Ingredients Company in Chilton, Wisconsin, produces *BriesSweet*, a certified organic brown rice syrup.

Oat Syrup

Oats, or waxy barley, provide a grain-based syrup that contains a significant amount of beneficial beta glucan. The sweetener OatsCreme is manufactured by American Oats in Minneapolis, Minnesota. The producer uses the sweetener in its own food product line, which includes a sports drink, and various nondairy products including frozen desserts.

This sweetener, made from grain, makes use of a combination of enzymes to convert a slurry to the level of desired sweetness. Most of the sweetness is provided by glucose. However, the other saccharides are larger and provide the viscosity and texture needed for frozen desserts. This sweetener, being exceptionally bland, contains an added flavoring agent. However, the product contains no added fats, sugars, or other ingredients. This syrup requires refrigeration.

Organic Hydrolysate-Derived Grain Sweeteners

Some grain-based sweeteners are composed of organically certified hydrolysates derived from oats, rice, or barley. The sweeteners are from grain that is certified to be GMO-free (grains that are not derived from genetically modified organisms). These sweeteners are manufactured by means of a proprietary enzymatic process. The sweeteners contribute moderate sweetness levels to products. Depending on the specific intended use, these products have a range of sweetness equivalent to dextrose. They have low-glycemic index rates.

All processed forms of sugar contribute approximately four calories per gram. All are primarily carbohydrates. They are simple ones, in contrast to complex carbohydrates from whole grains. Obviously, all of the traditional sweeteners are high in calories, low in nutrients, and do not differ dramatically one from another.

Chapter 3

CRYSTALLINE FRUCTOSE: A FRUIT-SUGAR PRETENDER

It is necessary to reinforce the idea that fructose is not a drug. It is only a natural food that in itself is deficient in vitamins, amino acids, and minerals. It is therefore a classic "empty calorie food." Yet it has advantages found in no other product.
—J. DANIEL PALM, PH.D., DEPARTMENT OF BIOLOGY, ST. OLAF COLLEGE, 1976

In the early 1970s, new sweeteners were introduced, primarily through health food outlets, consisting of 99.9 percent pure crystalline fructose (CF). In health-food trade journals, CF products were described as fruit sugar, found naturally in honey, berries, and fruits. CF was described as being nearly as sweet as sucrose in cold foods and beverages, as looking and tasting like ordinary sugar, but with half the calories.

FRUCTOSE'S SPECIAL PROPERTIES

What is this sugar? Fructose, also called levulose or fruit sugar, is a monosaccharide, and the sweetest of all commonly found natural sugars. It is found in nearly all sweet fruits, berries, some vegetables, and honey. *But CF products are made from cane or beet sugar.*

In 1792, a German-Russian pharmacist, J. T. Lowitz, probably identified CF when he described a type of sugar that crystallized only with difficulty. But fructose's discovery usually is credited to a French chemist, A. P. Dubrunfaut, who in 1847 successfully isolated fructose from cane sugar. By 1874, the sugar achieved some practical significance when E. Kuelz, a German, suspected that fructose might be suitable for diabetics. However, after Sir Frederick Grant Banting, a Canadian physiologist, discovered insulin in 1921, fructose's dietary use was nearly forgotten for three decades. It was produced by a complicated, expensive process using inulin, a substance found in the tubers of plants such as dahlias, Jerusalem artichokes, and chicory. Its use was limited almost exclusively to intravenous feeding.

In the late 1960s, leading European CF producers developed high-yield processes for economical large-scale production by synthesizing fructose from sugarcane and sugar beets. Commercially pure CF is produced by separating fructose from the glucose part in sucrose by means of chromatographic selective absorption techniques. The fructose, which is four times sweeter than glucose, is crystallized to CF. The remaining glucose is sold as a byproduct.

By 1970, commercial quantities of CF were marketed in Europe, notably in Finland, West Germany, Sweden, and Norway. In Finland, more than a hundred commercially processed food items were sweetened experimentally with fructose, in an attempt to learn if consumers found such foods acceptable. Among the treated items were jams, jellies, marmalades, soft drinks, ice creams, frozen foods, baked goods, confections, pickles, mustards, catsups, and even marinated herring. All of the products were judged satisfactory, and many were rated superior in taste to traditionally sweetened products.

Meanwhile, in the United States, CF's potentials were largely unnoticed and not developed by food and beverage processors. By 1975, CF began to attract attention. By then, an image had been established that CF was a "healthier" natural sweetening alternative for many general food and beverage applications, as well as potential applications for calorie-reduced foods that had come into vogue. The special physical, chemical, and metabolic properties of CF were extolled to processors, who began to view this sweetener as a particularly versatile and attractive raw material.

CF is the most water-soluble of all sugars. It dissolves readily even in cool media. CF is very hygroscopic, which makes it an excellent agent to prevent baked goods and confections from drying out. Used in highly sweetened foods and beverages, CF does not crystallize during shipment and storage of products. CF, one of the most chemically reactive of sugars, readily forms aromatically pleasant combinations and browning reactions in baked goods.

CF is also an excellent masking agent for the bitter aftertaste of saccharin, which intensifies the perception of sweetness through synergism. For example, 1 percent saccharin combined with 99 percent CF is five to seven times sweeter than sucrose. Saccharin is synergistic with sucrose, too. A 10 percent water solution of a mixture composed of 60 percent CF and 40 percent sucrose is about 1.3 times sweeter than a pure sucrose solution. By 1975, the potential uses for CF were described as "limited only by the creativeness of food technologists and dietitians," according to *Food Technology* (Nov 1975).

Cost was CF's main drawback. Its refining process is infinitely more complex and expensive than the refining process for sucrose. CF must be about 99.5 percent pure in order for crystallization to develop. No CF was produced in the United States. Hoffmann-La Roche became the sole importer of Finnish CF. But soaring sucrose costs by the mid 1970s made CF somewhat more competitive. At that point, the fructose craze began, and gained momentum.

SWEET SEDUCTION

Increasingly, CF was used with processed foods, including gelatins and frozen desserts, cake and cookie mixes, puddings, jams, jellies, and preserves; candies and chewing gums; salad dressings and mayonnaises; peanut butters; protein supplements; beverage powders; lemonade tea mixes; isotonic beverages for athletes; and breakfast cereals and their coatings for presweetened cereals. After successful test marketing, one prominent producer of frozen cakes launched a national distribution of six new types of cakes sweetened with CF.

By 1979, fructose was a household word due to books and media popularization. CF was central for diet plans purported to quell cravings for sweets, appease the appetite, and lose weight without dieting stresses such as abnormal hunger or energy loss. In February of that year, the "Fabulous 14-Day Fructose Diet Plan" appeared in the popular homemakers' magazine, *Family Circle* (see inset below). A fructose cookbook was advertised about the sensational all-natural sweetener, which was ideal for cooking and baking, a natural preservative, an insulin stabilizer, and a hunger reducer. Other cookbooks also included CF. At the 1979 Food Editors' Conference, Hoffmann-La Roche sponsored a seminar to extol CF's virtues. One food editor reported that, in general, the audience remained unconvinced that CF, at least ten times more costly at the retail level than sucrose, was especially beneficial for healthy people.

Health food stores, health food sections in supermarkets, and drugstores were targeted for marketing CF. In addition to the wide range of CF-sweetened products that were marketed, *Alive,* a magazine distributed in many health food stores, carried an advertisement in its autumn 1979 issue:

> Yes, we have fructose, the new sweetener you've been reading about. Fructose is an excellent source of energy for active persons such as athletes, long-distance drivers, and anyone subject to stress and fatigue . . . Our pure unflavored fructose may be your answer to a healthier diet.

THE "FABULOUS 14-DAY FRUCTOSE DIET PLAN"

At last, a diet for those who crave sweets! The secret is a supplement of fructose—the sweetest of all natural sugars—that quells the hunger and keeps up your energy. Plus a tempting low calorie 14-day menu plan that takes the guesswork out of dieting and lets you lose a pound of body weight—up to half a pound of actual fat—a day.

—J.T. Cooper, M.D. *Dr. Cooper's Fabulous Fructose Diet* (M. Evans, 1979)

Liquid fructose, formerly available only to industrial and institutional users, reached the retail level, packaged in easy-pour bottles, intended as a general table sweetener and for baking, canning, preserving, and other home uses. Honey-flavored syrup containing 90 percent CF was offered as an inexpensive honey replacer that would not crystallize or vary seasonally in composition, color, or flavor. The marketplace was flooded with many CF-sweetened products, including "all natural" soft drinks.

By 1979, the fructose craze reached such dizzy heights that Danny Wells, head of the Standards Committee of the National Nutritional Foods Association (NNFA), a trade organization of the health food industry, sent its members a letter cautioning against misrepresenting fructose, and warning them not to place CF on a "magestic plateau." Wells warned especially against irresponsible statements that described CF as a "harmless sugar," "an excellent sugar for hypoglycemics," or worse, that claimed, "even diabetics can safely use fructose." Wells suggested that retailers shun the fructose fad, and build sales based on sound nutritional principles. Wells' warnings were carried in the trade journal *Whole Foods* (May 1979), and were given serious attention by responsible NNFA leadership. At the organization's annual convention in July 1979, the program notes listed "The Fructose Debate" to provide an opportunity to educate its members.

Individuals within the health food movement engaged in discussion and soul-searching. Many questioned whether CF truly could be regarded as a "natural" sugar or whether it should be viewed as a processed carbohydrate, and as a refined sugar, derived from another refined sugar.

On the other hand, food processors continued to sell the natural image for CF. Their persuasive argument was that as a result of its natural occurrence in many sweet-tasting foods, fructose has always been part of the human diet. This notion is only partly true. Commercial CF may be identical to fructose chemically, as found, for example, in an apple or honey, but the commercial product is a substance in isolation. In food, it is accompanied by nutrients that aid in its metabolism.

The American Diabetes Association (ADA) issued a clear statement on this issue, of interest both to diabetics and non-diabetics (reported in *Processed Prepared Foods*, Feb 1979):

> Fructose in its refined crystalline state contains few minerals, no vitamins, or fiber in contrast to naturally occurring fructose, e.g., fruit and complex carbohydrates that do contain these substances. The effects of ingestion of large amounts of any refined carbohydrates on this aspect of nutrition must be considered.

THE FACTS BEHIND THE IMAGE

In May 1980, the Center for Science in the Public Interest (CSPI) petitioned the Food and Drug Administration (the FDA) and the Federal Trade Commission (FTC) to halt misstatements and exaggerations about CF's properties in advertisements and on labels, CSPI argued, in part, that manufacturers were taking advantage of "the sinking reputation of ordinary sugar" to promote CF-sweetened products as more healthful (reported in the *New York Times*, May 7, 1980).

Both federal agencies studied the question. The issue was a difficult one. Neither agency has ever established a definition of a "natural" food; neither has the health food industry defined it. "Natural" has been such a misused term that it is meaningless. In July 1980, in response to CSPI's petition, the FTC announced that it had begun an investigation and expected that several of CSPI's concerns would be met by the agency's planned trade regulation rule on food advertising, which would cover food products' energy and low-calorie claims. The FDA promised to have its field officers check labels.

In late 1980, the FDA received another complaint. The Sugar Association charged that certain claims made for CF-sweetened products were misleading. The association challenged the claims that CF is sweeter than sucrose, and that less CF is needed to obtain a similar sweetness level as sucrose in a given food. In a letter to the FDA, carried in *Food Engineering* (Mar 1979) the association said:

> It is difficult to make a sweeping generalization regarding the amount [of CF] necessary to make a product acceptable to the consumer . . . [and] it has not been shown that because one calorie sweetener is sweeter than another its preferential use will result in a lowered intake of calories.

In response, the FDA agreed. John M. Taylor, director of the agency's Division of Regulatory Guidance at the FDA, reported that a food processor using CF in a product would mislead the public with claims that "the greater sweetness of fructose will result in lowered intake of calories because of a lesser use level compared to other sweeteners," (quoted in *Food Engineering*, Oct 1980).

IS FRUCTOSE ANY BETTER FOR YOUR HEALTH?

Are claims justified that fructose is a "healthier sugar" or "the miracle sweetener" as the advertisements proclaimed? Hardly. Metabolically, CF is somewhat different from other sugars. During digestion in a normal healthy individual, sucrose is broken down into equal parts of glucose and fructose. These components enter the bloodstream through the small intestinal wall and the blood carries the sugars to the tissues and to the liver. They are converted to glycogen, and stored by the liver until needed by the body. Insulin makes it possible for glucose, the blood sugar, to enter nearly all of the body's cells and be utilized. Both glucose and sucrose are absorbed rapidly, and result in surges of high levels of glucose in the blood. This development places uneven and stressful demands on the insulin secretion system.

Fructose is absorbed more slowly, and goes directly to the liver, without insulin. The liver cells transform most of the fructose into glucose, which *then does require insulin for use by the body's cells. Therefore, it is incorrect to say that insulin is not required in fructose metabolism.* Almost all of the fructose eventually becomes glucose, but it trickles into the system and avoids large surges. The low amount of insulin required in fructose metabolism, and its slow absorption rate into the bloodstream, provide the basis for the special benefit claims made for CF. The ultimate insulin requirement is ignored.

One alleged but unproven benefit is CF's value in weight-reduction diets. Fructose is less likely than sucrose to cause blood sugar level fluctuations, which may trigger low blood sugar (hypoglycemia) with its accompanying tendency to cause overeating and result in weight gain.

Another purported benefit is for persons during extended periods of stress, such as drivers, pilots, athletes, or individuals engaged in food fasting. The reasoning is that fructose has a protein-sparing effect due to its slow absorption from the gut, but rapid metabolism in the liver. During exercise or fasting periods, the liver's glucose and glycogen stores are depleted. In attempting to replenish blood sugar, the body may use protein as the necessary raw material. Fructose consumption, it is argued, can provide a lasting supply of a readily available substance, and thus spare protein from being used for this purpose. The alleged benefit is that fructose, in slowing down insulin release, allows adrenalin to flow.

The most important claim, however, is fructose's special benefit to the nation's millions of diabetics. The slower uptake and the moderate blood glucose response are features that led to the notion that fructose is a better and easier sugar for diabetics to digest because they cannot manufacture enough insulin within their bodies to utilize glucose properly. These claims were reinforced by reports that fructose is used widely by diabetics in some European countries.

Most fructose studies and experiments for diabetics have been short term, or they lack essential data about effectiveness and safety. Scientific studies to evaluate CF for long-term dietary diabetes management are lacking. Studies with animals and humans have focused on tests with fructose and other non-glucose sweeteners in their pure forms, and as the sole item in the diet. According to the ADA, long-term realistic studies correlating fructose consumption with mixed meals typically eaten by diabetics are needed before any recommendation can be made. The ADA noted that the amount of fructose acceptable in a diabetic food plan is uncertain at present, and in the absence of sufficient evidence, approval of CF for diabetic use can be neither accepted nor rejected.

In well-managed adult diabetes, CF does not appear to have any dietary advantages over sucrose. In 1976, studies of blood sugar levels and urinary glucose excretion did not differ in nine adult diabetics, compared with three normal controls, when all subjects consumed breakfasts with similar amounts of sucrose or fructose. The researchers concluded that it seems unnecessary to have specially sweetened foods designed for diabetics.

Profound differences exist between the two main types of diabetes, type 1 and type 2. The effects of substituting CF for other carbohydrates in the diet also differ. In addition, obese adult diabetics may differ from lean young diabetics in their insulin-dependence. The advantages of using CF appear slight or negligible. CF use may be safe, provided the diabetic controls the total caloric intake.

Another consideration that tends to dampen enthusiasm for fructose substitution of sucrose was a finding in 1973 that carbohydrate restriction may not be as important in diabetic diets as previously believed. The newer emphasis in diabetic management is to control the total caloric intake to achieve ideal body weight. This means restricting all foods proportionately, not necessarily restricting carbohydrates disproportionately.

A report, Dietary Sugars in Health & Disease: Fructose, prepared in 1976 by the Federation of American Societies for Experimental Biology (FASEB) at the FDA's request, indicated that most American diabetologists were *not* recommending CF use to patients. FASEB concluded, "It is the prevailing medical opinion that there are no clinical advantages of substituting fructose for glucose either orally or parenterally [intravenously] in any disease state."

Dr. Victor Fratelli, assistant to the associate director for Nutrition and Food Sciences at the FDA, reported that the agency regarded the difference between the metabolism of fructose and glucose insufficiently significant to classify CF as a substance apart from sucrose. Fructose, which occurs naturally in foods, was granted GRAS (Generally Recognized as Safe) status for food use and was permitted whenever safe and suitable nutritive sweeteners are indicated. Because of this insufficiently significant difference between CF and other sugars, its value over other sugars either for diabetics or non-diabetics is questionable. Fratelli continued, in his contribution to FASEB report, "Any argument that one tries to develop that indicates these nutritive sweeteners are beneficial in weight reduction is very tenuous. What you are doing is substituting one carbohydrate for another."

June Biermann and Barbara Toohey, two diabetic authors, gave common-sense advice in their book, *The Diabetic's Total Health Book* (3rd edition, Tarcher, 1992):

> Fructose *cannot* be eaten freely without being counted. Indeed, one table-spoon of fructose is a fruit exchange without the fiber and nutritive advantages of fruit. A tablespoon of fructose does not seem like a good trade for a fresh, juicy peach or ten large sweet cherries, or a small crunchy apple. Fructose, in short, is not the free lunch you've been look-ing for. What is a diabetic to do, then, to satisfy the sweet tooth that some diabetics seem to have? Rather than trying to satisfy it, we think you should just yank the rotten rascal out by the roots. Get yourself to the point that you no longer like excessively sweet things. Change your taste.

This good advice is sensible for the general population as well as for dia-betics. Although CF's safety for hypoglycemics or its effectiveness for weight reduction are unproven, these features have been used as selling points for many food products sweetened with CF.

How valid is the claim for weight reduction with CF? Studies at Utah State University, reported in *Utah Science* (Fall 1980) showed that calorie-counting individuals are not likely to benefit by substituting CF for sucrose. The researchers concluded that the only guaranteed way to decrease calorie intake is to eat less (and exercise more). The researchers also found that con-trary to popular belief and advertising hype, CF does not sweeten all prod-ucts more efficiently than sucrose, and therefore would be undependable for calorie reduction.

CF use raised metabolic concerns. As early as December 1972, in *Diabetic Care*, the ADA cautioned diabetics that:

> Many of the abnormalities produced by feeding sucrose (including increased cholesterol, triglycerides, enlarged liver, damaged kidneys, impaired glucose tolerance, insulin sensitivity) are also produced, but even more extensively, by the fructose (and not by the glucose) part of the sucrose. The harmful part of the sucrose molecule is the fructose half. The safety of regular consumption of large amounts of fructose is unknown. Accumulation of fructose (and sorbitol, see Chapter 5) in nerv-ous tissues of untreated diabetics has been blamed for nerve damage.

In rat studies, fructose raised the serum cholesterol level, whereas glucose showed no such effect. Among potential adverse metabolic effects of high fructose consumption are its ability to induce gout in susceptible individuals and to raise fat levels (triglycerides) and cholesterol in the blood.

Metabolic disturbances may result in both normal and diabetic individuals when fructose is fed intravenously, either if infused rapidly or if used at high levels. Rapid infusions have caused nausea and epigastric pain. High infusion levels include a considerable rise in blood lactate and pyruvate levels, and can lead to metabolic acidosis, especially in uncontrolled diabetics. The ADA advised in "The Need for Special Foods & Sugar Substitutes by Individuals with Diabetes Mellitus," in FASEB's report to the FDA (May 1978) that "considering the potential adverse health effects, administration of [intravenous] fructose should be discouraged, particularly in diabetic patients."

Researchers suggested that the use of fructose offers no advantage in intravenous feeding. Yet physicians mistakenly may believe that no harm is done because fructose is utilized readily without extra insulin.

At times, health professionals use fructose intravenously to sober drunken patients quickly. Studies have questioned the effectiveness of this practice. Twenty males, aged eighteen to seventy years, were hospitalized for treatment of acute alcohol intoxication. In double-blind studies, the men were divided randomly into two groups. Blood samples were drawn from all men. Then, each man in one group was given 100 grams of fructose in 1,000 milliliters (ml) of water intravenously over one hour; in the other group, a similar amount of glucose was given in the same manner. Two hours later, blood samples were drawn again. The blood alcohol levels for the two groups did not differ significantly, nor did members of either group differ in their ability to walk straight lines. However, fructose did induce metabolic disturbances, by raising uric acid and lactate serum levels in all ten men in the group. The researchers recommended that fructose not be used to treat acute alcohol intoxication. Reports from elsewhere noted gout attack and lactic acidosis after fructose administration.

Other metabolic disturbances were reported with fructose consumption at high levels. Diabetics promptly spill sugar into the urine. Hypoglycemics, too, can suffer adverse reactions. Large single oral fructose doses (from 70 to 100 grams) by normal healthy people may result in gastrointestinal upset, including diarrhea, flatulence, and colic pains. Large individual differences have been found to exist in human tolerance to fructose.

Another health-related benefit ascribed to CF is a lower caries induction rate than sucrose. The evidence is equivocal. The claim is based on studies conducted in Finland from 1972 to 1974 at the Institute of Dentistry, University of Turku. CF totally replaced sucrose in the diet of human subjects. In a short-term study of only four days, a fructose-sweetened diet decreased plaque formation by 30 percent, compared to a similar diet sweetened with sucrose.

Although plaque is believed to be essential for caries production, visibly observed plaque is not necessarily cariogenic (leading to caries formation).

In two-year human feeding studies at Turku, thirty-eight subjects were placed on a fructose-sweetened diet, and fifty-two on a sucrose-sweetened one. The dental caries incidence dropped by more than 25 percent in those fed fructose. Results from this single study may be significant, but fructose is impractical and improbable as a total sucrose replacer.

Fructose is a fermentable carbohydrate. In four different animal studies, conducted from 1966 to 1974, fructose was found to be approximately equal to sucrose as a suitable medium for bacterial growth and caries formation. Possibly fructose is more cariogenic in experimental animals than in humans.

A FULL-PAGE ADVERTISEMENT FOR CRYSTALLINE FRUCTOSE

If it's sweet, juicy, chewy, fruity or baked—Krystar Crystalline Fructose can deliver better flavor, improved texture, longer shelf life and fewer calories, all at lower cost.

Created by [A.E.] Staley [Manufacturing], and available only from Tate & Lyle, Krystar crystalline fructose is today's perfect answer to the continuing consumer desire for innovative, lower-calorie food products. Equally, Krystar's unparalleled ability to enhance flavor and improve product quality, while also reducing costs, make it particularly attractive to manufacturers of baked goods, liquid and powdered beverages, dairy products, desserts, confections, processed fruits, and cereals.

In simplest terms: whatever you do with sucrose, you can do it better with Krystar, as a partial or full replacement. The standard result: a significantly improved product at a rewarding lower cost.

Tate & Lyle is now a world leader in the low-cost commercialization of fructose, and offers a complete line-up of Krystar in both pure crystalline and liquid forms: as always, you can rely on Tate & Lyle for a consistent, high-quality stable-cost supply anywhere in the world . . .

—*Food Technology,* March 2005
Note: Despite the repudiated health claims for CF, this sweetener is still being promoted.

Theodore Kourioudes, D.M.D., and his associates at the Dental Institute, University of Alabama in Birmingham, engaged in research funded by the National Institute of Dental Research, National Institutes of Health. They evaluated various sugars for their contributions to tooth decay in humans. The researchers found that fructose was equal to sucrose in attacking the smooth surface of the crowns of teeth. They reported their findings at a meeting of the International Association for Dental Research in Atlanta, Georgia on March 23, 1974.

In 1977, the main bacteria responsible for dental caries (*Streptococcus mutans*) was found to be transported and metabolized efficiently by fructose. Thus, fructose consumption can lead to caries formation. With increased use of fructose in many foods and beverages in the food supply, its advantage, if any, in lowering the incidence of tooth decay appears to be minimal.

THE BUBBLE BURSTS

By the early 1980s, it appeared inevitable that CF consumption would increase due to technological advances. The method of producing CF had been to use sucrose as the raw material. A new process, described by *Business Week* (May 12, 1980) as "startling," could convert corn into crystalline fructose. By using corn rather than sucrose as the raw material, *Business Week* predicted that fructose might "compete head on with cane and beet sugar." In 1981 a pilot plant was built in the United States, utilizing the new technique, and opened ahead of schedule in mid-1981. The future looked rosy for CF. The prediction was for future large-scale, efficient, and less costly domestically-produced fructose, leading to a food supply sweetened with CF.

The bubble burst. Due to other forces, crystalline fructose did not become a major player in the sweetener market. The phenomenal development of high-fructose corn syrups and the high-intensity, low- and non-caloric sweeteners became the major players in an ever increasingly crowded field of competitive sweeteners.

Chapter 4

HIGH-FRUCTOSE CORN SYRUP: A DANGEROUS SUPERSTAR

The industrial sweetener industry has changed permanently and significantly in favor of corn products at the expense of sugar.

—J. WILLIAM LEACH, FOOD AND BEVERAGE ANALYST, LOEB, RHOADES, HORNBLOWER & CO. *BUSINESS WEEK*, AUGUST 14, 1978

The advent of HFCS has made a basic and far-reaching change in the science of sweetening foods.

—ROBERT L. MARTIN, FOOD INDUSTRY ENGINEER, ADM CORN SWEETENERS, *DAIRY AND ICE CREAM FIELD*, APRIL 1979

In the mid-1970s, encouraged by United States Department of Agriculture (USDA) policy, American corn production soared and created problems of using bumper crops. The development of a new form of corn-based sweetener would utilize the surplus corn and supply processors of convenience foods and beverages with a new, inexpensive sweetener: high-fructose corn syrup (HFCS).

For many years, corn refiners supplied the food industry with corn syrups and dried corn syrup solids. Their share of the sweetening market from 1950 to 1976 increased from 10 percent to nearly 25 percent. But technical problems limited corn sweetener use. Cornstarch, broken down into the glucose molecule, is only half as sweet as sucrose. Scientists searched for economical ways to convert corn sugar (dextrose) into the much sweeter fructose.

"High-fructose corn syrup is one of the most successful new food products of the post-War era. It has led the way for the corn refining industry to become America's number one sweetener supplier," crowed Robert C. Liebenow, president of the Corn Refiners Association, Inc. (reported in *Prepared Foods*, Mar 1988). By 2004, the average American was consuming some 62 pounds of HFCS annually, turning this sweetener into yearly sales of $4.5 billion.

HOW HFCS IS MANUFACTURED

The technology for the manufacture of HFCS originated in Japan in 1971, and was brought to the United States by Iowa's Standard Brands. Early in its production, A.E. Staley Manufacturing and Archer-Daniels-Midland (ADM) Company also became participants.

At the time, the industry standard was an HFCS product containing 42 percent fructose. It was suitable for application with many food products, but not with beverages. "We wanted to get HFCS into soft drinks in a big way," admitted Martin Andreas, ADM's assistant to the CEO's director of marketing. Andreas described the interest as "one of the driving forces behind the U.S. acceptance of HFCS," as noted in ADM's brochure "The Nature of What's to Come: A Century of Innovation," published in 2002.

By 1975, ADM became interested in HFCS development, and the company's researchers worked to develop some method that would boost the fructose percentage to a level suitable for beverage applications.

John Long, Ph.D., a chemist at ADM, in perusing an oil and gas publication, noted a columnar machine, intended for petroleum refining by fractionating the oil, Long theorized that ADM could raise the sweetness level of the 42 percent HFCS product by running the syrup through such a columnar machine. After he persuaded ADM to purchase a machine, researchers primed it with 42 percent HFCS, and they were able to produce a 92 percent fructose concentration. This solution was too sweet and too expensive for soft drink application, so it was blended back with the original 42 percent concentration of fructose, with the hope of achieving a suitable sweetness level equivalent to liquid sucrose. The result was a 55 percent HFCS, which proved to be the suitable concentration for soft drink application.

Andreas presented the 55 percent HFCS to Shasta Beverages, a soft drink manufacturer located in California. Shasta's first purchase cleared out ADM's entire supply. Shasta executives held a press conference to announce the new development. The publicity nudged the two major soft drink producers, the Coca-Cola Company and the Pepsi Company to acknowledge HFCS. Both companies cautiously began to incorporate HFCS into their products, limited to only 25 percent of the total sweetening in their formulations of soft drinks, Andreas reported that "It took six or seven years to get them to go with 100 percent HFCS. But once you had the breakthrough, the momentum was undeniable," as quoted in ADM's brochure. HFCS accounted for 57 percent of all sweetener sales in North America.

HFCS is produced by processing cornstarch to yield glucose. Then, the glucose is processed to produce a high percentage of fructose. Three different enzymes are used in different stages of production in order to break down the cornstarch, which is composed of long chains of glucose molecules, into the simple sugars of glucose and fructose.

First, the cornstarch is treated with alpha-amylase (an enzyme) to produce shorter chains of sugar (polysaccharides).

Second, glucoamylase (another enzyme) breaks down the sugar chains even further, to yield glucose.

Third, glucose-isomerase (another enzyme) converts the glucose to a mixture of about 42 percent fructose, and from 50 to 52 percent glucose, along with smaller percentages of some other sugars.

Both alpha-amylase and glucoamylase are inexpensive enzymes. They are used only once, and then discarded. Glucose-isomerase, a more costly enzyme, is reused repeatedly, until it loses most of its activity.

The next step is to submit the sweetener to liquid chromatography, which converts the mixture to a much higher concentration of fructose—about 90 percent. Finally, this high level is blended with the original mixture to yield a final concentration of about 55 percent fructose. This sweetener, sold as HFCS, has the equivalent sweetness and flavor of sucrose from cane or beet sugar, but is cheaper to produce and easier to transport.

The successful development of HFCS manufacture came at an opportune time for corn growers. Soybean oil was competing with corn oil in margarine manufacture. HFCS took up the slack, as demands for corn oil-based margarine declined, At the same time, interest in lysine, an amino acid that can be produced commercially from corn residue after the glucose is removed, expanded in sales for use in animal feed and food fortification.

HFCS can be produced at three different levels of sweetness to meet various applications for food and beverage manufacturers. At 42 percent, HFCS is used in processed food and beverage products in which it will not mask flavors; at 55 percent, HFCS is the mainstay of the soft drink production; and at 90 percent, HFCS is a "super sweet" addition to reduced-caloric foods and beverages.

Due to rising sugar costs in the 1970s and the 1980s, HFCS rose to prominence as a cheaper alternative. Sales resulted, too, from aggressive promotion campaigns. "Fructose fest" luncheons were given to food editors and supermarket executives during 1980, with a menu consisting of "fructose" punch, salad with fructose dressing, ham and fructose glaze, fructose yams, fructose green beans, honey-flavored fructose corn bread, and fructose sundae. The fructose insinuated into all items on the menu was not CF from sucrose hut HFCS from corn. The National Corn Growers Association sponsored the luncheons as part of its public relations blitz during a lively competition waged between the corn and sugar interests, sparring to capture the sweetening market. Much to the chagrin of the sponsors, some reporters covering the

Fructose Fest were confused and described the luncheon items to their readers as if the items were sweetened with CF. By 1980, the public was confused about fructose. Many people thought that they were eating products sweetened with the much-touted CF. In reality, they were eating products sweetened with HFCS.

DESIRABLE ATTRIBUTES OF HFCS
FOR FOOD AND BEVERAGE PROCESSORS

For food and beverage processors, HFCS has desirable attributes. It is an exceptionally clear liquid, virtually water-white, and it has low viscosity. Although dry or granulated sweeteners are suitable for table use, liquid sweeteners are preferred for industrial uses. Processors of HFCS, hoping to invade the sucrose market, drew attention to HFCS's unique selling points in advertisements targeted at food and beverage processors. HFCS's color is lower than that of liquid sugars derived from beet or cane. HFSC does not produce floc (fine suspended particles) sometimes produced by sucrose. In acidic foods, HFCS has no inversion; sucrose can undergo chemical changes during processing that continue during storage and result in continual compositional changes that lower perceived sweetness, flavor, and appearance. HFCS penetrates products such as fruits and sweet pickles faster than sucrose, and produces full-bodied, firm-textured products with satisfactory sweetness and color. HFCS has a synergistic effect with saccharin. Used in combination, the overall sweetness level is retained, but requires less saccharin. In baked goods, HFCS can replace invert sugar completely, and can provide excellent browning effects. The clinching arguments were that HFCS is sweeter than sucrose and offers very substantial economic savings. In addition, because HFCS is not an artificial sweetener, the pitch to processors was that it "could help fend off consumer and health groups pressuring Americans to reduce their sweetener intake" (reported in *Business Week*, Aug 14, 1978).

In August 1978, the Food and Drug Administration (FDA) affirmed GRAS (Generally Recognized as Safe) status for HFCS containing 42 and 55 percent fructose. The agency held off approving HFCS containing 90 percent fructose. The agency reported that it needed additional data to affirm GRAS status for this form, which had minor uses in low-calorie foods.

In 1988, the FDA proposed a comprehensive evaluation of HFCS, but allowed the sweetener to remain on the market. By that time, there were disquieting reports, both in animal and human studies, suggesting health problems from high consumption of HFCS.

Once again, the FDA excluded HFCS 90 (containing 90 percent fructose) from GRAS status, the FDA reported that the agency still lacked sufficient information to assess the safety of residual processing materials in the final product as an ingredient in low-calorie foods.

In response to the FDA's general procedure to request input of public comments whenever a substance is under consideration for GRAS status, the Diabetes Research Center (DRC) of the American Diabetes Association (ADA) filed comment, charging that the safety of HFCS had not been established firmly for diabetic use.

In response, the FDA cited its Sugars Task Force Report that had stated that it could not find any basis in the scientific literature to conclude that increased fructose consumption by diabetics was potentially harmful. What the agency failed to admit was that such studies had not been conducted. The FDA also noted that the dietary guidelines of the ADA did not make any recommendation to avoid any *specific* sweetener due to safety concerns.

CLINCHING THE MARKET

By the mid-1970s, the traditional sucrose-dominated market was challenged by a combination of factors. Years of low prices and poor returns had slowed the international expansion of sugar production. Worldwide sugar demands had outstripped production capacity. Everywhere, sugar stocks were exceedingly low due to the greatly increased per capita sugar consumption. After an especially low 1973 and 1974 sugar harvest in western Europe and the Soviet Union due to poor weather, the supply dwindled further. The problem was exacerbated by general worldwide inflation and by speculators who had entered the sugar market. Also, many American farmers had switched from sugar beet production to more lucrative crops such as soy, wheat, corn, and tomato. The result was greater dependence on imported sugar.

In January 1974, raw sugar sold on the American market for about 11 cents a pound. The price began an upward spiral. By November of that same year, the price reached an all-time high of 71 cents a pound. The steep rise caused major worldwide upheavals within the food industry. At this particularly critical time, HFCS was 32 cents a pound; dextrose, 21 cents; and conventional corn syrups, 12 cents. Corn refiners were well positioned to compete in the sweetening market with their substantially lower-price products. Wide-scale commercial production of HFCS made this particular corn-based sweetener a formidable challenger to the traditional cane- and beet-based sucrose.

In the sweetener market, sucrose symbolized instability; HFCS represented security. Corn supplies were ample and available. Corn, the world's most abundant food crop, also was a basic U.S. crop. The American corn refiners utilized only about 6 percent of the domestic corn crop. Thus, corn sweeteners were not a major factor governing corn prices. Over the years, corn prices remained relatively stable. HFCS would protect the food industry against the vagaries of the world sugar market. Corn refiners claimed that they could produce enough corn sweeteners to replace all the sugar imported into the American market. It was expected that the price differential between HFCS and sugar would increase in HFCS's favor. This prediction was fulfilled. By 1980, the cost of HFCS was at least 10 percent lower than sucrose.

Sugar has few byproducts to reduce its production cost. Some molasses and furfural (an aldehyde used to make phenolic resins) are minor byproducts. Corn sweetener prices can be offset by up to 50 percent of the raw material costs by the sale of numerous profitable byproducts. Edible corn oil and corn germ are used in the human diet; premium protein ingredients from gluten seed and meal, as well as the soluble kernel portion, in livestock and poultry feeds; and cornstarch, in various food and industrial applications. HFCS could be a partial replacer for sucrose, at various ratios, with no perceived difference in the finished food product nor changed consumer acceptance. In some cases, HFCS could replace sucrose totally, pound for pound, on a dry weight basis. There were relatively few limitations. HFCS could not be used in dry desserts, or in candies because it would make such products sticky. It could not be used in ice creams because it would cause a lowered freezing point. However, university/industry-sponsored research programs fine-tuned the applications, and HFCS even became a total sucrose replacer in ice-cream manufacture.

HFCS, containing fructose at 42, 55, and 90 percent levels, rapidly achieved success in the sweetening market. In 1967, HFCS's annual per capita consumption was 0.1 pounds; by 1980, that number had increased to 18.9 pounds. The trade journal *Food Engineering* crowed in August 1979 that "the future growth of HFCS . . . seems almost unlimited."

GENETICALLY MODIFIED HFCS

In 1980, gene-splicing technology was applied to HFCS processing. A bacterium was found that was capable of producing an enzyme that could convert corn syrup into 100 percent fructose. Former methods allowed only up to 90 percent conversion. The newer process made it possible to produce fructose from corn in crystalline form. Then, efforts were directed for genetic modification by locating and transfering the enzyme's gene from that bacterium into another bacterium.

Soon, processors used HFCS in a wide range of products, including carbonated and non-carbonated beverages; jams, jellies, and preserves; salad dressings, pickles, and catsups; baked goods and icings; cereals; dairy products such as chocolate milk, eggnogs, flavored yogurts, ice creams and sherbets; dietetic and reduced-calorie foods; table syrups; and liquid table sweeteners. HFCS was used even in wines for attributes other than fermentation and alcoholic content.

A massive switch to HFCS occurred in 1980 when the two major cola beverage companies announced plans to use HFCS in their products, Sweetener use by these two companies represented two million tons of sugar annually. This news sent other processors scurrying to place HFCS purchasing orders as a hedge against possible shortages. HFCS producers retooled their plants to increase production for the anticipated sales to other soft drink manufacturers. By the mid-1980s, the anticipated annual market for HFCS was expected to reach 8 million tons.

As HFCS saturated the food supply, public confusion about fructose increased. The Sugar Association, in a complaint to the FDA, charged that several companies were making label claims that their products were made with fructose, although the products actually were sweetened with HFCS. By late 1979, the Federal Trade Commission (FTC) began to scrutinize various advertising claims made for fructose and for HFCS-sweetened products. The agency's investigation was spurred by a new petition from the Center for Science in the Public Interest (CSPI) that challenged advertisements of a specific soft drink, Shasta. The advertising copy read that the drink was "an alternative to ordinary sugared soft drinks," and claimed that ordinary refined sugar was replaced in the product "with simple sweeteners like fructose, a kind found in fresh fruit." CSPI noted that the drink was sweetened with 55 percent HFCS, and that the advertisement was deceptive on three counts: HFCS is not pure fructose; fructose is refined; and HFCS is not found in fresh fruits and honey. During the FTC's deliberations, relevant news broke elsewhere.

An inner office memo dated January 25, 1980 read, "Today Botsford Ketchum resigned the Shasta account." This prominent advertising agency had a six million dollar annual Shasta account. In a memo to Botsford Ketchum employees, the company's president wrote, (as quoted in the *Washington Post*, Feb 21, 1980):

> We believe in the principles we stand for and the people who have helped build this agency. We do not intend to change our course. Consequently, we believe Shasta will he better served by a different kind of agency and that our people can work better on other accounts.

The principle involved Shasta's advertising statements concerning fructose. The story, pieced together by the *Washington Post*, demonstrated that advertising agencies may depend on clients for technical information about products for their advertising copy. Botsford Ketchum relied on Shasta's supplied information about fructose. Eventually, through outside sources, the agency had concluded that better information was needed. The advertisements and television commercials had been cleared both by legal counsel and television network scrutiny. However, it was unlikely that either the agency's own lawyers or the networks' standards and practices departments were aware of the technicalities involved. After the case was publicized, Shasta changed its advertisements and commercials, and described its product as one that contained a high-fructose corn sweetener.

SOME HEALTH CONCERNS

Even when HFCS-containing products are labeled properly, is this sweetener safe for everyone? Individuals with at least two types of identified health problems need to avoid HFCS. Corn-sensitive individuals need to shun this sweetener because it is corn-derived. Diabetics should avoid HFCS because of its glucose content. All HFCS contains glucose, with some products having as much as 58 percent glucose. Glucose is the sugar that diabetics are least able to metabolize properly. In a 1980 press release, the ADA noted public confusion and warned diabetics to exercise extreme caution when purchasing foods with label claims that the products have been sweetened with fructose, because in reality, the sweetener might be HFCS.

At a 1980 seminar, the food industry, too, was cautioned by Dr. Howard P. Roberts, director of scientific affairs, National Soft Drink Association (and former director of the FDA's Bureau of Foods), who reported that HFCS is not pure fructose but consists of glucose, too. As reported in *Processed Prepared Foods* (Apr 1980), Roberts warned that:

> Industry should not be lulled into a false sense of contentment by thinking that increased use of corn sweeteners will alleviate the oversimplified criticism of sugar. Whether fructose comes from ingested sucrose or is ingested as fructose per se, it ends up as glucose in the body and the body cannot tell where the glucose originally came from.

By 1983, approximately 1.2 billion pounds of HFCS were being used in the United States to sweeten food and beverage products. Pepsi approved the use of 80 percent HFCS in its syrup used for its soft drinks, and Royal Crown, a 75 percent substitution in its canned and bottled colas. At the time, these were the largest percentages of HFCS use in formulations of the products of these two companies.

An advertisement for Archer Daniels Midland's HFCS, printed in *Food Engineering* (Mar 1983) announced, "Ten years ago it was difficult to find a single product sweetened with HFCS. Today, it's almost as hard to find one that isn't." The text continued to report that since 1970, annual HFCS consumption:

> ... has jumped from less than 1 pound to over 25 pounds per capita, a figure that food industry experts predict will increase 40 percent by 1987 ... [and that HFCSs have] fostered the growth of an efficient, new industry to support them. Soon, the capacity of this flourishing industry will reach 8 billion pounds per year.

By 1984, there was a potential for 100 percent substitution of HFCS for sucrose in soft drinks. The total HFCS shipments to processors were estimated at approximately 10.5 billion pounds annually. The prospect was favorable. The projection was for a year-to-year increase of some 700 million pounds, due mainly to the official approval of HFCS use in soft drinks. In addition, about 50 million pounds would be used in some dairy foods and with baked goods. At the same time, the domestic use of sugar was estimated to tumble 200,000 to 400,000 million tons less usage by 1985, mostly due to the increased use of HFCS in soft drinks.

Also, predictions from agricultural economists at the USDA's Economic Research Service (ERS) were promising. Robert Barry and Fred Gray, both from ERS, estimated in 1984 that HFCS use might reach 4.3 million tons annually, and would represent about 29 percent of all caloric sweetener consumption.

Increasingly, food and beverage manufacturers substituted HFCS for table sugar in their products, because of its relatively low cost, ease of shipment, and shelf life stability. Ultimately, HFCS would replace sucrose 100 percent in virtually all soft drinks. This replacement saved processors about 20 percent of manufacturing costs, and allowed them to boost portion sizes and still make profit.

With increased use of HFCS by processors, in an ever-expanding range of items, American consumption of HFCS rose to dizzying heights. HFCS consumption *increased more than a thousand percent* from 1970 to 1990, and continues to increase. By 2005, the average American consumed about 63 pounds of HFCS annually, in addition to other sweeteners. The United States is the only country where HFCS consumption is significant.

The rosy picture began to lose some of its color. By the late 1990s, the impact of high levels of HFCS consumption on health was beginning to appear. Apparently, this sweetener depleted the body's supply of several minerals: copper, chromium, and magnesium. The food and beverage industries had been asked to address the problem by Donald Best, technical editor of the trade journal *Prepared Foods* (Sept 1987), as the health problems were becoming evident. The headline of Best's article read, IS IT TIME TO ADDRESS THE COPPER-FRUCTOSE LINK? followed by Best's suggestion that:

> The food industry will soon have to confront recent studies linking high-fructose consumption to what some researchers believe may be the country's leading cause of ischemic heart disease—copper deficiency.

The Copper-Fructose Link

Fructose upsets the body's metabolism. It can cause depletion of vital minerals such as copper, iron, magnesium, zinc, and chromium. It interferes with the heart's utilization of these minerals. Also, such depletions can lead to type 2 diabetes, formerly observed in adults (and formerly termed adult-onset diabetes), but currently alarmingly prevalent in adolescent youths. Ironically, some health professionals formerly believed that fructose was safe for diabetic use because it does not raise blood sugar levels as high as other caloric sugars.

Animal studies showed that fructose interferes with dietary copper absorption. Both fructose and sucrose (consisting of linked fructose and glucose molecules) were found to aggravate the symptoms of marginal to severe copper deficiency. Dietary starch fractions were found not to be as damaging. Mortality rates increased 30 to 60 percent when copper-deficient animals were fed fructose or sucrose instead of starch.

Copper is essential for good health in animals and humans. In experiments, animals ranging from rats, to guinea pigs, to swine, when fed copper-depleted diets, developed symptoms similar to those in humans who are severely deficient in copper. The animals experienced rises in levels of blood cholesterol and blood pressure, damaged hearts and arterial muscles, neurological disorders, and changes in bone structure.

Several copper-dependent enzymes maintain the integrity of the cardiovascular system. Dietary copper deficiency compromises the functioning of these enzymes. For example, smooth heart and arterial muscles are bound by a proteinaceous connective tissue. Elastin, a component, consists of numerous protein subunits crosslinked by the enzyme, lysyl oxidase. Copper deficiency reduces the activity of this enzyme and weakens the elastin connective tissue.

Severe copper deficiency can weaken the heart muscle to the extent that the heart ruptures spontaneously. This tragedy has been observed both in humans and in animals.

At the Mayo Clinic in Rochester, Minnesota, a study showed human heart ruptures in a number of acute ischemic heart attack patients. When examined, the heart muscles in these patients were found to be low in copper.

Dr. Kenneth Allen and colleagues at Colorado State University in Fort Collins, Colorado, documented the structural abnormalities in the heart and aortic musculature of adult male rats maintained on marginal copper-containing diets since conception of the animals.

HFCS Makes Nutrient-Poor Diets Even Poorer

For a decade, Dr. Meira Fields, a biochemist in the USDA's Department of Metabolism and Nutrient Interactions, studied the effects of high-fructose diets on rats. Fields and her colleagues compared the effects of a diet low in copper and high in fructose with a diet low in copper but high in starch. The rats on the high-fructose diet developed high levels of blood sugar, cholesterol, and triglycerides; became anemic, and developed abnormalities of the heart and pancreas. The heart enlarged until it exploded. Fields reported that normally the rat lives for two years. However, after five weeks in this study, the male rats on the high-fructose, low-copper diet showed delayed testicular development. They died prematurely. The female rats were unable to produce live offspring. The rats on the starch/low-copper diet ended the study unscathed. Fields suggested that the study's findings had practical implications for humans. She and her colleagues recommended that Americans reduce their consumption of processed foods and beverages containing HFCS because this sweetener can aggravate the adverse effects of already nutrient-poor diets. Also, Fields noted that the medical profession regarded fructose as better than sucrose for diabetics. Yet every cell in the body can metabolize glucose, but all fructose must be metabolized in the liver. The liver of the rats on a high-fructose diet looked like the liver of an alcoholic, plugged with fat and cirrhotic.

After completing the rat studies, USDA researchers used swine for further investigation of the fructose-copper link. Much research on copper deficiency had already been conducted with swine. The cardiovascular system of swine is very similar to that of humans. Like humans, swine, too, develop cardiovascular problems when fed copper-deficient diets.

In the study, swine were divided into four groups. For ten weeks, the first group was fed a diet with 20 percent of calories derived from fructose, and was low in copper; the second, also with 20 percent of calories from fructose, but with an adequate amount of copper; the third, with 20 percent of calories from glucose and low in copper, and the fourth, also with 20 percent of calories from glucose, but with an adequate amount of copper.

The most significant result of this study was that the swine on the high-fructose and low-copper diet developed anemia and enlarged hearts that were in danger of rupturing. These signs were severe copper deficiency. It was not detected in the animals from the other groups. From this observation, the scientists expressed concern about the human health effects of ever-increasing amounts of fructose consumption in American diets.

Dr. Leslie Klevay, a pioneer in copper research at the USDA's Northern Regional Research Laboratory in Fargo, North Dakota, drew close parallels between animal and human data. Klevay documented a total of 28 anatomical and 15 chemical and physiological similarities between animals and humans with ischemic heart disease induced by copper-deficient diets. Klevay reported that the evidence suggests that *copper deficiency is the leading cause of ischemic heart disease in humans.*

The National Academy of Sciences (renamed the National Academies) estimated that an adequate dietary copper intake for humans is about 2 to 3 milligrams (mg) daily. Yet, research conducted by Klevay and others suggested that the average American consumes less than an adequate intake, at only 0.78 mg/day. Klevay estimated that 25 percent of the American population consumes less than 2.0 mg/day and 15 percent, only 0.8 to 1.0 mg/day.

Many people are low in copper due to eating large amounts of refined sugar and flour, both of which are stripped of copper as well as other nutrients. Many Americans do not eat foods that are good sources of copper, such as liver and oysters. Also, many Americans consume high levels of soybean constituents in numerous processed foods and beverages. Soybeans further deplete the body of copper.

Human studies of the fructose-copper link supplemented the animal studies. Dr. Sheldon Reiser, a specialist in carbohydrate metabolism at the USDA's research laboratories in Beltsville, Maryland, and his colleagues conducted a study that was reported in the *American Journal of Clinical Nutrition* (vol. 42, 1985). Reiser's team investigated the effect of fructose consumption on the copper status of twenty-four men who consumed a marginally low copper diet. The men were maintained on alternating diets. One diet contained 20 percent fructose, the other, 20 percent starch. The diets were designed to represent typical American diets. The researchers needed to terminate the study after four of the men developed cardiac problems, ranging from severe tachycardia (an abnormally rapid heart beat) to mild heart attacks within the first weeks of the study.

The Chromium-Fructose Link

Copper deficiency was not the only problem linked to fructose consumption. Dr. Richard Anderson, the lead scientist at USDA's Human Nutrition Research Center in Beltsville, had researched the health effects of HFCS in diets for two decades. He reported that low chromium levels are common in Americans. Low chromium levels, combined with high fructose consumption, can lead to higher blood levels of sugar, cholesterol, and triglycerides. High levels of all three substances in the blood are considered to be key risk factors in the development of diabetes and heart disease. Anderson demonstrated that diets high in HFCS lead to chromium depletion. This mineral is essential for the body's ability to utilize sugar, and to balance insulin levels. Anderson's research revealed that the chromium loss inflicted by HFCS was made even worse if it was eaten along with another, simple sugar such as glucose (a component of table sugar). This combination is all too common in the average American diet.

Anderson reported that chromium supplements, if given to people who show slightly elevated blood sugar, could be beneficial. The supplements could lead to a drop in blood sugar level in about 80 to 90 percent of such individuals. However, Anderson suggested that a better solution would be to have people reduce their intake of sweeteners such as HFCS and sucrose.

The Magnesium-Fructose Link

David Milne, a chemist at the USDA's Human Nutrition Research Center in Grand Forks, North Dakota, also conducted a human study with fructose consumption, with 500 young men. First, they were given a diet with 20 percent of the calories derived from fructose. Then, the men were switched to a diet with 20 percent of the calories derived from cornstarch. Copper intake was restricted in their diet to 0.5 mg/day, which was slightly more than half the level that Americans typically consume. On the fructose diet, the men's level of low-density lipoprotein (LDL) cholesterol rose. This undesirable form of cholesterol is thought to increase the risk of heart disease. When the cornstarch was substituted for fructose in the diet, the men's level of LDL cholesterol declined. Moreover, the high-fructose diet impaired the men's natural defense mechanism against destructive molecules (free radicals) that the body produces in response to environmental toxins such as cigarette smoke and ultraviolet light. Milne's studies extended to the effects of a high fructose diet on individuals with low magnesium intake. This mineral interacts with copper in the body. Like copper, adequate magnesium is important for a healthy heart.

The Metabolism-Fructose Link

Some of the human health problems induced by fructose, and especially from HFCS, were described in the January 1996 issue of *Food Technology*, in a letter from Russell M. Bianchi, of the Industrial/Technical Division of Liquid Sugars, Inc., in Oakland, California. Bianchi noted that both fructose and glucose have been stripped of any trace vitamin or mineral values that normally assist in metabolism. Initially, they raise the blood sugar level for energy, but within an hour after ingestion, they make the blood sugar drop, which leads to energy depletion. Thus, there is no real discernable energy benefit from simple carbohydrates such as fructose or glucose. Fructose has an additional metabolic disadvantage. This sugar is not even recognized at the time of ingestion, HFCS was Bianchi's main concern:

> HFCS is not recognized because its reversal molecule produced under chemical synthesis from corn causes the body to send the HFCS to the adipose tissue of the liver as fat or triglycerides. The resulting effect for digestive, cardiovascular, diabetes, and obesity problems has been discussed in the medical and scientific literature for some time, but the economic advantages of a cheaper sweetener system than sucrose has swept the evidence under the rug.

SOFT DRINKS AND HEALTH

"Sugar-sweetened soft drinks contribute 7.1 percent of total energy intake and represent the largest single food source of calories in the U.S. diet. Coincidentally or not, the rise of obesity and type 2 diabetes in the United States parallels the increase in sugar-sweetened soft drink consumption. Several studies have found an association between sugar-sweetened beverages and incidence of obesity in children. In one study, the odds ratio of becoming obese increased 1.6 times for each additional sugars-sweetened drink consumed every day . . ."

—Caroline M. Apovian, M.D., "Sugar-Sweetened Soft Drinks, Obesity, and Type 2 Diabetes," editorial, *Journal of the American Medical Association,* August 25, 2004

"Higher consumption of sugar-sweetened beverages is associated with a greater magnitude of weight gain and an increased risk for development of type 2 diabetes in women, possibly by providing excessive calories and large amounts of rapidly absorbable sugars."

—Matthias B. Schulze et al., "Sugar-Sweetened Beverages, Weight Gain, and Incidence of Type 2 Diabetes in Young and Middle-Aged Women," *Journal of the American Medical Association,* August 25, 2004

"Soft-drink consumption supplies the average teenager with over 10 percent of their [sic] daily caloric intake."

—Statement by Dr. William Dietz, in his testimony on the Center for Disease Control and Prevention's role in combatting the obesity epidemic, before the Committee on Health, Education, Labor and Pensions (U.S. Senate Hearings, May 2, 2002)

At the beginning of the twenty-first century it had become apparent that HFCS and other fructose-containing sweeteners used at high levels threatened human health. The numerous experiments conducted by USDA researchers such as Drs. Field, Klevay, Reiser, Milne and others all raised cautionary warnings. Donald Best, mentioned earlier as the technical editor of *Prepared Foods,* cautioned the food and beverage producers that the significant findings should not be ignored. He suggested that the sweetener industry should be identified as a group attempting to *find solutions* to the problem of dietary copper deficiency, rather than as a group that *causes* health problems.

HFCS as a Major Culprit in Weight Gain and Obesity

By 2003, HFCS was being singled out as one of the main factors in the alarming epidemic of obesity. In *Fat Land: How Americans Became the Fattest People in the World* (Houghton Mifflin, 2003) author Greg Critser accused HFCS as a major culprit. Critser blamed federal policy from the 1970s, with its encouragement of increasing American corn production. In turn, increased corn production gave food and beverage manufacturers a cheaper way to sweeten their products, and allowed them to "supersize" a number of sweet food products and soft drinks. In the 1980s, when food and beverage processors began extensive use of HFCS in their products, the relatively stable obesity rate began to rise. Of course, a rise in obesity at the same time that HFCS use increased does not, in itself, prove any cause-and-effect relationship. Many developments can occur at the same time, yet be totally unrelated. However, the cause-and-effect relationship of HFCS use and the increase in obesity was confirmed in several studies.

The USDA had gathered a body of evidence, through its various studies of human metabolism conducted by its own researchers that linked the rapid rise in obesity to the use of HFCS since the 1970s. Despite the implications of its findings, the USDA sounded no public warnings in its Dietary Guidelines for Americans, issued every five years, or in its Food Guide Pyramid revised repeatedly, concerning the health hazards of high levels of HFCS in the diet. The USDA merely issued vague advice about using added sugars 'moderately.' Clearly, the agency is conflicted. It promotes American agricultural crops such as corn and corn products. At the same time, the findings from many of its excellent research projects are in conflict with its policy of crop promotion. Nor were the disturbing USDA findings regarding HFCS and human health acted upon by sister agencies. The U.S. Health and Human Services (HHS) issued no warnings. Nor did its departments such as the FDA, Public Health Service (PHS), or Centers for Disease Control and Prevention (CDC) issue any warnings. HFCS remained as the 800-pound gorilla in the room: its presence known but unnoted as an important factor in the obesity epidemic.

By 2003, researchers at the University of Michigan reported that the fructose in HFCS elevates triglycerides dangerously—as much as 32 percent. This rise makes the body's fat burning and storage system sluggish, which leads to weight gain.

The continuing Nurses' Health Study II reported in 2004 that women who drink a lot of sugary beverages were at higher risk of weight gain and at higher risk of developing type 2 diabetes than women who do not drink these beverages. The study, conducted with more than 90,000 nurses, found that the women who increased their intake of sugar-sweetened beverages from one or fewer per week in 1991 to more than one a day in 1999, gained more weight than other women in the study. On average, these women gained more than ten pounds, between 1991 and 1995, and more than nine pounds between 1995 and 1999.

The weight gain comes primarily from excess calories. Dr. Frank B. Hu, associate professor of nutrition and epidemiology at Harvard University's School of Public Health, and co-author of the study, published the results in the August 25, 2004 issue of the *Journal of the American Medical Association.* Hu wrote, "The problem with soft drinks is that you don't feel like you are getting a lot of calories from them." He reported that soft drinks, containing HFCS, raise blood sugar and increase insulin dramatically, which stress the insulin-producing cells of the pancreas. There were confounding factors. The women in the study who drank most of the sugary drinks had other negative lifestyle factors. They tended to be physically less active, consumed more calories, and smoked more than those who did not consume the soft drinks.

The question of whether HFCS is metabolized differently by the body than other sweeteners remains unanswered. Although HFCS breaks down chemically, as does sucrose, into the same simple sugars of glucose and fructose, differences not yet understood may exist. In 2004, when this question was posed to Maureen Story, director of the Center for Food and Nutrition Policy at Virginia Polytechnical Institute and State University in Blacksburg, Virginia, she acknowledged that, to date, no study had been conducted to show conclusively how the body metabolizes HFCS.

It is known that fructose differs in human metabolism from dextrose (from corn) or sucrose (from sugarcane). Consumed dextrose or sucrose go through a complex breakdown process before their arrival in the liver. Fructose bypasses the breakdown process and arrives nearly intact at the liver. Fructose does not go through the intermediary breakdown step that sucrose and dextrose do. This unique feature of fructose, *intensified by its high concen-*

tration in HFCS, is known as "metabolic shunting" toward the liver, where it mimics insulin's ability to cause the liver to release fatty acids into the bloodstream. The liver uses fructose as a building block of triglycerides. This feature was discovered long after the fructose introduction into the human diet.

HFCS has hormonal links to obesity. Three hormones are being studied in obese individuals: leptin, insulin, and ghrelin. Leptin and insulin have three main functions as brain signalers. They help the brain to acknowledge satiety. They decrease appetite. They control body weight. Ghrelin causes the brain to feel a sense of hunger. Also, this hormone increases appetite.

Fructose consumption produces lower levels of leptin and insulin. Thus, fructose decreases the brain's feeling of satiety. Fructose consumption causes ghrelin levels to increase.

Obese patients, but not normal-weight patients, experience delayed decreases in ghrelin. It is thought that long-term fructose consumption may precondition the metabolism of a normal-weight individual to behave like that of someone who is obese. When fructose is replaced by glucose, the tendency to overeat decreases. Therefore, fructose's link with obesity may be related to its effects on the hormones that are responsible for feeling satiated: leptin and insulin.

In terms of satiety, fructose does not have the same effect on the brain as other sugars. This difference changes the normal metabolic functioning of the hormones involved. Fructose is more readily converted to fat by the liver than other sugars. This feature results in elevated fat levels (as triglycerides) in the bloodstream. Fructose does not activate the hormones responsible for regulating body weight, as do carbohydrates composed of glucose. Thus, high fructose consumption can lead to a greater intake of calories and result in weight gain. HFCS, used in soft drinks, may *stimulate* rather than *suppress* appetite.

Fructose became a popular choice for diabetics to help keep their blood sugar stable (because fructose does not stimulate the pancreas to produce insulin). However, fructose does not increase leptin production, but does suppress ghrelin production. It would appear that these features would make fructose undesirable for diabetics. One of the cardinal recommendations for diabetics is to control their weight.

Fructose malabsorption is another concern. A study, published by the American Dietetic Association (described in *Today's Dietitian*, Sept 2006) noted that one-half of the patients being studied had fructose malabsorption. Most patients complained of gastrointestinal distress. The researchers found that fructose was the main cause of the symptoms in patients with chronic diarrhea. The condition may be caused by overloading the intestine's ability to absorb carbohydrates due to excessive fructose consumption.

In 2000, as reported by Gail Vines in the *New Scientist* (Sept 1, 2001), researchers at the University of Toronto, Canada, fed a high fructose diet to Syrian golden hamsters. These animals were chosen because their fat metabolism is quite similar to human fat metabolism. Within weeks, the hamsters developed high triglyceride levels and insulin resistance. Insulin resistance is a condition in which the liver begins to interpret insulin as a signal to release more fats in the form of triglycerides. Current food choices, with frequent consumption of high-energy snacks, stimulate the pancreas to oversecrete insulin and expose the liver to long, uninterrupted bombardment with insulin. The liver then begins to interpret insulin differently, and release triglycerides into the bloodstream. The triglycerides overload fat cells, spill over as fatty acids strike at the pancreas' insulin-producing beta cells, cause insulin levels to drop, and blood sugar to spike. This development results in insulin resistance, weight gain, and increased risk of diabetes.

Preliminary human studies also demonstrated the health risks from high consumption of concentrated fructose. Dr. John Bantle, at the University of Minnesota in Minneapolis, fed two dozen healthy volunteers a diet with 17 percent of total calories from concentrated fructose. Bantle chose this percentage because he estimated that about 27 million Americans are what he termed "heavy users" of fast foods and of 32-ounce bottles of soft drinks. Such individuals who consume these soft drinks regularly have an intake of about 17 percent of their total calories from fructose. Bantle measured the blood fats and sugars of the volunteers on the 17 percent fructose diets. Then he switched them to a diet sweetened mainly with sucrose and measured their blood fats and sugars. The differences were startling. The triglyceride in the blood was about 32 percent higher in the fructose-sweetened diet than in the sucrose-sweetened one. Also, the fructose-sweetened diet made the triglyceride levels peak faster—shortly after the meal when such fats can do the most damage to artery walls. Bantle's findings, published in the *American Journal of Nutrition* (vol. 72, 2000) caused the journal's editor to caution that the deleterious changes caused by dietary fructose occur in the absence of *any* beneficial effect . . . and these abnormalities . . . appear to be greater for those individuals already at an increased risk for coronary artery disease" (emphasis supplied).

Consumption of HFCS increased more than 1,000 percent over the last thirty years, reported Staci Stone, R.D., C.D.N., in *Today's Dietitian* (Sept 2006). This phenomenal rise prompted some scientists to consider fructose consumption as an important, but overlooked factor, in the steady rise in obesity, due not merely to increased caloric intake, but perhaps more important through a variety of complex chemical reactions that this sweetener initiates in the human body.

In the mid-1970s, European researchers, J. Bremer and colleagues had begun to explore the cellular pathways that determine whether or not a cell burns or stores new energy. Two critical enzymes (acyl-COA and acylcarnitine) function as pathway regulators on the cell surfaces, and direct the inner cells either to store or burn a newly-arrived fat particle. Sugar and fats have different effects on these two enzymes, with fructose and glycerol as the main players. Fructose or glycerol, present in abundance, depressed the enzymes. This finding led the researchers to conclude that fructose and glycerol lower the rate of fatty acid oxidation.

Bremer's findings were ignored by American nutritional researchers for nearly a decade. Instead, the researchers were pursuing the subject of dietary fats, rather than dietary sugars. The emphasis on fats was established by the American Heart Association (AMA), which had concluded that dietary fat was the main culprit in cardiovascular problems. As a result, dietary sugars were ignored.

A study reported in the *American Journal of Clinical Nutrition* (Apr 2004) suggested that the consumption of HFCS in beverages may play a role in the obesity epidemic. The researchers noted that digestion, absorption, and metabolism of this sweetener differ from glucose. They suggested that HFCS use makes soft drinks sweeter, and consumers crave them more, and consume more of them.

HFCS LOSES "NATURAL" IMAGE

By 2005, the linkage of HFCS use and health problems including obesity caused some food manufacturers to return to their use of traditional sugars and other sweeteners. They had come to regard HFCS as not being a 'natural' sugar, according to Jim Tonkin, at Arizona-based Tonkin Consulting. In *Functional Foods and Nutraceuticals* (Jan 2005), Tonkin reported that "the health retail chains that have banned HFCS-containing products have strict criteria about what can be sold in their stores." According to Tonkin, the biggest asset of HFCS is its cost: only about 11 cents a pound. Tonkin added, "The only thing that would make the major soda bottlers change from HFCS is if there were a disastrous corn crop and the price of HFCS went through the roof." To date, corn crop failure has not been a critical factor, but an unforeseen development has occurred. Part of the corn crop is being diverted to produce a fuel substitute for gasoline, and soaring corn prices ripple through the food chain.

The World Health Organization (WHO) recommends that no more than 10 percent of daily calories should consist of added sugars. This translates to no more than 200 calories of added sugars for an individual eating a 2,000 caloric diet daily, or the equivalency of one 16.9-ounce HFCS-sweetened soft drink, or 3 ounces of plain M&Ms. Because sweeteners—so often in the form of HFCS—are found in so many processed foods and beverages, an individual can exceed the recommended limit very easily. By 2003, the average American consumed about 25 percent of daily calories from added sugars, mainly from fructose. The amount is two and a half times the recommended upper limit of WHO.

Chapter 5

SUGAR POLYOLS: CONSUMED BUT NOT TALLIED

Unfortunately, there are some negatives associated with sugar alcohols [polyols]. The most common side effect is the possibility of bloating and diarrhea when sugar alcohols are eaten in excessive amounts. There is also some evidence that sugar alcohols, much like fructose (natural fruit sugar) in fruit and fruit juice can cause a 'laxative effect.' Weight gain has been seen when these products are overeaten. The American Diabetes Association claims that sugar alcohols are acceptable in a moderate amount but should not be eaten in excess. Some people with diabetes, especially type 1 diabetics, have found that blood sugars rise if sugar alcohols are eaten in uncontrolled amounts.

—*NUTRITION ADVISOR* (NEWSLETTER), YALE-NEW HAVEN HOSPITAL,
NEW HAVEN, CONNECTICUT, MARCH 10, 2005

A group of non-glucose carbohydrates are termed variously "sugar polyols," "polyol sugars," "sugar alcohols," "rare sugars," "hexitols," "hexahydroxy alcohols," or "hexahydric alcohols." The "hex" prefix is given to sugar polyols because they are six-sided structures. Although some twenty sugar polyols have been identified, only eight of them are used as sweeteners: sorbitol, mannitol, xylitol, lactitol, maltitol, isomalt, hydrogenated starch hydrolysates (HSH), and erythritol.

Polyols are neither sugar (sucrose) nor alcohol (ethanol) as these words are used commonly, so the term "sugar alcohols" is misleading and confusing. In addition to this plethora of polyol terms, the Food and Drug Administration (FDA) decided to add yet another term. In formulating the Nutritional Labeling and Education Act (NLEA) in 1992, Virginia Wilkening, a nutritionist at the FDA, announced that the agency proposed to designate polyols as "simple sugars." The FDA classifies some polyols as GRAS (Generally Recognized as Safe), and others as approved additives.

POLYOLS: POORLY ABSORBED SWEETENERS

As nonglucose carbohydrates, polyols are utilized differently from sucrose in the body. Polyols are absorbed from the alimentary tract more slowly than sucrose, and are absorbed to a lesser degree than sucrose. Absorbed polyols are converted to energy by processes that require little or no insulin. The liver absorption of lactitol is less then 1 percent; mannitol, 50 percent; isomalt, from 50 to 60 percent; maltitol, from 50 to 75 percent; and sorbitol, from 50 to 80 percent. Liver absorption of erythritol is high, and xylitol absorption is variable.

Polyols are absorbed slowly and incompletely from the small intestine into the blood. What is not absorbed into the blood is metabolized to short-chain fatty acids and gases by bacteria in the large intestine. The gases are responsible for problems when polyol-containing foods or beverages are consumed at high levels. The gases produce flatulence, rumblings in the bowels, increased frequency of bowel movements, loose bowels, and osmotic diarrhea. Overconsumption of sorbitol- or mannitol-sweetened candies has resulted in numerous cases of hospitalization due to the diarrheal effect. The American Dietetic Association has cautioned against high consumption of polyol-sweetened food and beverage products.

In 1973 the FDA mandated that such products have a label warning that "excessive consumption may have a laxative effect." The laxative effect occurs if intake is more than 50 grams a day of sorbitol, or more than 20 grams a day of mannitol. However, some individuals may be affected at lower levels.

Due to the ever-expanding number of low-carbohydrate food and beverage products available in markets, the total polyol intake needs to be considered, because the total intake may be involved in the laxative effects. Other important factors to consider include the amount consumed in one sitting, the type of food or beverage, the individual response, and the possibility of adaptation over time. Even the circumstances under which the polyol is consumed may be important. For example, eating a product containing a high level of polyols as the sole breakfast food on an empty stomach may lead to worse symptoms than in eating the same product as part of a full meal.

In a study reported in 1996, conducted at the University of Salford, England, fifty-nine college students were given 100 grams of milk chocolate containing 40 grams of different types of sweeteners. The researchers compared the ability of polyols (such as maltitol, lactitol, and isomalt) with sucrose, in quantities of 30 to 40 grams, to stimulate symptoms of gastrointestinal upset. The study showed significant differences in the effects of various polyols. Maltitol, at 30 grams of ingestion, produced mild flatulence, accompanied by rumblings in the bowel, and colic. Lactitol, at 30 to 40 grams of ingestion, produced a significant increase in the incidence and severity of colic, gas, and increased laxation compared to sucrose. Reactions to isomalt were less severe than to lactitol, but more severe than to maltitol. The incidence and severity of the symptoms reported were dose-dependent for all three polyols.

IDENTIFYING POLYOLS ON LABELS

Consumers who wish to identify polyols used in products need to read labels of foods and beverages carefully. If present, specific polyols are listed by their names in the ingredient list. The Nutrition Facts panel gives the total carbohydrate content of a product including any polyols that are present. Also, a manufacturer may voluntarily add information about the number of grams of polyol(s) in a serving of the product. If the term "sugar-free" or "no added sugar" appears on a product label, the polyol content must be declared separately under "carbohydrates" on the Nutrition Facts panel. If the product contains more than one polyol the term "sugar alcohols" must be used on the panel.

Relatively new phrases that appear on the principal display panel of some products are "net carb," "low carb," or "impact carb." These terms are favored by processors, but have not yet been defined officially by the FDA.

Food processors calculate "net carb" by subtracting the grams of fiber and polyols from the total amount of carbohydrates present in the product. This calculation is controversial within the scientific community. Processors argue that polyols have fewer calories per gram because of their incomplete absorption, and because of the resulting lower energy density. Thus, it is argued, polyols should not be tallied as part of total carbohydrates. Processors use a similar argument for dietary fibers.

Formerly, polyols had been designated as sweeteners with the same caloric value as sucrose (4 calories per gram). In 1990, the European Union (EU) assigned a caloric value of only 2.4 calories per gram to polyols as a group. The American polyol interests urged the FDA to follow suit. The Calorie Control Council (CCC), an international association of manufacturers of low-calorie foods and beverages and reduced-fat foods, contracted with the Federation of American Societies of Experimental Biology (FASEB) to determine the best estimates of the caloric values of polyols. In 1995, FASEB concluded that polyols did have lower values than 4 calories per gram, and revised values for isomalt and lactitol, each with only 2 calories per gram; xylitol, 2.4; and HSH, 3. The old caloric value for sorbitol, which had been 4 calories per gram, was lowered to 2.6 calories per gram. Similarly maltitol—both in crystalline form and in solution—was lowered from 4 to 3 calories; and mannitol, from 2 to 1.6 calories. The lowering of caloric values assigned to polyols allowed processors to have their food and beverage products qualify for claims of "sugar-free" and "reduced calories" (or "lite") without any reformulation.

The CCC also requested FASEB to evaluate the available date of specific polyols. Earlier, the polyols had been reviewed by the FAO/WHO's Joint Expert Committee on Food Additives (JECFA) several times in the 1980s. This Committee reviews food safety data and establishes what it deems to be safe use levels. They may differ from what the FDA establishes as safe use levels. Also, in 1986, the FDA had contracted with FASEB to review the scientific data on the effects of certain polyols (sorbitol, mannitol, xylitol, and lactitol) that had been observed in animal experiments. In 1996, JECFA concluded that the earlier adverse findings in animal studies conducted with polyols in the 1970s were too sparse and not relevant to the toxicological evaluation of these substances in humans.

The FDA's Center for Food Safety and Applied Nutrition (CFSAN) formed a working group to evaluate systematically all available data for each polyol. In view of the rapidly expanding use of polyol, such data are vital. Yet, the United Stated Department of Agriculture (USDA) fails to track the per capita consumption of polyols in its statistics for sugars and sweeteners. The polyols are not listed among the caloric sweeteners, although they are caloric. Nor are the polyols listed among the "minor" sweeteners such as honey and maple sugar. According to Lyn O'Brien Nabors, an expert on sugars and sweeteners, and executive director of CCC, this association does not have per capita consumption figures for polyols, nor has Nabors recalled ever having seen such figures for polyols. Indeed, sugar polyols appear to be sweeteners that are being consumed increasingly in foods and beverages, but *are not being tallied in consumption data.*

Formerly, some polyols were used for special purposes in dietetic foods. Later, their use was extended to so-called sugar-free or no-sugar added products used by the general public. This pattern of extended use is similar to that of cyclamates, saccharin, aspartame, and others, which began with limited and specific uses, then greatly expanded to general use. (To learn more about these high-intensity synthetic sweeteners, see Part Three.)

"Polyols: A Global Strategy Business Report," (2004) published by Global Industry Analysts, Inc., in Fremont, California, revealed that consumption of a single polyol, sorbitol, was estimated to have reached nearly 500 million pounds of annual consumption in the United States; and globally, more than a billion pounds. Consumption of mannitol, another polyol, had reached over 20 million pounds of annual consumption in the United States. Its use with chewing gum accounts for several millions of these pounds. The global market for mannitol was estimated at nearly 50 million pounds annually, and growing significantly each year.

PROMOTIONAL HEALTH CLAIMS

Polyol-sweetened products have been promoted as being suitable for diabetics. Polyols cause less increase in blood glucose and insulin levels than do refined carbohydrates (table sugar and refined flour). Also, polyols, having fewer calories than sucrose, are promoted as sweeteners that may help diabetics achieve their weight goals. How valid are these claims?

The suitability of polyols for diabetics has been questioned by the American Diabetes Association (ADA). In 2004, the ADA noted the lack of any long-term studies comparing the effects of high- and low-glycemic diets in diabetic individuals. The ADA noted that "with regard to the glycemic effects of carbohydrates, the total amount of carbohydrate in meals or snacks is more important than the source or type."

Polyol-sweetened products have been promoted to the general public for weight management. It is reasoned that because such products will have fewer calories per gram, they automatically reduce the overall glycemic challenge of the diet. At present, researchers have produced no conclusive or convincing evidence that the glycemic index is related to weight control. (For the glycemic index, see Chapter 20.) Health experts caution that excessive energy *intake in any form* leads to weight gain. The *total* caloric content of the diet is important, and overconsumption of *all* foods, including ones containing polyols, should be avoided.

Certain polyols have been promoted for good dental health. Claims are made that products made with these sweeteners do not promote dental decay. A "Tooth-friendly/Smiling Tooth Program" with a smiling tooth pictogram is a registered trademark of Toothfriendly Sweets International (TSI), a non-profit association established in Switzerland in 1989. Later, the organization branched out to other countries. TSI is run by representatives of the dental profession. The mission of the organization is to reduce the incidence of dental caries globally by promoting good dental hygiene and encouraging "tooth-friendly" eating habits.

According to Diane B. McColl, counsel to TSI, the organization licenses use of the pictogram to national dental associations. Each program in different countries is funded initially by the licensing fees paid to the national dental association by food manufacturers for use of the pictogram in product labeling. The licensing fees are based on actual sales data supplied by the manufacturers. Once widespread public recognition and education are well established, the licensing fees are reduced and eventually are terminated. Among manufacturers participating are confectionery manufacturers and distributors, whose products are found to be toothfriendly.

Critics of the program charged that the claims made for the toothfriendly aspects of polyols are not supported by the evidence. Dental research indicates that plaque bacteria, exposed to sugar polyols over a long time as substitutes for nutritive sweeteners, may adapt their metabolic capabilities, and render the sugar polyols potentially cariogenic.

In 1983, Dr. John R. Edwards, chairman of the Chemistry Department of Villanova University in Villanova, Pennsylvania, noted that mannitol and sorbitol support the growth of *Streploccus mutans*. Neither polyol gives rise to dextran (glucan) in the plaque. When sucrose is eaten, the organisms can then make dextran, because the polyols have kept the cells alive. Xylitol is poorly metabolized and there is poor growth when, experimentally, tryptic soy broth (TSB) is supplemented with xylitol. However, the glucosyl-transferase (an enzyme) is still present in the xylitol-TSB grown cells, and they still can produce dextran when given sucrose. There seems to be an increase in the proteinases in xylitol-grown cells.

Despite these findings, in 1996, the FDA allowed a health claim for so-called "sugar-free" chewing gums to be promoted with the phrase "does not promote tooth decay." The agency proposed that this health claim be restricted to chewing gums. Interested segments of the food and beverage industries succeeded in having the FDA broaden the application of this health claim to include breath mints, hard candies, chocolate candies, and other polyol-containing products that were controlled by special dietary regulations.

WHY MANUFACTURERS FAVOR POLYOLS

Processors find many advantageous features in polyol use. Generally, polyols do not absorb water as sucrose does. As a result, food products containing polyols do not become sticky on surfaces as quickly as do products made with sucrose. Molds and bacteria do not grow as rapidly on polyols as they do on sucrose, so products have a longer shelf life with polyols than do those with sucrose. Used to sweeten medications, polyols generally do not react with pharmacologic ingredients as readily as sucrose does. Unlike some of the high-intensity sweeteners such as aspartame, polyols usually do not lose their sweetness when products are heated. They retain their sweetness in hot beverages and in foods that need to be heated in processing. However, polyols have a few drawbacks for processors. The polyols do not give a crisp brown surface to baked foods (the Maillard reaction). This property makes polyols unsuitable for use with some baked goods such as crusty breads for which browning is desirable.

Frequently, polyols are used in combination with other sweeteners, especially low-caloric ones such as high-intensity sweeteners. The polyols provide the bulk and texture of sucrose—qualities that are especially lacking in low-calorie sweeteners.

Originally, polyols were added to food and beverage products at very low levels, as sweetening and bulking agents. Over the years, their use has escalated enormously. This is reflected when, in January 1996, American Xyrofin (supplier of xylitol) announced plans to invest $25 million to build a new polyol manufacturing plant in Thomson, Illinois. The facility was described as the largest Xyrofin plant in the world, and the first one in the United States.

The use of polyols has expanded to include a very wide range of products, including baked goods, ice creams, fruit spreads, candies, and chewing gums. Because polyols also function well in fillings and frostings, canned fruits, beverages, yogurts, and tabletop sweeteners, their uses are constantly growing. Also, they are present in toiletries such as breath fresheners, toothpastes, and mouthwashes, as well as in pharmaceuticals such as cough syrups and throat lozenges. A few are used for intravenous solutions.

Individual polyols share some common characteristics, but do have differences. They will be discussed individually, with the first few in greatest usage.

SORBITOL

In 1809, the French chemist Joseph Louis Proust identified natural sorbitol, derived from sorbose, in the ripe berries of the mountain ash. It is a carbohydrate found in many berries, cherries, plums, peaches, pears, apples, seaweeds, algae, and is even detected in blackstrap molasses. Commercial sorbitol is made from dextrose. Sorbitol used to sweeten products is far more concentrated than naturally occurring sorbitol in fruits. For example, the amount of sorbitol used in a single sorbitol-sweetened mint is equivalent to the amount of sorbitol found in 3.5 ounces of cherries.

In 1929, sorbitol was granted GRAS status as a sweetener for special dietary foods intended for diabetics. Up to 7 percent sorbitol was allowed for this purpose in such foods and beverages. For many years, sorbitol was restricted to dietetic foods intended for individuals on sugar-free diets.

In 1989, sorbitol use was expanded when it was granted GRAS status for soft and hard candies, chewing gums, breath mints, and cough drops. This development meant that sorbitol was no longer limited for use in dietary foods intended for diabetics, but would became available for a variety of products consumed by the general public.

The Versatility of Sorbitol

With increased interest in sugar alternatives, processors viewed sorbitol as a potential sweetener for additional applications. They found that sorbitol was versatile. Among its many virtues, sorbitol could promote the retention of original food quality during shipment and storage. It could improve food texture, because sorbitol acts as a crystallization modifier, humectant, softening agent, controller of sweetness or viscosity, and an aid in rehydration. For these purposes, processors use sorbitol in baked goods, frostings and gelatin puddings; frozen dairy products; poultry, fish, meat, and nut products; snack foods; processed fruits; fats and oils; alcoholic and non-alcoholic beverages; and sweet sauces, seasonings, and flavorings. Among sorbitol's special uses, it acts as a release agent in candy manufacture by helping to slide products out of pans. Sorbitol added to formulas for cooked sausages and frankfurters helps to remove their casings. Sorbitol reduces charring and carmelization of processed meats when they are cooked in direct contact with heated metal, such as grill roller bars. Sorbitol leaves no bitter aftertaste, and it is used to mask this quality in saccharin-sweetened foods and beverages. Also, sorbitol provides body and mouthfeel in low-calorie drinks. Sorbitol tends to draw heat from the mouth as the sweetener is consumed. This feature results in a perceived cool sweet taste.

Compressed bite-size cereal cubes intended for astronauts are treated with sorbitol to prevent the cubes from crumbling and scattering in a weightless environment. Powdered sorbitol has excellent flow properties. In tablet manufacture, it is important to maintain uniformity in the weight of tablets. Sorbitol powder compresses readily, which gives a high-tablet performance, and reduces wear in the equipment.

With all these attributes, processors were more and more attracted to various applications with sorbitol. In 1992, the FDA was petitioned to use sorbitol at a 2 percent level to reduce the charring in pizza toppings and other cured meat products. The agency allowed sorbitol use in food products at various levels, and as high as 12 percent in non-specific products.

In April 1996, the USDA's Food Safety and Inspection Service (FSIS) proposed the use of sorbitol in cooked roast beef products as a sweetener and to reduce charring. In the following month, FSIS withdrew its final rule due to concerns raised by a mother in Tustin, California, with three children who suffered from multiple food allergies. She claimed that it was already difficult to plan and prepare adequate meals for her children given the number of foods they could not eat. Treated precooked beef would limit further food selections. She added that other parents would be unaware that their children might be negatively affected by the presence of substances hidden in prepared foods. Indeed, this is an issue with broad implications. Consumers are unaware of nontraditional additions in the food supply. For individuals with food allergies or sensitivities, such additions are especially worrisome.

Despite the mother's protest, a year later, the USDA proposed to allow the use of sorbitol up to 2 percent in a solution of ingredients that would be pumped into the beef prior to cooking. The final rule passed. It also removed an existing prohibition against the use of sorbitol in combination with corn syrup or corn syrup solids. The prohibition had been in effect since 1972. At the time, there were no effective laboratory procedures to measure the amount of sorbitol present, if used in combination with corn syrup. By the 1990s, methods for such detection were available.

Sorbitol may be synergistic with other sweeteners. This means that in combination, the sweeteners result in a higher level of perceived sweetness than by the sum of the individual sweeteners. Synergism provides sweetness at a lower cost, and sometimes achieves more stability. These are attractive features for food and beverage processors.

Dubious Health Claims

Some advertising and labeling of sorbitol-sweetened products, especially candies and chewing gums, have been misleading if not downright deceptive. One advertisement of a sorbitol-sweetened candy, cited in the *Consumer Affairs Newsletter* published by the City of Syracuse, New York (Feb 1979), declared:

> Sugarless candy . . . Free of sugar . . . Low in calories . . . Safe for diabetics . . . Can't hurt children's teeth . . . the secret of [brand name] amazing similarity to sugar-based candy is sorbitol, a safe, natural, nutritive sweetening agent extracted from the skins of fruits and berries. A completely safe, and . . . medically approved substance . . .

This advertisement should be parsed. "Sugarless" or "sugar-free" are misnomers for sorbitol-sweetened products. Sugarless is *not* free of sugar, but rather is free of sucrose. This misleading label and advertising term is tolerated by two federal regulatory agencies, the FDA and Federal Trade Commission (FTC). Some state and local authorities believe that the term is deceptive. The Connecticut Agriculture Experiment Station, with an admirable history of testing food products in Connecticut markets, has seized "sugarless" products for mislabeling. Connecticut authorities asserted in the 74th Report on Food Products in 1969 that "the sugarless statement is misleading. Sorbitol and mannitol, declared ingredients, are metabolized as sugars." Similarly, the Department of Consumer Affairs in Syracuse. New York, warned residents of the misrepresentation of "sugarless" products. Sorbitol has about 50 percent the sweetness of sucrose. As mentioned earlier, sorbitol has approximately 2.6 calories per gram, contrasted with 4 calories per gram of sucrose.

There is reason to believe that sorbitol contributes to tooth decay in individuals who consume it frequently. Several studies have indicated that in such individuals, the microorganisms in the dental plaque change, with an increase in the number of sorbitol fermenters. The end result is that more cavity-causing acid is produced when sorbitol is consumed.

"Can't hurt children's teeth" is untrue. Dental cavities are defined as localized progressive decay of the teeth, initiated by demineralization of the outer surface of the tooth due to organic acids produced locally by bacteria that ferment deposits of dietary carbohydrates. It is believed that *S. mutans* is the main bacterium responsible for human dental cavities, as mentioned earlier. *S. mutans* can transport and metabolize sorbitol as well as other carbohydrates. Admittedly, animal tests show that sorbitol is markedly *less* cariogenic than sucrose, and that dental plaque incubated with sorbitol produces *less* acid. Few bacteria in plaque are capable of fermenting sorbitol. However, incubated in test tubes with sorbitol as the primary carbohydrate source, *S. mutans* can grow rapidly and produce acid. Consuming sorbitol between meals, which frequently is the case with candies and chewing gums, *can* enhance *S. mutans'* ability to compete with other oral bacteria. In the absence of other fermentable carbohydrates, *S. mutans* is able to metabolize sorbitol. Also, there are other reasons why candies and chewing gums are undesirable, apart from the sugar issue.

"Sorbitol . . . extracted from the skins of fruits and berries" is misleading. It is true that sorbitol is a constituent in fruits and berries, but commercial sorbitol is prepared from glucose, a simple, inexpensive, readily available sugar (discussed in Chapter 2).

"A completely safe and medically approved substance" is unfounded. In addition to sorbitol's use as a sweetener, it has been used therapeutically as a carbohydrate source for intravenous feeding. It was discovered that sorbitol can affect the body's ability to absorb and utilize certain nutrients and drugs, either by inhibiting or enhancing them. This feature deserves attention, especially if sorbitol is used at high levels either as a sweetener or as a therapeutic nutrient.

Health Complaints

In one medical report, 30 percent of patients who consumed 10 grams of sorbitol orally suffered reduced absorption of vitamin B_{12} to within the range of pernicious anemia. This condition, inflicted from a single high sorbitol dose, was observed two or three days later. When the dose was increased up to 50 grams, nearly all the patients lost their ability to absorb vitamin B_{12} and the condition was no longer reversible. The experience was reported in *Connecticut Medicine* (Aug 1965). Similar inhibition of vitamin B_{12} absorption was demonstrated in laboratory experiments with pigs, rats, and guinea pigs.

Sorbitol also can affect the absorption of vitamin B_6. Sorbitol was found to *stimulate* production of some B vitamin fractions by affecting microorganisms in the intestinal tract, as reported in the *New York Times* (May 20, 1965).

At times, sorbitol is added to vitamins and other nutrients in pharmaceutical preparations to increase their absorption. This absorptive ability may be beneficial for certain nutrients, but undesirable for other substances. For example, if a soft drink sweetened with sorbitol contains synthetic colors, flavors, or other food additives of questionable safety, sorbitol's inclusion may result in greater absorption of toxic substances.

Sorbitol's ability to cause diarrhea is well known. In fact, medically, sorbitol can be used in large amounts as a cathartic. Use of sorbitol as a treatment for constipation in the elderly was found to be less costly than other laxations. Sorbitol's relatively slow absorption from the intestine may result in osmotic diarrhea and flatulence if individuals consume high daily amounts (from 30 to 50 grams), or single large doses (20 to 30 grams). The intolerance level varies among individuals. As little as 10 grams can cause bloating and flatulence; 20 grams can cause more severe symptoms of cramping and diarrhea. There is a correlation between the amount of hydrogen gas excreted in the breath and the severity of the symptoms. A condition has been dubbed "holiday diarrhea" because of overindulgence in sorbitol-sweetened candies during holidays.

SORBITOL LABEL WARNING IS INADEQUATE

"A half cup of ice cream, three tablespoons of jelly, five sticks of gum. That might be all it takes to produce gas, bloating, or diarrhea in some people who eat these foods when they contain sorbitol, a common artificial [sic] sweetener found in everything from carbonated beverages to baked goods . . . To alert people to the fact that sorbitol may produce undesirable symptoms, the FDA requires that when consumption of a product is likely to provide more then 50 grams of the sweetener over the course of a day, the following words must be on the label: 'excess consumption may have a laxative effect.' However, since most products contain much fewer than 50 grams of sorbitol in a day's 'supply' (you'd have to chew at least twenty-five sticks of gum to reach that level) food manufacturers are usually free to leave the warning out. Even if it is included, a caution about consuming 50 grams of the sweetener does nothing to help the person who suffers from as little as 10 grams . . ."

—*Tufts University Diet & Nutrition Letter,* September 1986

Numerous reports in medical journals describe cases of osmotic diarrhea induced from excessive consumption of sorbitol-sweetened foods and beverages. Commonly, cases concern young children who have overindulged with sorbitol-sweetened candies. A pediatrician at the Yale University School of

Medicine reported in *Connecticut Medicine* (Aug 1965) that within a fifteen-month period, ten children ranging in age from twenty to thirty-six months had been treated for diarrhea after having eaten large quantities of sorbitol-sweetened candies. This experience led to further studies at Yale with two groups of children. One consisted of five-to-six-year olds; and the other, children from twenty to thirty-six months of age. Each child was given one package of dietetic mints that contained a total of 9.3 grams of sorbitol. After the mints were consumed, the children and their stools were examined. None of the older children experienced any discomfort or change in bowel habits or stool consistency. The stools, examined twenty-four hours after the candy was eaten, contained less than 1 milligram (mg) of sorbitol per gram of wet stool and otherwise were normal. The younger children, however, developed diarrheal stools within two to five hours after eating the candy. Their stools were abnormal in sorbitol content, which measured 5 to 10 mg per wet stool.

Due to the difference in body size, young children may be at far greater risk than adults in eating the same amount of sorbitol. Young children do not have the fully developed detoxifying mechanisms of adults.

Naturally occurring sorbitol, found in apples, becomes concentrated in apple juice. Often, toddlers are given apple juice. Young children, aged one year to two and a half years, unable to break down the sorbitol in apple juice, suffer from diarrhea.

Lactose intolerant patients also may suffer from sorbitol and fructose intolerances. A majority of patients were found to benefit significantly from appropriate dietary measures and enzyme replacement for lactose intolerance, but only about half who were sorbitol intolerant benefited from dietary measures. At present, no enzyme replacement is available for sorbitol intolerance.

The risks of high levels of sorbitol consumption in adults also needs to be recognized. A physician reported in the *New England Journal of Medicine* (Feb 16, 1967) a case of an adult diabetic, who developed abdominal distension, gas, and diarrhea after eating sorbitol-sweetened candy.

Low sorbitol tolerance has been found to be prevalent. Gastroenterologist Maresh K. Jain and his colleagues at Misericordia Hospital in New York City tested forty-two healthy volunteers, aged twenty-one to fifty-nine years, for sorbitol intolerance. After an overnight fast, the volunteers ingested 5.5 grams of sorbitol—an equivalency of the amount of sorbitol present in only five sorbitol-sweetened mints. The sorbitol produced diarrhea, abdominal pain, or cramps in nearly half of the volunteers. Breath samples from all volunteers were collected at fifteen-minute intervals for four hours after the ingestion, and analyzed for hydrogen content, a test that reveals sorbitol intolerance. Seventy-four percent of the volunteers were judged to have biochemical sorbitol intolerance. Yet, not all those affected showed clinical symptoms of abdominal distension, pain, or diarrhea. Severe sorbitol intolerance, manifested in diarrhea, was identified in more then 16 percent of the volunteers.

In reporting the findings of this test to the ADA, Jain noted that with millions of diabetics in the United States and with more than 16 percent incidence of severe clinical sorbitol intolerance found in the study, a large number of diabetics could suffer from diarrhea by consuming 10 or more grams of sorbitol within a short period of time. Jain noted, too, that the sorbitol content is high in many dietetic foods consumed by diabetics, such as marmalades, chocolates, and chewing gums, to name a few. Jain conceded that a person is not apt to consume 100 grams of marmalade at a single meal, but might consume sorbitol at the same meal in several different dietetic foods. All totaled, the amount could be significant.

Sorbitol as a sweetener in foods may be an unrecognized cause of gastrointestinal disturbances in adults, and especially in diabetics. Jain observed that diabetics, compared to healthy people, are not necessarily more sensitive to sorbitol. However, because they tend to consume dietetic foods more often on the advice of their physicians, they are much more prone to develop gastrointestinal problems.

A study conducted in the mid-1970s of sorbitol intolerance in ten children suggested that their intolerance is greater than in adults. However, from Jain's study, he concluded that adults also have a fair amount of intolerance. He advised health professionals who treat diabetics with chronic diarrhea to inquire about their use of sorbitol-sweetened products. If sorbitol intolerance is detected, patients should be given a breath hydrogen test. If sorbitol intolerance is confirmed, health professionals should recommend that patients avoid sorbitol-sweetened products.

Sorbitol-containing chewing gums and candies should be banned for patients with eating disorders, according to Elizabeth S. Ohlrich and her associates at the University of Wisconsin Hospital and Clinic in Madison, Wisconsin. Daily use of these products was observed in nineteen out of twenty-one patients with eating disorders. Of these, thirteen reported bloating or intestinal gas; five reported occasional diarrhea or loose stools. The symptoms depended on the amount of sorbitol ingested in relation to body weight, making this sweetener especially potent in extremely low-weight patients. According to Ohlrich, laxative abusers may be especially vulnerable to sorbitol abuse if they discover that large amounts of sorbitol can have a laxative effect. Other eating disorder patients may abuse sorbitol-containing foods to avoid binge eating, alleviate tension, prevent vomiting, or suppress appetite.

Many so-called dietetic foods intended for weight-reduction regimens contain sorbitol and/or mannitol. The *Journal of the American Medical Associa-*

tion (Jul 18, 1980) reported the case of a healthy twenty-nine-year-old man suffering from diarrhea and cramps. In attempting to reduce weight, he had been consuming dietetic foodstuffs, many of which contained sorbitol. Each day the patient had chewed two packages of sugarless gum, had eaten two rolls of sugarless mints and two dietetic candy bars, which totaled about 50 to 55 grams of sorbitol daily. The diarrhea abated when the sorbitol-sweetened products were withdrawn. The internist who reported the case suggested that if physicians were aware of the problem, more sorbitol-induced diarrheal cases would be identified. The diarrhea had been merely uncomfortable for this patient. However, individuals with angina, diabetes, kidney problems, or other health conditions who consume large quantities of sorbitol, risk serious medical consequences.

Unknown Effects of Long-term Consumption

As mentioned earlier, the FDA, aware of the diarrheal problem from high consumption of sorbitol, mandated that products that might result in personal consumption of more than 50 grams of sorbitol carry the warning: "Excess consumption may have a laxative effect." However, the agency requires this caution on labels only for food products "whose reasonable foreseeable consumption" might result in a daily ingestion of 50 grams or more of sorbitol. The weakness in this policy is that no one food or beverage contains high levels. The real problem is the enormous escalation of sorbitol in many products, and the total intake from the food supply, especially for those individuals who are heavy users of highly processed foods and beverages.

On July 31, 1980, the Center for Science in the Public Interest (CSPI) petitioned the FDA to issue a regulation requiring *all* sorbitol-containing foods and beverages to carry the warning label. The agency took no action, but brought to public attention the labeling requirement.

Although sorbitol's ability to induce diarrhea is well defined, other possible health effects from high levels of consumption are not. Both animal experiments and long-range human feeding studies are few, and inconclusive.

Rats fed sorbitol at high levels (16 percent of the diet; 16 grams per kilo of body weight) after one year showed a tendency toward hypercalcemia (excessively high calcium levels in the blood and other symptoms of abnormality) with the appearance in some animals of bladder concretions (solid masses) and a generalized thickening of the skeleton. This study was cited by FASEB in its 1972 review.

Because sorbitol is used frequently by diabetics, any health effects on this group are of special interest. In other rat studies, high levels of sorbitol ingestion were related to vascular and nervous system complications, and to cataract formation. Diabetics frequently encounter all of these health problems.

Changes in aging may result from lifetime accumulation of sorbitol in cells. Sorbitol penetrates cell membranes poorly. But once it penetrates, sorbitol may become trapped intracellularly, and slowly leak out. The effect is an accumulation of sorbitol solution inside the cell, which results in increased osmotic pressure. For the diabetic, this development is of special concern. Osmotic pressure may relate to cataract formation, as well as damage to the vascular and nervous systems.

In studies conducted at the National Eye Institute of the National Institutes of Health, rabbit eye lenses incubated with a high-glucose medium absorbed sorbitol by osmosis. Leakage damaged the fibers and resulted in lens cataract formation.

It is important to emphasize that if these results can be extrapolated to humans, such possible complications might result from *high levels of sorbitol consumption* over a period of time. The ADA assured the public that there is no undue need for concern over possible complications of cataracts related to intracellular sorbitol accumulation, but cautioned that sorbitol should be used *sparingly*.

The ADA reported studies with well-regulated maturity-onset diabetic patients showing that sorbitol, substituted for table sugar or other sugars, offered *little if any advantage*. The ADA concluded that it appeared unnecessary to have specially sweetened foods designed for adults with this type of diabetes. The ADA also noted that the effects on diabetics from long-term consumption of large amounts of sorbitol has not been studied.

Present Status

High levels of sorbitol consumption may be cause for concern by everyone. The USDA reported that the total amount of sorbitol used in foods by 1970 was about seven times more than in 1960. Because the USDA stopped tracking polyol consumption, no current figures are available from this agency. Even when the USDA did track polyols, the daily average intake figures appeared to be unreliable and useless. FASEB, examining sorbitol in its GRAS review, expressed concern about an apparent discrepancy of monumental proportions. In its report Evaluation of the Health Aspects of Sorbitol as a Food Ingredient (Dec 1972), FASEB noted:

Even if all of the 105 million pounds were used in food, the per capita per day average intake of sorbitol would be only 654 mg rather than 30,191 mg given in the [National Research Council] table.

Also, FASEB noted that sorbitol begins to exert a laxative effect at levels that are about twice the estimated average adult intake level, and about equal to the estimated maximal adult intake level. The average consumption levels for children aged six to eleven months, and twelve to twenty three months are estimated to be close to, or in excess of a laxative level. However, because the reported average and maximal intake levels are known to be what FASEB termed "generous overestimates" FASEB concluded that "the use of sorbitol in food in the present or reasonably foreseeable amounts poses no problem in this regard." However, FASEB expressed concern:

> The actual consumption of sorbitol may be considerably higher than average consumption in certain segments of the population. These individuals, for dietary reasons, may select foods containing particularly high levels of sorbitol. Currently available food consumption data do not permit [FASEB] to determine the extent and significance of this problem in regard to sorbitol.

The Joint FAO/WHO Expert Committee on Food Additives (JECFA) reviewed the sorbitol safety data, and concluded that an acceptable daily intake (ADI) was "not specific" (that is, no limits placed on its use). This is the safest classification. Also, the European Commission's Scientific Committee on Food (SCF) did not set a limit on sorbitol use, and concluded that it is acceptable.

In 1999, once again, CSPI petitioned the FDA to require a more explicit warning label on processed foods and beverages that contain 1 or more grams of sorbitol or other sugar polyols. CSPI contended that sorbitol induces gastrointestinal symptoms in adults who consume between 10 and 50 grams and that children, due to their size and incomplete detoxification mechanisms, may be affected by lower amounts. CSPI claimed that the FDA's regulation, instituted in 1973, is not sufficiently stringent. The warning on the label for sorbitol is for a level of 50 grams. Yet children are affected at levels lower than 10 grams. Also, the warning fails to consider that total daily sorbitol intake may be from multiple sources of foods and beverages as well as from toiletries and medications.

The CSPI petition recommended that the label be modified to read: "NOTICE: THIS PRODUCT CONTAINS SORBITOL, WHICH MAY CAUSE DIARRHEA, BLOATING, AND ABDOMINAL PAIN. NOT SUITABLE FOR CONSUMPTION BY CHILDREN. TO PROTECT YOURSELF, START BY EATING NO MORE THAN ONE SERVING AT A TIME [OF A SORBITOL-CONTAINING FOOD]."

Although CSPI's petition focused mainly on sorbitol, the group also sought a warning label on products containing other polyols. Co-petitioners included Dr. Jeffrey S. Hyams, chairman of the Department of Digestive Diseases and Nutrition at Connecticut Children's Medical Center, as well as Dr.

Ray Breitenbach, a family physician and retired U.S. Air Force Lt. Colonel flight surgeon, who had written about the risks of eating sorbitol-containing candies. Dr. Hyams reported, "I know of people who have undergone extensive medical testing for abdominal pain and diarrhea when the problem was simply that they were ingesting excessive amounts of sorbitol."

For some adults, as little as 10 grams of sorbitol can induce adverse effects. Yet, there are products that contain more than 10 grams per serving, noted Hyams.

The FDA rejected CSPI's petition. Currently, the inadequate warning label from 1973 still prevails, despite the ever-escalating use of sorbitol.

The FDA has made seizures of sorbitol-sweetened baking mixes in several states. The amount of added sorbitol was found to be above the upper limit of 30 percent sorbitol permitted by GRAS affirmation regulations.

Sorbitol had been touted as a product "sweetening the foods of the 1980s" in advertisement directed to processors of foods and beverages intended for general consumption. Sorbitol continued to be promoted in the 1990s, and into the present. Although there is uncertainty regarding the amounts being used, what remains clear is that the number of sorbitol-sweetened products, resulting in high consumption levels, continues to be cause for concern.

MANNITOL

Mannitol, from mannose sugar, is found in many plants and plant exudates, especially in seaweeds, algae, fungi, and manna ash, also known as the European flowering ash. The manna ash and related plants produce a sweet, dried exudate known as "manna sugar" that has been used by Aboriginals in Australia as food during times of famine. Mannitol is utilized poorly by the body and is of limited nutritional value. However, commercial mannitol is made commonly from glucose or invert sugar.

Traditional commercial processing techniques used to manufacture mannitol were inefficient until recently. They exposed fructose and glucose to a metal catalyst and high-pressure by hydrogenation. (This process is similar to the one used for margarine manufacture.) The process was time-consuming. It produced chemical wastes. It was inefficient by converting only about 25 percent of the sugars into mannitol.

In 1995, Roquette America, Inc., petitioned the FDA to allow mannitol production by fermenting sugars or polyols with yeast. This improved process was followed, in 2003, by chemist Badal C. Saha and colleagues at the USDA's Agricultural Research Service (ARS) Fermentation Biotechnology Research Unit in Peoria, Illinois, where they attempted to produce mannitol more efficiently by feeding high-fructose corn syrup (HFCS) to the bacteria, *Lactobacillus intermedius*. After being in a deep-tank fermentor for a few hours, the bacteria converted 72 percent of the HFCS into mannitol. This process would be nearly three times more efficient, and also less costly, than traditional processing. The microbial conversion process, now patented, can use sucrose or other sugars. Ongoing research is being conducted by the USDA, jointly with the sweetener company zuChem, Inc., in Chicago, to scale up and refine the new process.

Commercial mannitol has fewer calories per gram than sucrose (1.5 grams and 4 grams, respectively). Mannitol is from 50 to 70 percent as sweet as sucrose.

Safety Concerns

In 1963, the FDA prohibited mannitol's use as a flavoring adjunct. Later, in 1973, the FDA proposed further limitations, but a trade group, the National Preservers Association, objected, and the proposal was not implemented. However, the FDA proposed to affirm mannitol as GRAS based on the findings of the Select Committee on GRAS Substances (1973) conducted by FASEB. Due to comments on the proposal that raised questions about mannitol's safety, the FDA withdrew its proposal to affirm mannitol as GRAS. Instead, the agency assigned an interim food additive status to the sweetener, "pending additional studies of the ingredient."

A Health Concern: Diarrhea

Like sorbitol, mannitol is absorbed poorly. It accumulates water during its slow passage through the intestinal tract. Even relatively small amounts of mannitol can cause diarrhea. The FDA requires a warning label, similar to the one with sorbitol, regarding the likelihood of diarrhea from high levels of mannitol ingestion. Although 50 grams of sorbitol may be required to induce diarrhea, only 20 grams of mannitol are required. CSPI petitioned for warning labels on all mannitol-containing foods and beverages, at the same time that the center petitioned for similar warning labels on sorbitol. The FDA's policy was similar with both sugar polyols. The agency merely brought to public attention its labeling requirements.

Traditionally, mannose sugar was used widely in southern Europe as a mild children's laxative. Many immigrants to the United States continued to import it for that use.

A Health Concern: Thymus Tumors

Aside from the diarrheal issue, other safety questions were raised about mannitol. Data from studies with mannitol demonstrated a significant incidence of benign thymomas (tumors in the thymus) and an abnormal growth of thymus gland tissue in female rats fed mannitol. While the FDA was evaluating this information, the agency received additional disturbing findings. Other studies showed an increased combined incidence of medullary hyperplasia and pheochromocytoma of the adrenal glands in a certain rat strain (Fischer) fed a diet of 10 percent mannitol. The same effect was not observed in other rat strains (Sprague-Dawley and Wistar). Medullary hyperplasia is an abnormal increase in normal cells in normal arrangement in the central portion of the adrenal glands. Pheochromocytomas are tumors of chromatin tissues of the adrenal medulla or sympathetic paragonpha. The notable symptom is hypertension (high blood pressure) caused by increased secretions of epinephrine and norepinephrine (two hormones).

After evaluating the new data FASEB reported in 1986 that "there was a statistically significant increased incidence of adrenal medullary hyperplasia and pheochromocytoma in rats fed high levels of sugar alcohols, including mannitol." However, FASEB downplayed any importance of the findings, and concluded, "The existing data provided no satisfactory mechanistic explanations of these adrenal medullary lesions, which are commonly found in aged rats maintained on standard laboratory diets."

Following FASEB's report, the FDA announced that it would review the safety data for mannitol. The FDA conducted a protracted review of mannitol and other sugar alcohols. By December 1994, the agency reported that it was reviewing additional data from animal studies of these substances to determine whether any regulatory action would be appropriate for any or all of the sugar alcohols. Meanwhile, mannitol continued to be listed on an interim basis for food use.

A Health Concern: Enhances Growth of *S. Mutans*

Mannitol, like sorbitol, is a fermentable carbohydrate in the mouth, but to a lesser extent than sucrose. Although few bacteria in plaque can ferment mannitol, *S. mutans* can transport and metabolize mannitol efficiently. In test tube experiments, when mannitol was the sole carbohydrate source, *S. mutans* grew rapidly and produced acid. Ingestion of mannitol between meals, such as consumption of mannitol-containing candies or chewing gums, can enhance *S. mutans'* ability to compete with other oral bacteria. In the absence of other fermentable carbohydrates, *S. mutans* can ferment mannitol.

A Health Concern: Intravenous Feeding

Mannitol has been used as an intravenous osmotic diuretic to reduce intercranial pressure. For this purposes it can be lifesaving. However, mannitol used for intravenous feeding has been associated with a wide range of pathological findings. In 1971, one report noted various manifestations of disturbed metabolism, resulting from intravenous infusion with mannitol. The conditions ranged from acidosis, dehydration, kidney stones and kidney failure, to death. Some of the conditions were accompanied by symptoms of nausea, confusion, and unconsciousness.

In 1979, another danger of intravenous mannitol infusion was reported in a case study by a physician who administered repeated high doses (2 grams per kilogram every four hours) to a child with Reyes syndrome. He noted sharply increased osmotic pressure within the child's skull. If the high dosage of the infusion had been continued, death might have ensued.

Animal studies showed that a single, repeated, and massive infusion of mannitol in dogs resulted in structural and functional changes in the kidneys and brains of the animals. Long-term mannitol therapy resulted in serious kidney damage.

A Health Concern: Laxative Use of Mannitol

A letter to the *Journal of the American Medical Association* (Aug 5, 1988) reported that oral mannitol was used as a colonic cleaning agent to prepare patients for surgery and for roentgenographic and endoscopic procedures, and as an hyperosmotic agent to treat constipation. One case described a previously unreported hazard of pneumatic explosion of the colon and death, following the use of oral mannitol as a cathartic agent in an individual who had suffered from chronic constipation. "Although oral mannitol has been routinely used by some as a mechanical cleaning agent," warned the journal, "extreme caution should be taken when this agent or other fermentable hyperosmotic laxatives are used to treat severe constipation, particularly when statis [blockage] might contribute to gas production and accumulation." This warning was sounded by Major Frank M. Moses, medical chief at Walter Reed Army Medical Center in Washington, D.C. Moses noted that other polyols used as cathartics also are fermentable hyperosmotic laxatives.

Uses in the General Food Supply

Mannitol use, originally for dietetic applications, has developed for additional uses in the general food supply. Mannitol is used in many so-called sugarfree confections, and as a release agent in the powdery coating of chewing gums. It is used in solid chocolates, confectionery coatings, and panned sweets. It is used in many pharmaceuticals, such as breath fresheners, as a binder in antacid tablets, cough and cold remedy tablets, children's aspirin tablets, and some medication pills.

At times, mannitol is used in combination with other polyols such as sorbitol. (Mannitol and sorbitol are related as isomers—substances with the same chemical formula but with different shapes.) Mannitol and sorbitol were the earliest, and most widely used bulking agents. Also, early on, mannitol was used to mask the bitterness of saccharin. Presently, mannitol in powder form is used to improve the stability and to mask the odor of fish oil in omega-3 products. Mannitol (and sorbitol) products are available to food and beverage processors in a wide range of particle sizes for baked goods to provide benefits as a humectant, to extend the shelf life of baked products, to enhance their texture, and to act both as a bulking agent and as a sweetener.

XYLITOL

Xylitol is a monosaccharide five-carbon polyol. It occurs naturally in many fruits and vegetables, and during normal metabolism is produced by the human body. However, commercial xylitol is produced from xylose, a wood sugar widely distributed in the xylan (cell walls) of plant materials, especially in birch, maple, and cherry woods. Xylose is found, also, in waste products such as wheat straw; leaves; cottonseed hulls; almond, peanut, and coconut shells; sugarcane bagasse; and in wood fiber waste from paper mills.

Intense-Sweetening Power

The sweetening power of xylitol was discovered as early as 1891 by a German chemist, Emil Fischer. However, xylitol's commercial development as a sweetener was developed a half-century later. Faced with sugar shortages during and after World War II, production of xylitol from plentiful sources of birch tree bark was begun in Finland. After xylitol extraction, the waste bark was utilized further by feeding it to cattle. For many years, Finland would remain the main source of commercial xylitol. For other countries, importation of xylitol was expensive, and the sweetener was not cost competitive with domestically available sweeteners.

The USDA's ARS attempted to develop a process that could utilize domestic wastes to produce xylitol. The researchers found that they could turn corn fibers—a waste product from ethanol production—into xylitol. This development would lower production costs, and increase market sales. The new process, reported in 2000, yields xylitol from ethanol waste by using a strain of yeast that converts xylose, the wood sugar, into xylitol. To overcome glucose repression—whereby glucose slows or shuts down some microbial metabolism—two groups of yeast were used. The first group consumed all of the glucose in the fermentation vat. Then, the second group of yeast was free to convert xylose to xylitol. Also, the researchers discovered that a xylose-related sugar, arabinose, induced no repression of xylitol production. The researchers suggested that by means of genetic engineering, the yeast might be able to produce xylitol from arabinose as well as from xylose.

Xylitol is about the same as sucrose in its sweetness and bulk. The FDA assigned an interim value of 2.4 calories per gram for xylitol. Having a caloric value about 40 percent lower than sucrose permits manufacturers of xylitol-containing products to make a label claim of reduced-calories. Xylitol has a much lower glycemic index rating than sucrose. (See Chapter 20 for the glycemic index.)

Another favorable feature reported about xylitol is its good taste, with no unpleasant aftertaste. Xylitol produces a cooling sensation in the mouth. In crystalline form, xylitol dissolves quickly. It is very hygroscopic and tends to absorb moisture. It does not undergo browning.

Retards Cavity Formation

Early on, in examining xylitol's potential as a sucrose substitute, Finnish dental researchers made a startling discovery. In 1976, headlines concerning xylitol were ecstatic, from print media as widely divergent as the *Wall Street Journal*, the *National Enquirer*, and *Food Processing:* FINN RESEARCHERS HAIL SWEETENER XYLITOL AS 'MIRACLE' THAT CAN HEAL TOOTH DECAY; MIRACLE SWEETENER ENDS TOOTH DECAY; and FIVE STICKS A DAY KEEPS THE DENTIST AWAY were the respective headlines.

The enthusiasm was generated by results of the first xylitol studies, known as the Turku Sugar Studies, of Dr. Kauko Makinen, a biochemist, and his colleague, Arje Sheinin, D.D.S. They had divided 125 dental students from the Finnish University of Turku into three groups. The first consumed foods in which xylitol totally replaced sucrose; for the second, fructose totally replaced sucrose; and for the third, sucrose was eaten at an average level. After one year, the xylitol group had 90 percent fewer new cavities than the sucrose group, and 30 to 40 percent fewer cavities than the fructose group.

In another Turku experiment, a hundred students were divided into two groups. Both groups had free choices of food selection. But one group chewed about five sticks of xylitol-sweetened chewing gum daily; the other, sucrose-sweetened chewing gum. After a year, the xylitol group had an average decrease of one cavity per person; the sucrose group, an average increase of three cavities per person. In some students on xylitol, the decay process appeared to be reversed, which suggested a possible therapeutic effect of xylitol.

The study demonstrated the role of fermentable carbohydrates in human caries formation, and the fact that oral bacteria do not ferment xylitol. Apparently, the breakdown of carbohydrates to acids in the mouth is arrested, partly because xylitol, itself, does not break down in the mouth, but does so in the stomach. Also, by raising the plaque pH level above the acid range for prolonged periods, xylitol inhibits the action of *S. mutans*, and thus retards cavity formation.

In press meetings, Makinen's statements were uncharacteristic of most scientific researchers. "It's miraculous," Makinen was quoted as saying to the news media. He claimed that xylitol "goes beyond" other noncariogenic sweeteners that purportedly do not promote decay. Xylitol actually prevents it and will even heal incipient cavities.

The 'miracle' sweetener generated enormous interest. At the time, the segments of American industry that would benefit most were the manufacturers of chewing gums, candies, and chocolates, with a combined annual $3.5 billion market, according to *Chemical & Engineering News* (Sept 12, 1977).

Launch of a Long-range Study

The National Institute of Dental Health (NIDH) announced that it would launch a three-year study with about a thousand American school children to confirm the Turku findings. Both American Chicle and Life Savers decided to hold back cautiously, and await the outcome of the study, but Wrigley decided to introduce a xylitol-sweetened chewing gum. United States law did not permit advertisement of xylitol's cavity-fighting ability during the trial period of the study. Wrigley made no dental claims, but merely described xylitol's sweetening ability and its agreeable cooling perception in the mouth.

In November 1977, the NIDH launched the study. Sticks of xylitol-sweetened chewing gum were distributed to schoolchildren on Long Island. The chewing gum was 50 percent xylitol, a level five times higher than in the Wrigley product. The children were instructed to chew three sticks daily, for a period of three years.

After day three, with only nine sticks chewed, parents were notified to return the remaining supply of chewing gum. The experiment was halted, unexpectedly and abruptly.

Disturbing Findings

This action was triggered by news from the Huntingdon Research Center in Great Britain. Ongoing animal safety studies with xylitol, funded by Hoffmann-La Roche, the American distributor of imported xylitol, were showing disturbing results. Preliminary findings from a two-year mouse study showed that a substantial number of males fed high doses (10 to 20 percent levels) of xylitol developed urinary bladder stones late in life. Of these animals, some developed inflamed bladders and bladder tumors. In a two-year rat study, with animals fed at similar levels of xylitol, no bladder stones or tumors developed. However, some male rats, fed at the 20 percent level, developed growths on their adrenal glands. In some cases, malignant tumors developed in the adrenal glands.

The FDA announced a review of the British findings, but took no action to revoke xylitol's food uses. Some responsible manufacturers, including Wrigley, voluntarily withdrew xylitol from their American products. Other companies continued to promote it.

The reality should have sobered health professionals, had they pondered the implications of the study. An anticavity substance would be carried mainly in a medium that should be used sparingly, if at all. Instead, with a new image of chewing gum as a prophylactic delivery system, it would appear virtuous to chew gum frequently. The emphasis was wrongly placed. Instead of seeking ways to make highly processed foods and beverages more acceptable, funding and efforts should have been directed to encourage people to eat basic foods, dense in nutrients, with no added sweeteners. Such foods are not only life-sustaining, but they are noncariogenic.

In hindsight, clearly the promotion of xylitol in the late 1970s preceded its safety evaluations that followed. Finnsugar Xyrofin, the world's largest manufacturer of commercial xylitol, voluntarily limited its marketing activities in the United States, pending results of safety tests.

In 1986, the FDA commissioned FASEB to review all relevant data regarding xylitol. The following year, Finnsugar Xyrofin submitted studies to the FDA to clarify questions raised by FASEB.

Among the studies evaluated, one was a sixty-three-week rat feeding study with xylitol. Adrenal medullary tumors had been observed in the animals. These effects also had been noted with sorbitol combined with xylitol in animal feeding studies. The petition contended that the increased incidence of adrenal medullary tumors in rats fed xylitol "is attributed to a biological mechanism not operative in humans and thus does not provide a meaningful basis for evaluating the safety in humans" as reported in *Food Chemical News* (Oct 26, 1987). The petition continued:

> The results demonstrate the xylitol-induced hyperabsorption of calcium is causally related to the observed proliferative changes in [the] adrenal medulla. Because xylitol does not enhance calcium absorption in humans, and pheochromocytomas are not reported to occur more frequently in hypercalciuric and hypercalcemic individuals than in the normal population, the increased incidence of adrenomedullary tumors in rats ingesting high dietary doses of xylitol, other polyols, and lactose does not, therefore, provide a meaningful basis for extrapolation regarding human safety.

FASEB claimed that no mechanistic explanation existed for the occurrence of adrenal lesions in rats fed polyols, and the findings left certain questions unanswered.

Another finding was from a two-year feeding trial, also with rodents. Male mice given up to 20 percent xylitol in their diet developed more crystalline calculi in their bladders than did mice fed up to 20 percent sucrose in their diet.

IS XYLITOL OR SORBITOL AN INDIRECT LINK WITH CATARACTS?

The possibility that xylitol or sorbitol might influence cataract formation was discussed by an ad hoc study group of FASEB, requested by the FDA. The consensus was that exogenous xylitol and sorbitol have *no specific* or *direct* influence on cataract formation. (Exogenous xylitol and sorbitol would be from sources such as food, taken into the body rather than ones produced within the body.) This view is supported by the fact that the intact eye lens is nearly impermeable to xylitol and sorbitol. *Indirectly,* however, a possibility exists. Glucose, resulting from the metabolism of xylitol and sorbitol in the liver, could contribute to hyperglycemia in a poorly controlled diabetic. In this case, there is an elevated glucose level in the aqueous humor and lens of the eye, which may result in a conversion of the glucose (via the enzymes aldose reductase and reduced nicotinamide adenine dinucleotide phosphate) to sorbitol in the lens. These events are considered to be a major factor in cataract development in diabetics.

Additional Health Concerns

The European Commission's SCF designated xylitol as "acceptable" for special dietary uses. FAO/WHO's JECFA recommended a specification for lead contamination of xylitol, and assigned a "not specific" ADI for xylitol as a sweetener.

As early as 1971, the FDA had proposed to revoke xylitol's status as a regulated food additive. The agency had been concerned about problems that had been noted with xylitol's use in intravenous feeding solutions given to humans. Some individuals had suffered kidney failure. In a few instances, with quite high dosage levels, adverse effects such as kidney, liver, and brain

HOW XYLITOL IS METABOLIZED

Xylitol is not metabolized via the main metabolic process for sugar breakdown (glycolysis) but by an alternate process known as the pentose shunt pathway. When high amounts of xylitol are administered, transketolase, an enzyme in the pentose shunt pathway, becomes overloaded. Excessive xylitol may interfere with ribose, an essential RNA building block. Increased RNA breakdown, and especially breakdown of its component, purines, has been confirmed. Also, another breakdown product, uric acid, is found at elevated levels in human and animal blood after xylitol ingestion. Both breakdown products, purines and uric acid, are associated with gout.

disturbances were observed. In Australia, some deaths were reported in patients who had received xylitol intravenously,

The FDA proposal remained in limbo for two decades. Ultimately, in January 1993, the FDA decided to withdraw its proposed revocation of xylitol's status as a regulated food additive. By that time, the agency regarded the original data to be outdated, and no longer valid for a final decision. Xylitol would remain as a regulated food additive for special dietary foods. Xylitol has never achieved GRAS status.

REINTRODUCTION OF XYLITOL

Following the fiasco in 1977, use of xylitol in the United States abated. After a long hiatus, several factors combined to reintroduce xylitol. The sweetener had cleared safety hurdles with FASEB, JECFA, and the EEC. The FDA had established xylitol's legal status. The sweetener was being used in many other countries. Newer processing techniques made xylitol's production more cost competitive with other sweeteners. Some consumers were suspicious of synthetic sweeteners, and kept seeking the Holy Grail for sweeteners from "natural" sources.

Finnsugar Xyrofin decided that the time was propitious to reintroduce products in the United States that conformed to the limitation of products permitted under the regulation, such as xylitol-containing chewing gums, chewable tablets, and confectionery products for special dietary use. Concurrently, the benefits of xylitol to consumers were being extolled. Dental schools participated in research. Results of their findings with xylitol were publicized to convince consumers that xylitol was highly beneficial for dental health. Several American dental associations endorsed xylitol.

One highly publicized study was conducted for two years at the Vivieska Health Center in Finland. Children aged eleven years and twelve years, who had consumed 7 to 10 grams of xylitol daily in chewing gum, had 30 to 60 percent reduction in new dental caries, compared with the control group of children who did not chew gum. The study was continued for a third year with a group of children who were considered to be at high risk for caries development. In this group, those who chewed xylitol-sweetened chewing gum developed 50 to 80 percent fewer new caries than the control group of children who did not chew gum.

In evaluating this study, it is necessary to pose a question: how much of the benefit can be attributed to xylitol? Other factors need to be considered. Throughout the study, all participating children maintained an existing caries prevention program, based on fluoridated water and fluoride-containing toothpaste. How much of the benefit was achieved by fluoride and by a diet comprised of low-cariogenic foods and beverages?

A forty-month cohort study with fourth grade students in Belize used xylitol-containing chewing gum. Nine treatment groups consisted of a control group (no chewing gum); four groups consuming xylitol-containing chewing gum (at a range of 4.3 grams to 9 grams daily); two groups consuming xylitol/sorbitol chewing gum (total polyol consumption at a range of 8 grams to 9.7 grams daily); one group consuming sorbitol-containing chewing gum (9 grams daily); and one group consuming sucrose-containing chewing gum (9 grams daily). Compared to the no-gum control group, those using sucrose-containing gum showed a marginal increase in the rate of caries development (relative risk 1.20). The group chewing the sorbitol-containing gum showed a reduced rate of caries development (relative risk 0.74). The four groups consuming various amounts of xylitol-containing gum were the most effective in reducing the rate of caries development (relative risk from 0 .48 to 0.27). The most effective gum was the one containing 100 percent xylitol as a sweetener (relative risk 0.27). The chewing gum consisting of sorbitol combined with xylitol for sweetening was less effective than with xylitol as the exclusive sweetener, but still reduced the rate of caries development significantly, compared with the groups using no-chewing gum or sorbitol chewing gum.

Other recent dental studies with xylitol have been conducted. One study, with more than 2,600 children in San José, Costa Rica, suggested that xylitol added to a fluoride-containing toothpaste acts synergistically and increases the efficacy of dentifrice to prevent caries formation.

Additional studies, conducted at university dental schools in Michigan and Indiana examined the effects on dental plaque from the use of xylitol combined with sorbitol in chewing gums and mints. Use of the products showed significant decreases in plaque accumulation.

Factors that implicate tooth decay include susceptible teeth, the presence of cariogenic mouth bacteria, and fermentable carbohydrates in the diet. If all three factors are present simultaneously, the cariogenic bacteria break down the fermentable carbohydrates and produce acid, which attacks susceptible tooth enamel. One may not be able to avoid the problem of susceptible teeth, but the mouth bacteria and fermentable carbohydrates in the diet are within control. By selecting nutritious food and severely limiting—or even better, avoiding—fermentable carbohydrates such as sugars, most tooth decay is controllable.

Xylitol Intolerance

During the Turku studies, some Finnish students who chewed xylitol-sweetened chewing gum and also ate large amounts of xylitol in prepared foods, suffered from diarrhea. This side effect was noted, too, in 1977 by a researcher at the National Institute for Dental Research, of the National Institutes of

Health, who reported that in some persons even *moderate* xylitol doses have a cathartic effect. A single diarrheal dose is usually from 30 to 40 grams. However, wide individual differences exist in xylitol intolerance, and its sustained use may lead to adaptation so that higher doses may be tolerated.

Diarrheal effects were reported in animal studies, too. In 1979, rats fed xylitol at high levels developed severe diarrhea and gas. This study, conducted by Dr. Marleen Wekell, a nutritional science professor at the University of Washington in Seattle, demonstrated how a substance such as xylitol can adversely alter the bacterial composition of an animal's intestinal tract. Symptoms of diarrhea and gas were attributed to the prolific growth of *Clostridium perfringens*, a disease-causing bacterium normally found only at very low levels in healthy rats. *C. perfringens* causes similar intestinal distress in humans, and is one of the bacterial species implicated in metabolizing harmless substances into carcinogenic ones. Because the formation of some carcinogens may depend on the gut's bacterial environment, this finding underscores the critical role of diet in health. The role of sugars needs to be examined within this framework.

GLOBAL XYLITOL CONSUMPTION

By 1998, the annual global consumption of xylitol was estimated at 480,000 tons. This translates to 960 million pounds. Its greatest use was in chewing gums. The figures were gathered by Global Industry Analysts in Freemont, California, a publisher of business research. The information was included in its comprehensive report, *Polyols: A Global Strategic Business Report*, released August 1998.

Despite the legal status of xylitol's restricted use as a food additive for dietetic foods, it is being used by the general public. It is available in individual packets as well as in bulk packaging—intended for everyone. The pattern recalls the consumption of cyclamates and saccharin: restricted to dietetic use, but flaunting the regulation, expanded to general use. (To learn about these sweeteners, see Chapters 11 and 12.)

Health Claims

Xylitol is considered to be acceptable for use by non-insulin dependent diabetics. Xylitol is metabolized largely independently of insulin. However, xylitol's caloric value must still be considered in the diet.

A newly discovered use for xylitol-containing chewing gum has been found as a relief for otitis media (OM) in children. This infection in the middle ear is a prevalent disorder and reported to be an increasing problem in the United States, Canada, England, Australia, and elsewhere. Xylitol has been found capable of inhibiting the growth of *Streptococcus pneumoniae*, a major causative factor in OM. However, xylitol-containing chewing gum only treats the symptoms, but does not address the basic cause. Commonly, the condition is treated with antibiotics and, if persistently recurring, with tubes inserted in the eardrums. The tubes may result in a permanent hearing loss from 3 to 5 percent. If the tubes are inserted two or more times, the permanent hearing loss increases an additional 3 to 5 percent with each insertion. Some dentists claim that many OM cases are caused by an overclosed bite in the oral cavity, and results in a failure of the eustachian tubes to open properly. In turn, fluid drainage from the middle ear is obstructed, and puts extreme pressure on the eardrum. The chewing of gum may bring some temporary relief, but dental intervention is more effective. According to dentists, there is a need to build up the lower primary molars in order to open overclosed bites. Dentists who have used this procedure report a 90 to 98 percent success rate, without use of eardrum tubes or antibiotics, and without inflicting trauma or hearing loss.

Other claims made for the benefits of xylitol chewing gum are impressive, if true. Among the claims are the following:

- Xylitol does not give rise to acid. It is not fermentable by bacterial commonly found in the mouth. Xylitol actually helps to remove acid from the mouth. If xylitol-sweetened chewing gum is used after sucrose has been consumed, the pH is raised to a safe level. Saliva flow is stimulated. This development helps to rinse away excess sugar residues and neutralize acids that have been formed. The natural remineralization mechanism of saliva is enhanced.

- In the presence of low concentrations of fluoride, damaged tooth enamel is repaired by the improved saliva and reduced plaque formation. The resulting enamel is mineralized optimally and is more resistant to acids than the originally intact enamel. Hence, xylitol-containing products assist the mechanism by which the body repairs damage to teeth from acid attack.

- Xylitol is effective in increasing salivary flow to aid in the repair of damaged tooth enamel. Xylitol can remineralize demineralized teeth. Xylitol is effective in bestowing a low decay rate, and the effect lasts in the mouth even years after xylitol use is discontinued.

- Dental plaque, grown in the presence of xylitol, is less adhesive and less sticky than other plaque, and may be removed more easily by brushing and by the natural defense mechanisms in the mouth. (Note that this claim is a qualified one. The dental plaque is not rendered *totally* nonadhesive, nor *totally* nonsticky by xylitol, but *relatively less adhesive and sticky.*)

- Xylitol may reduce nasal, sinus, and oropharyngeal infections. Also, it is effective against *Helicobacter pylori,* a microorganism implicated in periodontal disease and bad breath as well as gastric and duodenal ulcers, and stomach cancer.

- Xylitol may relieve dry mouth.

- Among the non-dental benefits claimed for xylitol is that it helps the reversal of bone loss in osteoporosis.

Currently, xylitol is being used in chewing gums and confections such as gumdrops and hard candies. It is used also in pharmaceuticals and toiletries, such as throat lozenges, cough syrups, children's chewable multivitamin tablets, toothpastes and mouthwashes. It is used in infusions for parenteral nutrition, as well as in dietetic foods. There are a number of producers of xylitol. The American Xyrofin in Schamburg, Illinois provides xylitol for chewing gums such as Breath Assure, Trident, and Advantage. Acology in Cape Coral, Florida, provides xylitol flavorings and flavor enhancers in Flavor-Sweet. Xlear in Orem, Utah provides Perfect Sweet, Miracle Sweet, Healthy Sweet, and makes available single-serve packets consisting of 100 percent xylitol. RBV Leaf in Holland produces XyliFresh chewing gum.

LACTITOL

Lactitol was identified as early as 1920. However, use of this polyol in foods was begun only in the early 1980s. Lactitol is manufactured by reducing the glucose portion of the disaccharide lactose (milk sugar) by hydrogenating it under high pressure. Unlike the metabolism of lactose, lactitol is not hydrolyzed by the enzyme, lactase. Lactitol is neither hydrolyzed, nor absorbed in the small intestine. Rather, it is metabolized by bacteria in the large intestine, where it is converted into biomass, organic acids, carbon dioxide, and a small amount of hydrogen. As one would expect, the end result can be intestinal distress. Products that contain lactitol must carry a warning label that "excess consumption may have a laxative effect."

In the large intestine, the organic acids from the metabolized lactitol are metabolized further. Lactitol is only about 30 to 40 percent as sweet as sucrose. Although the EU had provided a nutrition labeling directive assigning a caloric value of 2.4 calories per gram to *all* sugar polyols, both Canada and the United States made further refinements. Canada has assigned a figure of 2.6 calories per gram to lactitol; and the United States, 2 calories per gram. At this level, food manufacturers can make a "non-caloric" claim for lactitol-sweetened products. The FDA allows a non-caloric claim for a polyol if its caloric value is below the threshold that the agency established to regard a sweetener as being caloric.

Weighing the Evidence of Safety

The safety of lactitol was reviewed. In 1983, C. W. Chemie Combinatie Amsterdam petitioned the FDA for lactitol use, but the agency took no action. Nearly a decade later, the Dutch company withdrew its petition in the summer of 1992. At the time, the FDA's CFSAN had questioned lactitol's safety. Data showed a significant increased incidence of Leydig cell tumors in male Wistar-type rats fed diets containing 10 percent lactitol as well as 10 or 20 percent lactose during their lifetime. Leydig cells are in the testes and considered to be the main source of testicular androgens and possibly other hormones.

The FDA withheld GRAS status for lactitol until CFSAN could complete a review and make a determination. Two scientists defended lactitol's safety.

Dr. Ernest E. McConnell, a toxicologist and pathology consultant from Raleigh, North Carolina, reviewed the submitted data and concluded that neither lactitol nor lactose, nor their constituent sugars or metabolites are directly responsible for elevation of the Leydig cell tumor incidence. McConnell suggested that the significantly depressed weight gain that the experimental animals experienced was due to the high levels of lactose used in the animals' diet. McConnell thought that the levels were sufficient to upset the normal homeostasis of the animals and resulted in non-physiologic effects.

Another defender was Dr. Charles C. Capen, professor and chairperson at the Department of Veterinarian Pathobiology at Ohio State University, who also reviewed the data. Capen concluded that the weight of the evidence supported the conclusion that development of benign testicular tumors derived from Leydig cells in male rats fed high lactitol levels did not indicate a carcinogenic response. Nor is lactitol genotoxic, according to Capen, as reflected by a standard battery of in vitro (test tube) assays. Capen claimed that interstitial cell adenomas are common benign spontaneous tumors found in many strains of male rats, which suggests a genetic susceptibility. Capen noted that by comparison, this type of tumor is extremely rare in the testes of men, and there is no epidemiologic evidence to suggest that the incidence is increased by the consumption of lactose, lactitol, or any other dietary constituent. Capen reported that no malignant tumors developed in mice of either gender following the chronic feeding of lactitol. In his judgment, the tumors developed through chronic stimulation of a uniquely sensitive endocrine cell population in rats by hormonal imbalances that resulted from an increased intestinal absorption of calcium.

In addition to the issues raised in the FDA's review, the safety of lactitol, based on animal and human studies, was reviewed by several international agencies, including JECFA in 1983, and EEC in 1984. The JECFA approved lactitol, with a recommended ADI as "not specified," signifying that no limits were placed on its use. ("Not specified" is the safest category for a food ingredient in JECFA's categorization.) Many countries that lack agencies to review food additive safety adopt JECFA's decisions.

Lactitol has been approved for use in food products in a number of European countries within the EU, as well as in Switzerland, Canada, Australia, Israel, and Japan. In the United States, a self-affirmation petition for GRAS status was accepted for filing in September 1993 by the FDA for lactitol's use in chewing gums, hard and soft candies, and frozen dairy desserts. More recently, Purac Biochem submitted a self-affirmation GRAS petition for lactitol, which was accepted for filing by the FDA. A self-affirmation GRAS petition, if accepted by the FDA, allows a manufacturer to produce and sell a newly introduced substance intended for use in food manufacture as specified in the petition. This procedure allows manufacturers to decide that the substance is safe for its intended use(s). The manufacturer is expected to offer proof of safety, if challenged.

The self-affirmation petition was devised by the FDA in recent years. It is intended to speed up the lengthy and costly procedure previously required for a manufacturer to petition the FDA for GRAS status. However, the new procedure relaxes regulations. Many self-affirmed petitions go unchallenged, yet proof of safety may be of doubtful worth.

Features and Uses

Lactitol is used as a bulk sweetener combined with other sweeteners, in a wide variety of calorie-reduced, low-fat and/or sugar-free foods, including chocolates, baked goods, sugar-reduced preserves, and sugar substitutes.

Food processors report that lactitol, as a white crystalline powder, gives a sweet clean taste that resembles sucrose. Lactitol is one of the least hygroscopic polyols, and it helps maintain the crispness in products such as cookies and chewing gums. Also, it extends their shelf life. Unlike some synthetic sweeteners, lactitol remains stable in food products that are cooked. Lactitol's cooling effect is rather mild, and far less pronounced than sorbitol or xylitol. Lactitol is compatible with low-caloric sweeteners commonly used in low-calorie and sugar-free foods.

Like other polyols, lactitol is promoted as a suitable sweetener for diabetics. Lactitol does not induce an increase in blood glucose or insulin levels. Hence, foods containing lactitol to replace sugar are regarded as helpful for diabetics to control their blood glucose, lipids, and weight. All three features are important in diabetes management.

Like some other polyols, lactitol is promoted as a substance that does not promote tooth decay. Lactitol is not metabolized by oral bacteria that break down sugars and starches to release acids that can erode tooth enamel and lead to caries formation.

The demand for low-calorie food products is rising. According to the CCC, in its brochure on lactitol, originally printed in 1994, and revised in 2003, "With the relatively new introduction of lactitol, many innovative products are on the horizon." We can anticipate expanded use and consumption of lactitol-containing products.

MALTITOL

Maltitol is a crystalline polyhydric polyol obtained by the hydrogenation of maltose, a disaccharide consisting of two glucose units linked by a bond. It is possible to produce maltitol powders with different contents and product compositions by using different processes, such as crystallization and solidification. Both Mitsubishi in Japan and Roquette America, Inc., manufacture maltitol from starch.

Hurdles Before Approval

In 1987, the Japanese company Towa Chemical Industry Co., Ltd., attempted to defend its self-affirmation petition for GRAS status of its maltitol product that contained not less than 89.5 percent maltitol. The remainder consisted of sorbitol, maltotrititol, and hydrogenated oligosaccharides.

Dr. F. Pellerin, from France, objected. In his opinion, the FDA should require a higher minimum percentage of maltitol. Towa rejected Pellerin's objection, and contended that the regulation that it sought would establish the definition and the usual name for the product, maltitol, used as a food ingredient. Towa noted that no food additive or GRAS substance is required to be, nor can any be, 100 percent "pure" in the sense that it contains only those molecules by which the additive or GRAS substance is named. Towa cited sorbitol as an example. The GRAS affirmation for sorbitol refers to specifications of the Food Chemicals Codex, which requires not less than 91 percent sorbitol, and allows for the inclusion of small amounts of mannitol and other polyols. Towa reported that the FDA has established that a product can be called "sorbitol" even if only 90.1 percent of the molecules in the product are pure sorbitol molecules. Towa charged that Pellerin had provided no data to support any claim that the Towa product was unsuitable nor had it provided any data whatsoever. Pellerin's objection was part of the process the FDA has established whereby any individual or organization can file comments for the agency to consider during its deliberations before arriving at a final decision on a submitted petition.

The petition for GRAS status for maltitol remained in limbo. Six years later, in 1993, the FDA's CFSAN placed Towa's petition in "reject status." According to the agency, this status signifies that "the data and information currently available in the petition are not sufficient to permit the agency to affirm the petitioned substance as GRAS." The FDA raised concerns about deficiencies in the submitted studies to support the petition, especially a lack of "published key studies." After additional studies had been submitted, the FDA advised Towa that the petition was shifted to "review status."

Later, in 1993, the FDA expressed "increasing concern" about the safety of *all* polyols. The CFSAN formed a sugar alcohols' work group to "evaluate systematically all of the available data on each of the sugar alcohols." Maltitol was one of the polyols singled out, because one of its major metabolites was sorbitol. Carl B. Johnson, a member of the sugar alcohols' work group, noted that:

> "... in light of the continuing concern that sorbitol and maltitol could be associated with increased incidence of pheochromocytomas (tumors of chromatin tissues of the adrenal medulla or sympathetic paragonpha, with notable symptoms of hypertension as reflected in increased secretion of epinephrin and norepinephrin) in laboratory animals, we recommend the submission of quality published long-term feeding studies ..." Johnson added, "depending on the outcome of our review of available data, we reserve the right to request additional safety data if, in our judgment, it is required to support the safety of ... maltitol."

These findings were worrisome because increased incidence of pheochromocytoma in rats also had been found with mannitol use.

In 1994, results of a long-term maltitol toxicity study in rats were sufficient to detain approval of the self-affirmed GRAS petition submitted by Towa for maltitol.

The FDA had submitted the study to the FAO/WHO's JECFA for review. The group found that benign and malignant pheochromocytomas were present in male and female rats in the group fed high maltitol levels, and an increased frequency of slight to moderate adrenal medullary hyperplasia was found in all groups fed maltitol. Also, there was a slight increase in the incidence of mammary gland adeno-carcinomas in female rats with two different dose levels of maltitol. The significance of this finding was unclear, and possibly was unrelated to maltitol. However, the moderate adrenal medullary hyperplasia recalled similar findings with mannitol.

The FDA considered that the effects observed in long-term toxicity/carcinogenicity tests to be of serious concern, and that "the interpretation of these data is of major importance to the safety evaluation of maltitol." Because of the "data deficiency," once more the FDA rejected Towa's petition, and reported that in its present form GRAS status would not be granted unless amended to provide the requested data and that "these data are judged adequate to support safe uses." The protracted procedure to obtain GRAS status for maltitol continued to remain in "review status."

JECFA reviewed the safety data and concluded that maltitol is safe. The committee established an ADI as "not specified" signifying that no limits were placed on its use. In addition, the European Commission's SCF concluded that maltitol was acceptable for use. Like JECFA, it did not establish any limitation for maltitol's use.

In 1999, the FDA accepted for filing a petition for self-affirmation of GRAS status for maltitol. The petition described maltitol's numerous benefits for processors, as a flavoring agent, formulation aid, humectant, nutritive sweetener, processing aid, sequestrant (chelating agent), stabilizer, thickener, surface-finishing agent, and texturizer. The petition specified maltitol's uses at levels up to 99.5 percent in hard candies and cough drops; 99 percent in sugar substitutes; 85 percent in soft candies; 75 percent in chewing gums; 55 percent in non-standardized jams and jellies; and 30 percent in cookies and sponge cakes. Obviously, there had been an escalation of maltitol uses in processed foods and other consumer items such as chewing gums and pharmaceuticals.

Caveats to Health Claims

As with other polyols, maltitol can have a laxative effect when it is consumed at high levels. A warning statement on labels of products, similar to the one for other polyols, was recommended in the GRAS petition for foreseeable consumption of maltitol of more than 100 grams per day. Maltitol is promoted as a sweetener that is noncariogenic. It resists metabolism by oral bacteria that break down sugars and starches to release acids that can lead to tooth enamel erosion and cavity formation. The American Dental Association (ADA) officially acknowledged the usefulness of maltitol (as well as other polyols) as a sugar alternative as part of a comprehensive program that includes proper dental hygiene. The FDA approved the use of a phrase for a health claim on labels "does not promote tooth decay" for sugar-free foods sweetened with maltitol.

Maltitol is promoted as a sweetener that may be useful for diabetics because it does not raise blood glucose or insulin levels. In recent years, this feature has been somewhat toned down, with provisos and qualifiers. For example, the CCC noted in its brochure on maltitol in 2005:

Recognizing that diabetes is complex and requirements for its management may vary between individuals, the usefulness of maltitol should be discussed between individuals and their health care providers. Foods sweetened with maltitol may contain other ingredients that also contribute calories and other nutrients. Those must be considered in meal planning.

A Niche Sweetener Favored by Processors

Processors find that maltitol has many attractive attributes that allow its use in a diverse range of food applications. Its taste is similar to sucrose, with about 90 percent the sweetness of sucrose, but with only 2.1 calories per gram, compared to 4 calories per gram of sucrose. Maltitol is quite nonhygroscopic, and it is heat stable. It has only a slight cooling effect. It does not brown foods. It can be used to replace sugar in some baked goods, and can replace fat because it provides a "creamy" texture to foods such as brownies, cakes, and cookies. Maltitol's crystalline form, low hygroscopicity, high melting point, and stability make it particularly useful with high-quality chocolate coatings, confectionery, bakery chocolate, and ice creams. Before the development of maltitol, the production of sugar-free or no-sugar added chocolate proved difficult to achieve, due to the lack of a polyol with the physical, chemical, and sweet-tasting characteristics desired for such products.

Maltitol was found to be suitable for granola bars, jams with no added sugars, pie fillings, salad dressings, and spreads. Although maltitol is compatible with other sweeteners, the addition of other low-calorie sweeteners is not needed if maltitol is used, because of its sweetness.

Towa Chemical Industry Co., Ltd., continues to market maltitol.

Along with other polyols, the use of maltitol continues to escalate. As noted by the CCC in 2005 in its brochure, "with the increasing demand for products reduced in calories and fats, maltitol's use is expected to increase."

ISOMALT

Isomalt, a polyol, is derived from isomaltulose, also known as palatinose. It is a disaccharide found in small amounts in honey and sugarcane extract. Commercial isomalt, however, is made from sucrose.

Isomalt was discovered by chance in the late 1950s by a sugar processor in Mannheim, Germany. The company found that a microorganism, commonly found in its sugar beet refineries, was capable of rearranging the structure of sugar molecules and could give the molecules different properties. By using sucrose, commercial isomalt could be manufactured by using an enzyme (glycosyltransferase) from bacteria in a two-step process. After hydrolysis, the resulting isomalt is a mixture of two isomeric disaccharide polymers. It consists of 25 percent sorbitol, 25 percent mannitol, and the remaining 50 percent consists of glucose. After research and development, the company produced an odorless, white crystalline sweetener and bulking agent. The commercial isomalt is known as Palatinit and it is available to processors from Palatinit of America, Inc., in Morris Plains, New Jersey. This company is a subsidiary of Südzucker Group, Europe's largest sugar producer.

Cooperatively, the two groups worked to develop a family of isomalt sweeteners from isomaltulose for use in numerous sugar-free products. Different isomalt versions meet specific requirements. Isomalt ST is used in hard candies and chewy candies. Being low in hygroscopicity, this sweetener does not cause the candies to become sticky or to require that they be wrapped individually. Also, this sweetener is used for certain types of baked good that do not require browning. It offers bakers an alternative to bulk sweeteners used in sugar-free products. Isomalt helps foods retain their crispness because of its low-water absorptiveness.

Isomalt LM is used especially for chocolate manufacture. It serves as a sugar replacer in many cocoa-based products such as chocolate coatings, chips, and fillings. This sweetener does not produce the mouth-cooling effect common with many polyols.

Isomalt DC is used for tablet manufacture by pharmaceutical companies, as well as for nutritional supplements. This sweetener dissolves readily in the mouth when tablets are chewed.

Isomalt GS is used for coating chewing gums. This sweetener intensifies other flavors, and retains flavors longer as the gums are chewed.

Few Safety Concerns

Safety tests showed that isomalt, at dietary levels up to 10 percent, displayed no toxicologic effects on the development or reproduction of test animals, even in generational studies.

The FAO/WHO's JECFA reviewed available research on isomalt and concluded that it was safe. JECFA set an acceptable daily intake (ADI) for isomalt as "not specified"—JECFA's safest category. This designation allowed for unrestricted use of isomalt.

The European Commission's SCF in its 1985 assessment of sweetening agents, found isomalt acceptable for use without establishing an ADI.

In 1990, EEC's committee of toxicological experts drawn from its member countries, allowed isomalt use in all food applications and in some beverage applications, too.

At the recommendation of the Food and Contaminants Committee, isomalt has been used in the United Kingdom since 1983. Since the early 1980s, isomalt has been approved for marketing in other European countries, including

Germany and Switzerland. Globally, isomalt is used in more than twenty countries.

In 1990, the FDA accepted for filing a petition for self-affirmation of isomalt as GRAS. Subsequently, isomalt has been used in the United States.

In 2005, there was interest in expanding isomalt uses. Palatinit of America, Inc., filed a novel (that is, new) food application for palatinose in Germany for approval in the EU.

Like all polyols, isomalt has low absorption and can cause a laxative effect if it is consumed at a high level. As much as 40 percent of isomalt is digested in the small intestine. The remainder, including the nonabsorbed mannitol and sorbitol components, is fermented by intestinal microflora in the colon, which produces methane and hydrogen gases. Consumed at high levels, isomalt will produce gas, bloating, cramps, and diarrhea. The manufacturer of Palatinit advised food and beverage processors who use this sweetener in their products to inform consumers of the possible laxative effect, by printing an advisory on labels.

It has been found that isomalt, consumed up to 35 grams at one time, or up to a total of 60 grams over a day, appear to be tolerated. An average piece of isomalt-containing hard candy has about 3 grams of isomalt. Thus, an individual would need to consume more than a dozen hard candies to induce a laxative effect. Oddly, children appear to be less sensitive to the laxative effect of isomalt than adults. This finding is unlike the findings with sorbitol and mannitol.

Appealing to Consumers

Isomalt, consumed at low level, is promoted as being beneficial to the gut. Isomalt has been found to be a prebiotic that promotes an increase of beneficial bifidobacteria in the large intestine. Isomalt's water-binding characteristic may influence the structure of the gut's content. If the consistency of the feces is too soft, isomalt can cut down the food intake into the gut and allow time for adaptation. Similar to dietary fiber, isomalt is broken down by gut bacteria to short-chain fatty acids (SCFAs) and gases. SCFAs decrease acidity in the large intestine. Some SCFAs may benefit epithelium health in the large intestine.

Isomalt is promoted as having general benefits to consumers. Because of its low glycemic response, isomalt is less likely to result in any sharp increases in blood sugar or insulin levels as sucrose does. (To learn about the glycemic index, see Chapter 20.) Hence, isomalt is viewed favorably for diabetic use. Also, because isomalt has fewer calories than sucrose, it is used in calorie-reduced foods.

Isomalt is promoted for dental health. Like other polyols, claims are made that isomalt is a sweetener that is "toothfriendly" and does not promote tooth decay. Claims go still further. Isomalt, like xylitol, is reported to help repair early dental cavity lesions by remineralization. Such promotion is used in sales pitches, but scientific researchers are more cautious. They are more likely to describe isomalt and other polyols as having low cariogenicity (ability to damage the teeth) rather than noncariogenicity. Also, they are more apt to say that bacteria present in the mouth do not *readily* convert into decay-causing acids in the presence of isomalt. Researchers caution, too, that long-range studies have not been conducted,

A series of in vitro tests (test tubes) and in vivo tests (live animals) with four palatinose (isomalt) compounds A, B, C, and D showed them to have low cariogenicity. In mouthrinsing studies, palatinose compounds A, C, and D caused only minor pH changes of the dental plaque, compared to sucrose. In vitro studies showed that palatinose compound D, when used in combination with sucrose or glucose, had no ability to inhibit the acid formation produced from these two recognized cariogenic sugars. Acid production resulting from palatinose compound D was very low, compared to the acid production from sucrose or glucose. However, acid production from palatinose compound B was of the same order of magnitude as that from sucrose or glucose, and palatinose compound B showed no ability to inhibit the acid production from these two sugars.

In animal studies, rats fed a diet containing palatinose compound C induced caries in the sulcus (the space between the teeth and gums). Although the damage was low compared to rats on a sucrose diet, researchers cautioned about a possibility that the oral flora might acquire an increased ability to ferment palatinose.

In one modest study with humans, fourteen male volunteers were given between-meal snacks for four weeks. One snack was sweetened exclusively with isomalt; another, exclusively with sucrose. The third snack was sweetened with 70 percent isomalt and 30 percent sucrose; and the fourth snack, with 50 percent isomalt and 50 percent sucrose. The group eating snacks sweetened exclusively with isomalt displayed the lowest amount of plaque deposit on teeth of any group. However, the researchers noted that the long-term effects of isomaltulose on oral microflora have yet to be considered.

Since 1996, the FDA has allowed manufacturers of sugar-free products sweetened with isomalt to make the health claim "does not promote dental caries," providing the product does not reduce the acidity in the mouth to less than 5.7 pH during its consumption or for up to thirty minutes after its consumption. Acidity is one factor in plaque formation and caries development.

Appealing to Food Processors

Isomalt has characteristics that appeal to food processors both as a sweetener and as a bulking agent. Isomalt has similar properties as sucrose, from which it is derived. However, isomalt has only half as many calories as sucrose (two calories per gram for isomalt; four, for sucrose). Isomalt has about 45 to 65 percent the sweetness of sucrose. Isomalt does not change the taste of food. It gives sugar-free products a similar volume, texture, and appearance as sucrose. Isomalt is synergistic with other sweeteners, and may be used with products, in combination with other sweeteners. By combining sweeteners, processors can use less, and cut costs. The downside of isomalt for processors is that this sweetener does not brown or carmelize in baked goods as does sucrose. Isomalt cannot be used in beer or other yeast-fermented products. Yeast breaks down sucrose readily, which is advantageous, but isomalt remains stable and does not break down. Despite these few limitations, isomalt is versatile.

Isomalt has a wide range of applications with wellness and sports beverages; in breakfast and meal-replacement drinks; as a sweetener in instant tea and coffee products; in nutritional and cereal bars; in toffees, lollipops, fudges, and wafers; and in sugar-free chocolates. Isomalt is used, too, in over-the-counter medications such as cough drops and throat lozenges.

Advertisements for isomalt products targeted to processors in trade journal announce that isomalt is "the sugar that isn't," and "the only sugar replacer derived from real sugar." One isomalt advertisement quotes from the February 1997 issue of *Focus Group Study*, a publication that reports on the findings from focus group sessions: "The fact that the ingredient was a sugar derivative was appealing. If it was natural, they felt that it could not be bad or dangerous."

HYDROGENATED STARCH HYDROLYSATES

Hydrogenated starch hydrolysates (HSHs) are syrups made from hydrogenated glucose, maltitol, mannitol, or sorbitol. They are polysaccharides, produced by the partial hydrolysis of starch from corn, wheat, or potato. Then, the substance is hydrogenated at high temperature and pressure to produce the syrup. HSHs were developed originally in Sweden in the 1960s, and since then they have been used in many countries by food and beverage manufacturers. By varying the manufacturing process, different end products can be created to meet specific needs.

If the HSH contains 50 percent or more of hydrogenated glucose, it is known as hydrogenated glucose syrup, or sorbitol syrup. Some of the end products do not contain a single polyol as a major component, but are mixtures of polyols. For such products, a general term, hydrogenated starch hydrolysates, is used. The term HSH can be applied to any polyol processed into a syrup, but in practice, only sorbitol, mannitol, and maltitol are cited by their common names. Depending on the specific syrup, an HSH product may be from 40 to 90 percent as sweet as sucrose.

Formerly, a value of not more then 3 calories per gram was assigned to HSH products. Later, the EU designated a lower value of 2.4 calories per gram (compared to 4 for sucrose).

Safety Status

Despite the fact that polyols are calorie sweeteners, illogically, the FDA does not regard them as sugars. Processors who use HSH as sweeteners can use label terms such as "reduced-calorie" and "sugarless" on their products, and promote these features in advertisements. However, processors are not allowed to use the phrase "no sugar added" for products containing HSH.

The safety of HSH products and their components was challenged in 1993. Roquette America, Inc., had filed a self-affirmation petition with the FDA seeking GRAS status for one of its products, Lycasin, a hydrogenated glucose or maltitol syrup. The FDA rejected the petition, citing deficiencies in eight out of ten safety tests submitted for approval. The identified deficiencies were: too small a group of animals in tests; only one dosage of Lycasin administered; a lack of gross or microscopic examination of some tissues; and failure to provide raw data to verify the results. In addition, the FDA found flaws in key studies, making it impossible for the agency to assess the safety of long-term exposure to the product. The FDA assigned Roquette's petition to "reject" status.

Ultimately, the safety of HSH products and their components satisfied the FDA, and were granted self-affirmed GRAS status. The products can be used lawfully in the United States for the petitioned uses. HSH products are approved elsewhere, including Canada, Australia, and Japan.

Health Claims

As with all polyols, HSHs are absorbed slowly in the digestive tract. Gradually, a portion of HSH is hydrolyzed enzymatically in the body to sorbitol, maltitol, and glucose. A portion of HSH in a food reaches the lower part of the digestive tract, where it is metabolized by bacteria. This action results in a reduced availability of calories and this is the reason that HSH can be designated as a reduced-calorie sweetener. However, HSH should not be consumed at a high level. It is estimated that from 30 to 60 grams of HSH in a meal can result in a laxative effect.

HSH is promoted for diabetic use. Because HSH absorption is slow and incomplete, the rise in blood glucose and insulin levels associated with glucose is reduced significantly when HSH is used as an alternative to sucrose as a sweetener. The reduced caloric value of HSH meets major goals in diabetic management: blood glucose control and weight control. HSH-containing products are promoted as ones that make possible a wider variety of reduced calorie and sugar-free choices for diabetics. However, diabetics need to be cautioned that HSH-containing products also may contain other ingredients that *do* contribute calories as well as other nutrients that need to be considered in the total diet. Many of these food products are ones that are not nutrient-dense, and should be limited or even avoided.

HSH-containing products are promoted for dental health. Because HSH resists metabolism by oral bacteria, it is considered to be noncariogenic. Therefore, it is used and promoted in many "sugarless" products, including chewing gums and candies.

Functional Roles

HSH syrups (as well as maltitol and sorbitol syrups) serve a number of functional roles in food and beverage manufacture. They are useful as bulk sweeteners and bulking agents. They serve as sugar-free carriers for flavors, colors, and enzymes. They are excellent as humectants that do not crystallize. This feature makes them useful as sugar replacers in a variety of frozen desserts. They can be used to make sugar-free confections, and the same processing systems can be used to produce sugar-containing candies. HSHs blend well with other sweeteners and flavors, and they can mask unpleasant off-flavors such as bitterness.

Recent research showed that more than 100 million Americans consume low-calorie products. More than half of them would like to have additional low-calorie products available. The main interest is for more desserts and sweets, including baked goods, candies, chocolates, and ice creams. HSH products are used in many of these products. It is reasonable to expect a continued expanded use of HSHs to meet the desires for such products.

ERYTHRITOL

Erythritol is a naturally occurring four-carbon polyol found in various plants, including melons, grapes, and pears, as well as in mushrooms, seaweeds, and animals. However, commercially produced erythritol hardly fits the advertising hype as being "part of the human diet for thousands of years." Like other polyols, the erythritol added to foods and beverages, is produced chemically through hydrogenation, and is a processed sweetener. Wheat or cornstarch is hydrolyzed to glucose, and then, by means of yeasts and molds, fermented to a broth from which erythritol is ultrafiltrated and crystallized. The resulting product is a white and odorless powder with a clean taste. Erythritol is about 60 to 80 percent as sweet as sucrose, and it provides 0.2 calories per gram (compared to 4 calories for sucrose), thus making products sweetened with erythritol "non-caloric." However, in advertisements, erythritol is promoted as having "zero calories"—a phrase that stretches the fact.

Erythritol is the newest of the polyols to be manufactured and marketed for use as a sweetener in the United States. It has been described as "a product that represents a very significant advance in the polyol sweetener sector. It provides fewer calories than other polyols (and) does not cause laxation," according to the CCC in *Reduced-Calorie Sweeteners: Erythritol* (2004).

Safety History

Erythritol has been available in Japan since 1990. The Japanese government deemed it safe, and it became a popular sweetener for candies and chocolates. The Mitsubishi Chemical Company developed an exclusive patented process to manufacture erythritol. In 1997, Cargill Food and Pharma Specialties in Wayzata, Minnesota began a joint venture with Mitsubishi to produce this sweetener in Blair, Nebraska. The plant, located at an existing Cargill corn wet-milling complex that produced HFCS and other corn products, served as an appropriate site for an expansion opportunity. Cargill has chosen to name its erythritol product Eridex. An erythritol product, Cerestar, is available from Cerestar USA, Inc. in Hammond, Indiana, as well as Cerestar International Sales, in Brussels, Belgium.

Data were submitted to the FDA for evaluating the safety of erythritol in order to achieve GRAS status. Critics raised questions regarding some physiological responses to erythritol. They claimed that the sweetener, used at high levels, might stress or damage the kidneys. Also, they claimed that the potential amounts of its consumption might have been grossly underestimated.

The petitioners' expert panel reported that it had used intake estimates for erythritol in providing reasonable "worst case" estimates of human consumption, calculated from its intended uses. The expert panel concluded that the toxicological and clinical studies provided a clear and strong basis for concluding that erythritol was safe. No toxicity was observed in the long-term feeding studies, which included an examination of organ systems.

The FDA was satisfied that erythritol was safe for its intended uses, at varying levels, as a flavor enhancer, formulation aid, humectant, nutritive sweetener, stabilizer, thickener, and texturizer. In January 1997, the FDA accepted for filing a self-affirmation GRAS petition submitted by a consortium of erythritol manufacturers: Cerestar Holding BV of Vilvoorda, Belgium; and Mitsubishi Chemical Corporation and Nikken Chemical Company, both from Japan. In addition to the United States and Japan, erythritol has been approved for use in Canada, some European countries, Australia, New Zealand, Korea, Taiwan, Singapore, Russia, Israel, and South Africa.

Advantages Over Other Polyols

Erythritol has versatile qualities that make this sweetener attractive to processors. It can be used for many purposes. It has excellent crystalline properties. It is nonhygroscopic and moderately soluble in water. It is stable at high temperatures and in a wide range of acidity. Manufacturers of erythritol cite certain advantages of this sweetener over other polyols. It has the lowest caloric value of any polyol. Clinical studies showed that erythritol has a digestive tolerance two to three times better than xylitol, lactitol, maltitol, and isomalt; and three to four times better than sorbitol or mannitol, both of which require warning labels about their laxative effects.

Unlike other polyols that are transported into the gut through passive diffusion, what is not absorbed is sent to the lower gut. Erythritol is absorbed rapidly in the small intestine due to its small molecular size and structure. According to clinical studies in Europe and Japan, more than 90 percent of ingested erythritol is absorbed but not metabolized. Some 90 to 95 percent is excreted unchanged in urine within a twenty-four-hour period. This digestive pathway allows less than 5 to 10 percent of ingested erythritol to reach the large intestine and be fermented into volatile fatty acids or to be metabolized into carbon dioxide. Thus, even food products that contain substantial amounts of erythritol are not likely to cause the gaseous and laxative effects as experienced after ingesting high amounts of other polyols.

Used in combination with high-intensity sweeteners such as aspartame, sucralose, or acesulfame-K, erythritol can improve the flavor profile, provide body and mouthfeel, and mask bitterness or astringency. Erythritol has a cooling effect in the mouth, which makes it attractive for use in chewing gums by enhancing a perception of a taste of freshness.

Niche in the Marketplace

Erythritol may be appropriate for diabetics. Single dose and fourteen-day chemical studies showed that erythritol did not affect blood serum glucose or insulin levels. Clinical studies with diabetics suggested that erythritol might be a suitable sucrose replacer in foods formulated specifically for diabetic use. However, diabetics need to consider the dietary impact from other ingredients used in such products.

Products made with erythritol are promoted for weight control because this sweetener is so low in calories. However, the total caloric content of an erythritol-containing product may not necessarily be low in calories due to other ingredients used in the product.

Erythritol it regarded as noncariogenic. Some research suggests that ery-thritol helps reduce the presence of oral bacteria capable of fermenting carbo-hydrates that lead to dental enamel erosion and caries formation. The FDA has approved a health claim for sugar-free foods containing erythritol. "Does not promote tooth decay" may be printed on the labels of such products.

Erythritol has found a niche in the marketplace. It can be found in many applications, including bakery and dairy products, desserts, confections, bev-erages, tabletop sweeteners, candies, chocolates, fondants, fudges, chewing gums, toiletries, and pharmaceuticals. It is reasonable to assume that this newest-to-be-introduced polyol will continue to be used increasingly, even in a very crowded competitive market of sweeteners.

Part Two

HIGH-INTENSITY PLANT-DERIVED SWEETENERS

Chapter 6

LICORICE: A FLAVORANT CONVERTED INTO A SWEETENER

Snack time, dinner time, sweet time, any time! Use Magnasweet anytime and you'll get a boost in flavor every time. Magnasweet natural flavor enhancers bring out the magical essence in a wide variety of foods. You can soften harsh notes, brighten subtle under-tones, or mask artificial tastes . . . it only takes a few parts per million to give your products a powerful but inexpensive flavor boost . . .
— ADVERTISEMENT FOR MAGNASWEET IN *FOOD ENGINEERING* (JUNE 1969)

Licorice is extracted from a woody-rooted shrub, *Glycyrrhiza glabra*. It grows four to five feet high and has feathery leaves and light-blue flowers. It grows wild in the subtropical regions of the Middle East, southern Europe, and west Asian countries. The plant's large branching roots grow down as far as three feet, and grow out laterally as many as twenty feet. The roots contain two major biologically active components, glycyrrhizic acid and glycyrrhetinic acid, as well as numerous other active plant components. The sweetness in natural licorice is extracted from the two major acids.

The plant needs to grow four or five years before the roots are hand-harvested, dried, and sold. Licorice processors boil the roots, extract the sweet principles, and convert them into different forms such as solid dark blocks, semifluids, syrups, and powders.

The powdered root extracts are used for flavoring and flavor enhancement.

Licorice has had a venerable history of use as a flavoring agent. The strong dark-colored sweet flavor of licorice was prized by entire civilizations long before the Christian era. The Chinese who may have been the first to use licorice, called it *gancao* which translates to "sweet grass." In Sanskrit, licorice was termed "sweet stalk." The Greeks named it "sweet root." Licorice use was limited to the role of a flavoring agent, not one as a primary sweetener. Also, because licorice contains active principles, it was used medicinally.

LICORICE'S SURPRISING RANGE OF USES

Say "licorice" and the response may be "candy." Children associate licorice candy with its ability to color saliva. But candy is only one of many applications. According to Mafco Worldwide in Camden, New Jersey, a leading licorice supplier, about 80 percent of its product, Magnasweet is used universally by the tobacco industry. Licorice is used to flavor cigarettes, cigars, pipe and chewing tobaccos, and snuffs. Licorice may comprise as much as 10 percent of the ingredients in some brands of chewing tobaccos. In addition to flavoring the tobaccos, licorice helps keep them moist.

Many pharmaceuticals contain licorice as a flavorant, flavor enhancer, or masking agent for bitter drugs, cough drops, and herbal supplements. Licorice may replace saccharin in low-residue diet preparations, breath sprays, mouthwashes, laxatives, and chewable vitamins.

Food processors discovered that licorice has foaming and emulsifying action in water, and they began to add licorice to cake mixes, ice creams, ices, candies, baked goods, gelatin desserts, meat sauces, seasonings, and fruit and vegetable products. Although licorice foams, it does not ferment.

Licorice is fifty times sweeter than sucrose, and it is synergistic. Combined with sucrose, licorice yields a perceived sweetness one hundred times greater than sucrose by itself. Ammoniated glycyrrhizin, a derivative of glycyrrhizic acid, exerts an even greater synergistic effect.

Food and beverage processors utilize this synergism by using licorice to intensify flavors such as maple, vanilla, anise, root beer, rum, walnut, butterscotch, chocolate, honey, and pickling spice mixes. By adding some powdered or liquid extract of licorice root, they can reduce the amount of costly ingredients. For example, a relatively small amount of licorice greatly intensifies the chocolate characteristic in a product. In some chocolate-containing products, licorice may replace up to 20 percent of costly cocoa. Another money-saving feature of licorice is its ability to mellow a general harshness present in synthetic flavors that are less expensive than natural ones.

Ammoniated glycyrrhizin can be produced by repeated crystallizations, until it is converted into a colorless substance. This significant development attracted the attention of processors who regarded this form as a potential sweetener and sweetener intensifier—new roles—in addition to its traditional uses as flavoring agent and flavoring intensifier. Licorice's potential as a natural sweetener was given consideration in the wake of the cyclamate ban in 1969. At the time, the largest licorice producer enjoyed a twentyfold increase in orders, for applications ranging from salad dressing and toothpaste, to baked goods, cured ham, and bacon. The threatened saccharin ban in 1977 gave further impetus to interest in licorice's sweetening ability.

LICORICE USE IN FOODS AND BEVERAGES

The amounts listed as "average maximum parts per million" (ppm) are not tolerance limits. In actual usage, often these levels are higher.

Item		Approximate average maximum ppm
Licorice Extracts	gelatin desserts	4
	beverages	33
	ice creams, ices	39
	syrups	50
	baked goods	84
	candies	130
	chewing gums	29,000*
Licorice Extract Powders	beverages	110
	ice creams, ices	200
	baked goods	200
	candies	6,500
	chewing gums	22,000*
Licorice Root	baked goods	75
	beverages	130
	candies	460
	chewing gums	3,200*

*The swallowed saliva that results from the chewing of these gums results in a sizable amount of ingested licorice, especially for individuals who chew gum frequently.

—Data from *Chemicals Used in Food Processing*, Pub No 1274, Washington, DC: National Academy of Sciences/National Research Council, 1965.

LICORICE'S EFFECTS ON THE BODY

As part of the entire Generally Recognized as Safe (GRAS) review in the 1970s, the FDA requested the Federation of American Societies for Experimental Biology (FASEB) to evaluate the existing literature on the safety of licorice and its derivatives. FASEB concluded that the compounds were safe when used as food flavorings at the levels being used (1977), and should be affirmed as GRAS, with specific limitations on their use. On August 2, 1977, the FDA issued a proposed rule in the *Federal Register* to affirm the GRAS status for licorice compounds used as flavoring agents, with specific maximal use levels for various food categories. Nothing was mentioned about licorice compounds used as sweeteners and sweetener enhancers. The FDA proposal was based on an assumption that the sole applications for licorice compounds would make their level of use self-limiting once a desired effect was achieved for flavoring purposes.

This was not the case. Increasingly, in addition to the traditional uses of licorice compounds, food and beverage processors used them as sweeteners and sweetener enhancers with sucrose or saccharin. In 1979, for example, possibly as a hedge against future action against saccharin, Alberto-Culver Company test-marketed a saccharin-free product, described as a low-calorie granulated sugar replacer. The label stated that the available carbohydrate was 87.3 percent. The company admitted that this percentage included not only dextrose, which was listed on the label, but also the "natural flavoring." Hidden in this term was ammoniated glycyrrhizin.

The unanticipated expanded use of licorice compounds as sweeteners and sweetening synergists made any self-limiting feature ineffective. The FDA recognized that the food level of use for licorice was outstripping the assumed limitations of the 1977 proposal. In 1979, the FDA proposed an amendment to licorice's GRAS status, and to limit its uses.

The curbing action was prudent. Glycyrrhizic acid, an active principle in licorice, is related both chemically and structurally to adrenal gland hormones (desoxycorticosterone and aldosterone). Glycyrrhizic acid can produce steroidal effects, estrogenic effects, and other biological actions. Aldosterone, produced in the adrenal gland, is the body's chief steroid regulator of electrolytes, and it has a powerful effect on the amount of potassium in the bloodstream. Licorice lowers the amounts of aldosterone and renin (an enzyme produced in the kidneys). The glycyrrhizic acid in licorice prevents the enzyme from converting the steroid hormone cortisol into cortisone. The body regulates these two substances, which act in tandem in a complex biochemical mechanism. Even small changes in the amount of one of these chemicals can alter the other severely. High licorice consumption leads to sodium retention and potassium loss—two features that are involved in high blood pressure.

High licorice consumption can interfere with prescription drugs, by decreasing their efficacy. Cardiac glycosides, such as digitalis, are used for heart conditions. The glycyrrhizic acid in licorice can interfere with the action of such drugs, as well as others such as stimulant laxatives, anticoagulants, steroids, insulin, corticosteroids, and potassium-depleting drugs. The glycyrrhizic acid can increase the activity of certain drugs, such as diuretics and lithium. Such increased potency can be dangerous. The glycyrrhizic acid also potentiates hydrocortisone activity in the skin. Licorice poisoning increases in hypertensive people who are taking drugs to control high blood pressure.

MEDICINAL USES OF LICORICE

Due to the biological activity of some constitutents in licorice, it has been used medicinally in many applications. In the early 1990s, the National Cancer Institute (NCI) launched a designer foods program to examine compounds naturally present in foods that might help prevent disease. Licorice was among them. The NCI funded the consulting firm, Arthur J. Little, Inc., headquartered in Cambridge, Massachusetts, to gather technical data about phytochemical research. Alegua Carugay of Arthur J. Little, reported that licorice contained over 200 phytochemicals, of which twenty-nine were thought to have cancer-preventive properties. They included antioxidants and flavonoids.

Licorice has been used for chronic inflammations of the respiratory tract; as an expectorant and to increase the bronchial secretion and transport of mucus; for liver function and chronic hepatitis B; for allergies; as an antibacterial agent; as an adjunct to avoid sepsis in burn patients; as an antiviral agent to inhibit the growth of herpes simplex; to retard the progression of HIV, and to improve blood parameters in AIDs treatment; and as an antitumor and anticancer agent. Licorice extracts are used for some ulcers, such as peptic, gastric, duodenal, and aphthous. However, licorice use in ulcer therapy has reported side effects including cardiac asthma and swellings in 20 percent of treated patients. For some health conditions, licorice needs to be used in a deglycyrrhizinated form (97 percent of the glycyrrhizic acid is removed).

Glycyrrhizic acid is being investigated for its ability to kill herpes virus. Researcher Ornella Flores and associates at New York University in New York City exposed white blood cells to glycyrrhizic acid. Some of the cells had been infected with Kaposi's sarcoma-associated herpes virus; other of the cells were not infected. The glycyrrhizic acid started a chain reaction in the infected cells and led to self-destruction and death of the herpes virus. The glycyrrhizic acid was selective, and had no detrimental effect on the uninfected cells. The results suggest that development of a drug based on glycyrrhizic acid might be able to search out and destroy latent herpes viruses in people before the viruses cause symptoms. The research was reported in the *Journal of Clinical Investigations,* March 2005.

Compounds in licorice root have been found to exhibit potent antibacterial activity against *Streptococcus mutans,* a common oral pathogen that causes tooth decay. This finding has roused interest in toothpaste companies for its potential use. Four flavonoids already had been isolated from licorice root. More recently, two pterocarpene compounds glycyrrhizol A and B, were isolated by Wenyuan Shi and colleagues at the Univeristy of California in Los Angeles. The researchers found glycyrrhizol A to exhibit the stronger anticariogenic activity (*Journal of Natural Products,* vol. 69, 2006).

High licorice consumption leads to hypokalemia (potassium depletion) with muscle weakness, fatigue, and edema. Skin and serum discoloration have been reported from eating licorice pastilles in large amounts. High licorice consumption may be a factor in sexual dysfunction and decreased libido. A Finnish study in 2001 with more than a thousand women and their infants showed that pregnant women who had consumed high levels of licorice candy were very apt to give birth prematurely, and place their off-spring at unnecessary health risks.

THE HAZARDS OF OVERINDULGENCE

The safety margin established for licorice use may be inadequate for a segment of the population. Limitations are based on *average* usage and fail to include persons with idiosyncratic dietary habits. Licorice "freaks" are not uncommon, and from time to time, case histories are reported in medical journals describing the adverse health effects from high licorice consumption. Some of these reports predate the era of increased licorice use as a sweetener and sweetener enhancer.

One case, reported in 1968, was of a fifty-eight-year-old man who daily, for seven years, had eaten two to three licorice candy bars. He developed high blood pressure and paralysis of his extremities. The syndrome disappeared after licorice was eliminated from his diet.

Another case reported in 1970 concerned a fifty-three-year-old man who had eaten about 1.5 pounds of licorice candy (about 700 grams) over a nine-day period. He suffered shortness of breath, ankle and abdominal swellings, weight gain, headaches, and weakness. Although previously he had an excellent health record, his respiratory distress required hospitalization for a developing heart problem. The physician who reported this case felt that the medical community should be aware that overindulgence in licorice-containing products may induce congestive heart failure.

An eighty-five-year-old man was admitted to a hospital in 1980, suffering from a progressive generalized weakness and inability to rise from a sitting position. He had experienced this weakness for ten days. He could not raise his arms above a horizontal position, had moderately swollen ankles, and profound muscular weakness. The man had chewed eight to twelve ounces of tobacco daily, and swallowed the saliva. The tobacco that the man had been chewing contained licorice. He had engaged in this practice for half a century. It was estimated that he had been consuming from 0.88 grams to 1.33 grams of glycyrrhizic acid daily, which was within a range known to produce health problems including muscular weakness, hypertension, and potassium deficiency. The potassium deficiency in this man was aggravated further by his low-potassium food choices. Being toothless, he had been eating canned soup and soft vegetables for more than a year as his sole dietary intake. Potassium-rich fruits and berries were missing in his diet.

Men with sexual dysfunction should avoid licorice. An Italian study, reported in the *New England Journal of Medicine* (vol. 34, 1999) demonstrated that licorice consumption lowered testosterone slightly in men. On the basis of this finding, the researchers recommended that licorice should be avoided by men with low libido or other sexual dysfunction, as well as those with hypertension. They suggested that health professionals should question men with these conditions about their consumption of licorice confections. Later, the same Italian researchers demonstrated that licorice decreased plasma testosterone in healthy young woman during the luteal phase of the menstrual cycle, and reported their findings in *Steroids* (vol 69, 2004).

Additional research, conducted by Iranians, reported in the *Journal of Pharmacy and Pharmacology* (vol. 33, 2003), showed the effect of licorice root extract on healthy male volunteers. Their results confirmed the earlier Italian study with men and showed decreases in serum testosterone levels from licorice. The effect was credited to the active agent, glycyrrhizin, with hydroxysteroid dehydrogenase, the enzyme that catalyzes the conversion of androstenedione to testosterone.

In western Europe, a popular alcoholic licorice-containing drink is Un Boisson de Coco. Persons who habitually drink one to three liters daily have been reported to show muscular weakness, paralysis, tetany (muscular twitchings and cramping), and hypokalemia (low blood potassium level).

Obviously, licorice use in the food supply needs careful monitoring and limitations. Any increased use of licorice compounds, especially to serve as sweeteners and sweetener enhancers, is fraught with hazard.

Chapter 7

STEVIA: SWEETENER
OR DIETARY SUPPLEMENT?

*The FDA serves as the pharmaceutical industry's watchdog
which can be called upon to attack and destroy a potential
competitor under the guise of protecting the public.*

—JAMES P. CARTER, M.D., *RACKETEERING IN MEDICINE: THE SUPPRESSION
OF ALTERNATIVES* (HAMPTON ROADS PUBLISHING CO, 1992)

The story of stevia in the United States encompasses tradition, science, economics, and politics. In one sense stevia is a success story, as a sweetener derived from protein rather than carbohydrates in a plant, and brought to successful commercial development. However, in another sense, stevia is a failure story, with powerful competing sweetener interests thwarting attempts to allow it to be marketed.

Stevias are annual or perennial herbs, sometimes shrubs. They grow wild. The genus *Stevia* is relatively large, comprising more than three hundred species. In Mexico alone, there are some seventy species; in Paraguay, among some fourteen known species, only one, *Stevia rebaudiana*, native to the northeastern section of the country, has captured attention.

Stevia's use in Paraguay dates back to pre-Columbian times. Traditionally, its leaf was used as a sweetening agent, and known by the indigenous people as "honey leaf." The leaf was used, too, for medicinal purposes.

In 1899, Moises Bertoni, a South American naturalist and director of an agricultural college in Paraguay, was introduced to the sweetness of stevia's leaves. He discovered that the plant was unknown to the scientific community.

At first, the plant was named *Eupatorium rebaudiana*. Later, to honor Bertoni, it was renamed *Stevia rebaudiana bertoni*. It is the only known species in the stevia genus that is utilized commercially. The first cultivated stevia crop was harvested in 1908. Plantations were established in South and Central America, and later, in Israel, Japan, China, Thailand, and the United States.

Currently, it is the only high-intensity protein sweetener that has been researched, developed, and available globally. In the United States, it is licensed *solely* as a dietary supplement. The bizarre story about this classification is discussed later.

In 1899, stevia was introduced in developed countries where it was dubbed "the sweet herb of Paraguay." In 1905, researchers began to investigate the plant's sweet principles. As early as 1909, the principles were extracted. By 1931, scientists had isolated and identified stevioside as the molecule responsible for the plant's sweetness. In the 1950s, the sweet principles were characterized. By 1963, investigators identified other active molecules in the plant.

In concentrated extract form, stevia can be from 150 times to 4,000 times sweeter than sucrose; and in leaf form, approximately ten times to thirty times sweeter. If stevia is tasted in a concentrated raw extract form it has a licorice taste. However, this taste is absent when the stevia extract is diluted for normal use. As a sweetener, stevia is practically noncaloric. Ten leaves contain only one calorie.

REPORTED HEALTH ADVANTAGES OF STEVIA

Traditional use of stevia gave primary emphasis to its health benefits rather than its sweetening ability. Because the stevia plant is indigenous to Paraguay, some of the research related to its health effects have been conducted in that country.

For more than 1,500 years, stevia has been used in the region, especially among the Guarini Indians. For more then a half century, in recent time, stevia has been used commonly in Paraguay with diabetics. Research confirmed that stevia helps to normalize blood sugar.

In 1921, before the widespread use of saccharin and cyclamate in the United States, stevia's health benefits and commercial possibilities led the American Trade Commissioner George S. Brady to recommend stevia's use as "an ideal and safe sugar for diabetics."

In 1966, Dr. Olivido Miguel, who had been professor of pharmacology at the Paraguayan National University, described the beneficial relationship of stevia with the body's regulation of blood sugar. He noted no intolerance, nor any toxicity from a dry extract of stevia. Miguel reported that diabetics experienced a feeling of well-being unknown to them up to that time in the course of their sickness.

Another Paraguayan study, presented before the Seventh Congress of the International Federation of Diabetes held in Bueno Aires, in August 1970, reported on stevia's beneficial effects on hypoglycemics. The sweetener regulated blood sugar. Even when stevia was used in a wide range of administered amounts—all in very small quantities—the sweetener was beneficial and the results were lasting.

Physicians in Paraguay, as well as in Brazil, China, and Thailand, have long made use of stevia for diabetic patients. Its use has been based on their own clinical experience as well as after having read available medical reports.

In many Latin American countries, in addition to Paraguay as well as in Asia, stevia has been used as a tonic to stimulate mental alertness and to counter fatigue. Stevia has been reported to facilitate digestion, improve gastrointestinal functions, and to regulate arterial pressure. It has been used to regulate the liver, pancreas, and spleen. Also, stevia has been reported as an aid in weight loss. Stevia does not feed candida growth of yeast infections. Stevia retards the growth of dental plaque and cavities. There have been no reports of any toxic effects from stevia use.

Scientific reports establishing stevia's safety have been published since 1931. Various toxicity tests indicated that the compound was nontoxic, nonteratogenic, nonmutagenic, noncariogenic, and devoid of contraceptive activity.

STEVIA'S SUCCESS OUTSIDE THE UNITED STATES

No discussion of stevia would be complete without its role in Japan. Both the Paraguayan experience and the Japanese experience need to be appreciated as background before discussing stevia's fate in the United States.

In post-World War II, preliminary research in Japan resulted in propagation of the stevia plant through cuttings. As a result, the Japanese began to use stevia as a sweetener in various commercial products.

In the mid-1960s, the Japanese government banned the use of artificial sweeteners. The official policy resulted in having the population turn to natural sweeteners that would not be detrimental to health.

In 1970, Mideo Fujita and Tomoyoshi Edahiro, researchers from the Japanese National Institute of Health, investigated stevia and one of its constitutents, stevioside. Extensive short- and long-term safety tests with animals produced no abnormal changes in their feed intake, cell or membrane characteristics, enzyme or substrate utilization, or chromosome characteristics. The substances did not induce cancer, fetal abnormalities, or tooth decay. Extensive hematologic and histologic tests and autopsies revealed no problems.

In 1977, M. Yabu and colleagues at the School of Dentistry, Hiroshima University in Japan, found that stevia was not a nutritional source for oral bacteria. On the contrary, stevia might possess properties that suppress bacterial growth, and might be effective in cavity prevention.

After extensive testing by the Japanese government as well as other scientific groups, Japan officially declared stevia safe and legal to use. Since 1970, stevia has been the noncaloric sweetener of choice in Japan. Stevia extracts are permitted for general use as a sweetener and as a flavor enhancer. About 40 percent of low-calorie food products sold in Japan are sweetened with stevia. A variety of juices, soy sauces, pickles, frozen desserts, soft drinks, chewing gums, toothpastes and mouthwashes are sweetened with stevia. The Japanese versions of products familiar to Americans, such as Coca-Cola's Diet Coke, are sweetened with stevia. Beatrice Foods, a large American conglomerate, uses stevia as a sweetener in its processed products exported to Japan. Globally, Japan leads in stevia use as a sweetener. After more than three decades of its widespread use in Japan by the general population, there have been no reports, either epidemiologic or clinical, of adverse effects on humans resulting from stevia use.

The Japanese investigations of stevia have been notable in the extensiveness of their research. They advanced the original studies conducted in the 1950s, when stevioside had been identified as a sweet constituent in stevia plants. In the 1970s, Japanese researchers at Hiroshima University and at Hokkaido University isolated additional sweet compounds in the plants: *Rebaudioside* A, B, C, D, and E; steviol bioside; and ducoside. All of the sweet compounds in stevia are diterpene glycosides. *Rebaudioside* A has a sweeter and pleasanter taste than stevioside. Depending on the concentration levels, these compounds are far sweeter than sucrose, yet they have only a miniscule caloric value compared to sucrose. (For the relative sweetness of sugar and sweeteners, see Appendix C.)

In the early 1970s, a group of Japanese food companies formed a consortium to develop stevioside and stevia extracts commercially for use in their products. At present, four Japanese companies compete to produce the greatest number of stevia products.

At first, Japanese scientists were most interested in pure stevioside. However, the interest then shifted to an interest in mixtures of diterpene glycosides from the stevia plant because the extracts have a sweeter, more sucroselike flavor than pure stevioside. As a result, many Japanese producers began to use the mixtures.

Stevia became widely used throughout Asia. It is reported to be used extensively in China, which has become its major global supplier. Elsewhere, stevia is permitted to be used in Switzerland, some Eastern European countries, Israel, and South Africa. Application to legalize stevioside use is pending in Australia.

In 2000, the European Union (EU) banned stevioside use due to a study that found it potentially toxic. Later, after evaluation, the study as found to be flawed and was widely repudiated. Newer research, conducted at Leuven Catholic University in Belgium, exonerated stevioside. The findings were distributed to all EU members, as well as to federal agencies worldwide. The newer findings helped to legalize stevioside use in many markets.

The WHO/FAO's Joint Expert Committee for Food Additives (JECFA) reviewed data and established a recommended daily intake (RDI) of steviol at 2 milligrams per kilogram of body weight. The JECFA requested additional research on the effects of low and high concentrations of steviol in consumers with hypo- or normotension; insulin-dependent and noninsulin-dependent diabetics; and more stability studies and better specifications of the steviol glycoside mixture.

Stevia has a great potential in the European market, especially with EU countries. One factor is the cessation of sugar subsidies.

In the late 1990, the Singapore Environmental Technology Institute (ETT) established a joint venture with Royal-Sweet Asia, Ltd. (RSA) and with the National Research Council of Canada, to build what ultimately will be a $50 million full-scale sweetener manufacturing plant in Singapore. The present total market for generic stevia sweeteners is about 2,000 tons annually, with Asia accounting for about 90 percent of the world's consumption. Initially, RSA's new plant will produce 500 tons per year, with an expectation that the plant will be enlarged to produce double that amount within four years.

RSA's parent corporation is Royal Sweet International Technologies, Ltd. (RSIT) in Vancouver, British Colombia. The Canadian company has patented a method for water extraction of stevia, without use of chemical solvents. The resulting product is regarded as "all natural." The company has isolated from the stevia plant the specific stevioside that has the best sweetness profile: *Rebaudioside* A, resulting in better tasting and less bitter aftertaste. Chinese-grown stevia has 6 to 10 percent *Rebaudioside* A in total glycosides; the Canadian, about 17 percent. The company's patented seeds can be electromapped. If the seeds are used illegally elsewhere, they can be identified.

At one time, RSIT had a partnership with Monsanto Chemical Company, the producers of NutraSweet (the high-intensity synthetic sweetener) for research and development of stevia. However, the collaboration ended bitterly and RSIT extricated itself only after a prolonged legal battle.

Ultimately, Monsanto retained rights to shares in RSIT's Asian stevia ventures. Meanwhile, Monsanto launched neotame, a spinoff dubbed "super-aspartame," discussed later in Chapter 14.

RSIT also worked closely with the Southern Crop Protection and Food Research Center, a governmental agency located in London, Ontario. Jim Brandle, a plant geneticist and his colleagues, are attempting to develop stevia cultivars that will thrive in southern Ontario, a land of harsh winters, and hot summers with long bright days. These conditions are thought to be excellent for producing stevioside in the leaves of the stevia plant. Brandle suggests that stevia would be a good alternative cash crop for Canadian farmers who now grow tobacco. As a cash crop, stevia would be quite competitive with tobacco, and more profitable than wheat, corn, or canola (rapeseed).

In 1993, Canadian government researchers collaborated with scientists from Thailand to do basic research on stevia. John Salminen, head of the additives and contamination section of Health Canada (the Canadian counterpart to the U.S. FDA) reported that no problems with stevia safety has come to his attention, but to date the Canadian government has not received any application for stevia's use. Salminen said, "If we do, we would have to look at the scientific safety data carefully." He added that in any evaluation, he would be open to including the decades of Japanese experience with stevia. This openness and inclusiveness on the part of a Canadian official is in stark contrast to the closed, exclusionary mentality displayed by U.S. officials, which will be discussed later.

To meet expanding market demands for stevia, interest in growing the plant has expanded.

As early as World War II, England had experimented with growing stevia as a substitute for the limited supply of sugar and other sweeteners due to tight rationing. After the war ended, and restrictions were lifted, England abandoned the program. Also, the expanded use of inexpensive cyclamates and saccharin contributed to the demise of interest in stevia as a marketable sugar substitute.

Even agricultural officials in the United States have shown interest in stevia as a potential crop. In the early 1980s, researchers at the University of California at Davis had experimented with stevia as a viable agricultural crop. Their preliminary trials demonstrated that the production of stevioside from stevia could be equivalent to the sweetening power of 28 tons per acre of sucrose from sugarcane. The September–October 1982 issue of *California Agriculture* announced that a limited number of root cuttings of stevia were available for research purposes, and that the California Department of Agriculture had published "Experimental Cultivation of Rebaudi's Stevia in California," available to interested persons.

The Paraguayan government noted that the U.S. Drug Enforcement Administration (DEA) strongly supports the idea of replacing marijuana production with other commercially profitable crops. The Paraguayan government suggested that the stevia plant is a viable alternative. This suggestion is not apt to be accepted by the U.S. government in view of FDA's policy (discussed later) including its former ban on imports of stevia. (The ban is now lifted.)

If, at some future time, the United States changes its present policy with stevia, the plant could become a lucrative domestic crop for many farmers. It grows well in a range of climates. It is grown commercially in Mexico to our south, and in southern Ontario, Canada, to our north. Traditionally, the USDA seeks out new crops for American farmers to consider, stevia has promise. However, the USDA would need to harmonize its efforts with those of its sister agency, the FDA.

With expanded interest in stevia uses, currently this plant is cultivated in at least a dozen countries worldwide, including Japan, China, Taiwan, Thailand, Korea, Brazil, and Malaysia. However, the best tasting stevia is reported to be from the Guarini plantations in Paraguay.

Due to the success story of stevia outside the United States some observers in Japan predicted that stevia will become the main natural sweetener globally. Also, they view stevia as representing the first successful development of a high-intensity protein sweetener that made its way into large-scale commercial production. For various reasons, numerous other promising high-intensity protein sweeteners have not been developed, and remain in limbo. They will be discussed in a later chapter.

According to Linda and Bill Bonvie, authors of *The Stevia Story* (B.E.D. Publications, 1997):

> The FDA's stevia policy is filled with contradictions and intrigue, secret trade complaints, search and seizures, and is generally intimidating. The actions which, in the minds of many knowledgeable individuals, smack of a conspiracy between regulators and certain powerful commercial interests to keep this centuries-old sweet herb, which is used throughout the world, away from American consumers.

Another observation was made by Kathi Keville in her article "The Herb Report: Stevia" (*The American Herb Association Quarterly*, Spring 1994):

> Considering the investment U.S. manufacturers have made in artificial sweeteners like aspartame, they are unlikely to invest money in getting FDA approval for a nonpatentable substance like stevia.

ENFORCEMENT ACTIONS AGAINST STEVIA SALES

The FDA has had a long history of denigrating stevia. In the late 1980s, the agency launched a vigorous campaign to pressure herb companies to stop using stevia, which the agency called an unsafe food additive. It was reported that FDA's campaign was in response to complaints that it received by producers of NutraSweet. Some American food and beverage processors were showing increased interest in having stevia available as an additional sweetener that could be chosen among other sweeteners already available. Stevia seemed particularly attractive as an "all natural" sweetener that blended well with other sweeteners. Also, processors recognized that more consumers were trying to avoid products with sucrose, and stevia was attractive as a sugar substitute. Another factor was the growing popularity of the low-carbohydrate, high-protein diets which discouraged use of both caloric and synthetic sweeteners. Some American processors initiated arrangements that would assure a growing market for stevia-sweetened products.

The FDA launched an all-out assault on companies dealing with stevia, by using embargoes, search-and-seizure operations, and ultimately, an import ban, which the agency instituted in May 1991. According to Zoltan P. Rona, M.D., "The FDA banned stevia imports for use in foods reportedly at the request of an aspartame manufacturer." Dr. Rona was quoted in *Health Naturally*, August–September 1991 issue. He also charged that the FDA implemented the ban because of the agency's strong loyalties to Monsanto, the manufacturer of aspartame.

Even the food trade journal, *Food Product Design* noted in its October 2001 issue that "proponents of approving stevia as a food ingredient in the United States say that the FDA is kowtowing to the special interests of the synthetic sweetener industry."

The FDA import ban was applied to the use of stevia in foods. Justification for the ban was based on a study that had been conducted at the University of Illinois, in which a genetically altered synthesized version of stevia extract allegedly caused precancerous changes in a strain of bacteria. A follow-up study pointed to flaws in the study, and threw its conclusions into serious doubts. Nevertheless, the FDA used this flimsy evidence to impose the import ban. Critics charged that the agency was using the flawed date to justify its actions, and that the agency, in bowing to the pressures from corporations that produced synthetic sweeteners, was anxious to suppress potential competitors. The import ban created supply shortages of stevia, and would continue with ever-dwindling supplies for four years.

In September 1985, the FDA relaxed its imposed stevia import ban. The agency announced that imports could be resumed, provided that stevia was regarded as a dietary supplement, but not as a sweetener. Like the Dutchess in *Alice in Wonderland*, the meaning of a word is whatever the FDA chooses to say it is.

The problem was not with stevia, which was permitted to be sold as a dietary supplement under the Dietary Safety and Health Education Act (DSHEA). The FDA decided that stevia products could be marketed solely as a dietary supplement, without any statement or even a faint hint about stevia's sweetening quality. Problems arose when producers, distributors, and sellers stated or implied that stevia could be used as a sweetener. If the stevia was used by itself it was considered to be a dietary supplement. However, if the stevia was an ingredient in a food or beverage product, the FDA would regard it as an illegal food additive, subjected to federal regulations for food additives. The agency would declare that such a product was adulterated and subject to seizure.

The FDA regulations deem a food to be adulterated, among other reasons, if it is a dietary supplement or contains a dietary ingredient that "under conditions of use recommended or suggested in labeling" present a significant or unreasonable risk of illness or injury. Thus, the issue became one of classification and labeling.

The regulations define "labeling" as "all label and other written, printed, or graphic matter upon any article or any of its containers or wrappers or accompanying such articles," according to the FDA. Materials include books or articles written by third parties. Thus, books become part of labeling.

THE FDA AS KEYSTONE COPS

In April 1998, the FDA announced that it would monitor the use of publications used in connection with the sale of dietary supplements, and added that the agency "intends to monitor the use of 'third-party' publications to promote the sale of dietary supplements and, if necessary, will develop appropriate regulatory guidance to ensure that the information is balanced and truthful."

Intent on crushing the growing interest in stevia—a threat to the popular high-intensity sweeteners that monopolized the sweetening market—the FDA decided on a bold move. It would act against the Stevita Company in Arlington, Texas. Stevita was both producer and distributor of stevia. The company had a modern plant located in Brazil, and also was a major stevia distributor in the United States. The FDA already had taken a series of actions against Stevita, including the issuance of Warning Letters, impoundings, recalls, and relabeling demands. Joseph R. Baca, Dallas District Director of the FDA had warned Stevita that by laboratory analysis, the agency had confirmed the presence of stevia in some of the company's products. Baca claimed that these products were being promoted in settings that intimated that stevia was not merely a dietary supplement. Baca cited as an example, "This literature pictures a drink appearing to be coffee or tea surrounded by jars and packets of Stevita's stevia." Baca cited "offending" statements, regarding stevia such as "Stevia extract is 200 to 3,000 times sweeter than sugar—but it is not sugar!" and "Just use it right out of the jar." Apparently, the most offensive statement was that the product was "tabletop ready!" However, the main problem, according to Baca, was that the stevia products were being "actively promoted, through labeling in the form of promotional literature, as conventional foods." Stevita was selling three different books about stevia. In the FDA's view, the books constituted labeling.

For any FDA watcher, this was déjà vu. In the 1960s, the FDA had used books as labeling, even with foods. The popular *Folk Medicine* by D. C. Jarvis., M.D. (1961, reissue edition, Fawcett, 1985) described the health benefits of apple cider vinegar and honey. The FDA agents had seized copies of the book displayed in natural food stores if they were in proximity to bottles of apple cider vinegar and jars of honey, declaring the book as "labeling" for unproven health claims. Arbitrarily, the FDA decided on the amount of space that would be permitted between the book display and the foods, in order for the books not to be considered as labeling. The FDA agents actually used tape measures to assess the distances! The action was so ludicrous that it caused one wag to ask rhetorically if the FDA would seize copies of the Holy Bible as labeling if the books were in close proximity to milk and honey.

Two weeks after Baca visited Stevita, the FDA decided to take action. On May 19, 1998—to borrow a phrase—a day that would go down in infamy—FDA Compliance Officer James R. Lanar faxed a letter to the Stevita Company announcing the probable impoundment and destruction of some 2,500 copies of the offensive books that discussed stevia and were being sold by Stevita. This warning signaled the crackdown on books considered as labeling. Furthermore, the faxed letter stated "upon visiting the Stevita company, investigators would conduct a book inventory" and "witness the destruction of the cookbook, literature and other publications for the purpose of verifying compliance." Book destruction? Shades of Nazi Germany?

Oscar Rodes, president of the Stevita Company, estimated that destruction of its inventory of books would cost the company a sum in excess of $10,000. There would be no compensation, nor any recourse.

The offensive literature included three different books about stevia printed by third-party publishers. The books contained general information about the history, scientific studies, and use of stevia. One of the books was a cookbook. Another book not only discussed stevia but was a political exposé of the FDA, and listed names of officials, dates, and agency actions that defied rational explanations.

Two hours after the arrival of the faxed message, FDA agents arrived at the Stevita Company. They announced that they were there to observe the destruction of the offensive books and other literature related to stevia.

Rodes, who had not yet been able to contact his lawyer, later reported wryly in the August 17, 1998 issue of *Insight*, "I told them I did not have a permit for burning from the city of Arlington, so I asked them whether it would be okay just to put [the books] in a dumpster."

Meanwhile, Rodes handed a video camera to one of his associates, and told her to tape the proposed destruction of books. After she activated the camera, the agents hesitated. One of them said that he had been told to *mark* the printed materials to invalidate their use. After marking six copies of books, the agents decided that they needed to contact their supervisor. For two hours they attempted, unsuccessfully, to reach a designated individual. Without further action, they left the premises.

In the end, the FDA backed away from its enforcement actions against the Stevita Company. The company had attempted to make its labels conform to FDA's demands. The month following the fiasco at Stevita in Arlington, Texas, on June 28,1998, the FDA told Rodes's attorney that "products may be import-ed and distributed as labeled." Further, "[the] FDA has no issues with your client's distribution" concerning two of the books the agency had intended to destroy. Nothing was mentioned about the cookbook.

The incident prompted one wit to pose a hypothetical case, printed in the same issue of *Insight:*

> Suppose a dietary-supplement producer, in a lighthearted mood, labeled his product 'Witch's Brew' and promoted it by giving away copies of Shakespeare's *Macbeth*, would the cauldron scene, demonstrating uses of herbal supplements unapproved by [the] FDA, be considered as 'offending' literature or just as a cookbook?

The FDA's attempted seizure at Stevita caused Betty Martini, a long-time foe of aspartame and associated with Mission Possible International, wrote a letter to *Townsend Letter for Doctors and Patients* (Jan 1999):

> In a country founded on freedom you can go to the library or buy a book on how to make a bomb, or buy trashy pornography, but it's illegal to tell the consuming public the history of the stevia leaf, and the fact that it is a sweetener and has health advantages.

REGULATORY WAR AGAINST STEVIA CONTINUES

At the same time that the FDA was waging war against stevia producers, dis-tributors, and sellers, with harrassments due to the agency's policy of import ban, Warning Letters, search and seizures, threats of book destruction, and other actions that would discourage stevia's sales and use, the agency was waging war against stevia on yet another front. The FDA was adamant in maintaining its stance of refusal to file any petition for self-affirmation of GRAS (Generally Recognized as Safe) status for stevia. Repeatedly, the agency continued to place obstacles in the regulatory path for stevia.

Several interested groups petitioned the FDA to file for GRAS status for stevia. In October 1991, the American Herbal Products Association (AHPA) in Austin, Texas, sent the FDA a petition consisting of several hundred pages supporting stevia's safety, and requested "concurrence and acquiescence" to allow foods and food products containing stevia leaf to be marketed in the United States. The AHPA's petition was supported by a safety review of stevia gathered for the Herb Research Foundation (HRF) by Dr. A. Douglas Kinghorn, professor of pharmacognosy at the University of Illinois in Chicago. Kinghorn was considered to be a leading authority on plant-derived sweeteners, and had published extensively on stevia's toxicology, pharmacology, and use.

The FDA, in classifying stevia as a "food additive," required premarket approval, including extensive toxicological and safety studies before the substance could be sold in the United States. Under the provision of the 1958 Food Additives Act, substances that were "in common use in food" prior to 1958 are exempt by being "grandfathered" from the Act's provision.

The AHPA's petition included statements by USDA botanists in 1918 and specimens studied and reported by the USDA in 1921 and 1939. The petition cited studies by the National Institutes of Health (NIH) in 1955. All of these studies had been conducted prior to the 1958 Act. The petition included statements of the Spanish conquistadors in reference to stevia, and also cited documents in the National Archives in Asunción, Paraguay.

The FDA was unimpressed by the Paraguayan documents. The agency rarely recognizes the validity of safety tests conducted in other countries. This narrow-minded stance is supercilious, arrogant, and insulting.

In 1992, the AHPA submitted more than 300 additional articles to the FDA attesting to stevia's safety. The FDA refused to file either petition. An act of filing renders the documents accessible for public review. The FDA insisted that filing the petitions would depend on data to demonstrate that stevia had been used "by a significant number of people for a substantial period of time" prior to 1958. This ploy was another obstacle tossed into the regulatory path. When the FDA was pressed to define what it considered a "significant number of people," Eugene Coleman, chief of the Direct Additives Branch at the FDA, responded. As reported in *Better Nutrition* (Dec 1998), Coleman said, "This may sound flippant but we would know that number when we see it."

In 1992, the HRF in Boulder, Colorado filed a Freedom of Information Act request concerning contacts between the FDA and the NutraSweet Company for the time period during which the FDA was conducting a safety review of stevia.

In 1993, once again, the FDA refused to file AHPA's petition. The agency reported that the petition contained "mostly anecdotal and speculative information." The agency claimed that the stevia plant was "rare." The FDA wanted to know how a rare plant could have been in general use. The AHPA responded by citing twenty pages of statements from the Brazilian and Paraguayan health departments, as well as scientific and scholarly sources that were readily available to U.S. researchers.

The FDA remained unimpressed. "We have not evaluated the petition because we have safety concerns." As evidence, the FDA produced some limited studies showing that stevioside, a glycoside in stevia, contains a component, steviol, that caused cell mutation in test animals. Kinghorn reviewed the studies and suggested that the test findings did not warrant the FDA's conclusions based on the data. He noted that the studies involved chemically pre-treated rats' livers. Although rats' intestinal microflora are capable of converting stevioside into the potentially toxic steviol, there is no proof that the human digestive tract is the same as the rat's. Kinghorn added that "other substances found in the diet are known to cause disease-promoting damage to cells with no apparent impact on our health" (*Healthy and Natural Journal*, Apr 1999). As examples, Kinghorn noted that the FDA has approved potentially mutagenic caffeine and saccharin, substances that many people consume daily. Also, an earlier study, published in the September 1993 issue of *Environmental Health Perspectives'* supplement, had shown that neither stevioside nor steviol caused mutations in human cells.

In 1998, a study published in *Drug and Chemical Toxicology* had examined steviol toxicity in relation to hamsters' growth and development. The study showed that high doses were toxic, but the amounts were eighty times higher than the FDA deemed safe and allowed for stevia's use as a dietary supplement. One of the study's researchers, Maitree Suttajit, professor of biochemistry at Chiang Mai University's Medical School in Thailand, reported that it would be virtually impossible for humans to consume even the lowest level of steviol that had been used in the test, due to the intense sweetness of the substance.

The Thomas J. Lipton Company also was unsuccessful in having the FDA file its petitions for GRAS status of stevia. FDA's Dr. George Pauli repeated the mantra that the petition failed to prove either widespread historical use or to present a persuasive body of safety data.

Apart from the several petitions, Dr. Ryan Huxtable, professor of pharmacology at the University of Arizona in Tucson, noted the long history of stevia use in South America and in Japan, without any reports of adverse effects from its use in humans. Huxtable added that animal tests showed that at high levels, stevia can interfere with energy metabolism. Whether that takes place in humans is unknown. Of course, due to stevia's intense sweetness, it is used at exceedingly low levels.

In January 1994, the FDA announced that it refused to file AHPA's submitted petition for stevia on the basis that more information was needed. The AHPA hoped to resubmit its petition by June 1994.

Even though the AHPA submitted additional date, the FDA responded by citing some highly suspect animal study published in an obscure journal. The study claimed that stevia interrupted the fertility cycle in some test animals. It was the kind of research that the FDA would normally not accept if some company submitted it as part of its submitted data. Yet, the FDA saw fit to use this study to bolster its own position. Furthermore, the study had been published in Brazil. As noted previously, usually the FDA dismisses foreign-derived data. In this case, the FDA saw fit to use the study for its own purpose. Even if the study was of dubious worth, the FDA used it as its linch-pin argument to prop up its rejection of stevia as a safe additive.

In 1994, passage of federal legislation would affect stevia's status, and ren der all past GRAS petitions inconsequential. The U.S. Congress attempted to reform the FDA's chaotic practices in regulation and control of vitamins, minerals, and dietary supplements as if they were dangerous drugs. In 1994, Congress passed the DSHEA and declared that the legislation protects the right of access by consumers to safe dietary supplements necessary in order to promote wellness. Rebuking the FDA, Congress added "a rational federal framework must be established to supercede the current ad hoc, patchwork regulatory policy on dietary supplements," and added, "the federal government should not take any action to impose unreasonable regulatory barriers limiting or slowing the flow of safe products and accurate information to consumers." These statements seemed highly pertinent to stevia.

Using DSHEA, the FDA decided to classify stevia as a dietary supplement, even though every analysis has noted that stevia has no nutrients and contributes practically no calories to the diet. Its sole merit is its sweetness with foods (apart from its medicinal uses). The FDA prohibited any mention of stevia as a sweetener. This action would protect the interests of manufacturers of synthetic high-intensity sweeteners.

CLASSIFICATION HOBBLES STEVIA

Under DSHEA, stevia can be marketed under less stringent guidelines for dietary supplements. Unlike foods or food additives, dietary supplements do not have to be proven safe or effective before they are sold. However, the FDA can take action if a marketed dietary supplement is shown to be unsafe.

The FDA permits stevia to be considered as a dry herb. It is used legally in numerous herbal tea blends and shakes.

The FDA's policy is irrational. The agency prohibits stevia's low use as a sweetener because the agency claims that the substance is unsafe as a sweetener. Yet, the FDA allows stevia's unrestricted use as a dietary supplement, with no reliable data regarding its potential use at extremely high levels. As a dietary supplement, Americans can buy stevia in capsules of 200 milligrams (mg), 300 mg, or even 1,000 mg, and consume as many capsules as desired, with no regulations restricting its use for safety reasons. However, if permitted as a sweetener, Americans would be consuming stevia in exceedingly small amounts due to its intense sweetness.

There has been an estimate of the economic fallout of stevia's classification as a dietary supplement rather than as a sweetener. The regulatory environment has shrunk the stevia market by about 500 percent, according to Steve May, chief operating officer at Wisdom Natural Brands, in Mesa, Arizona, the largest stevia processor in the United States. May estimated that "the market would be about $100 million larger if the government allowed its use as a sweetener." May was quoted in *Functional Foods and Nutraceuticals*, March 2005.

May estimated that the retail market for products containing stevia to be about $20 million annually in the United States but he did not expect the herb's regulatory status to be changed in the near future. The FDA requires industry to file a petition requesting a change in the regulatory status of a substance. According to May:

> These can be very costly . . . Current law also denies any economic recovery mechanism for the company that pays the costs of approval of a natural product. So, while the patent laws encourage companies to develop chemical products and submit them for approval, the law provides an enormous disincentive to bear the cost of the food additive approval process for stevia. I do not know of any serious effort to change the current law that limits stevia use to the confines of the Dietary Supplement and Health Education Act.

Despite the prohibition of promoting stevia as a sweetener, some sellers are circumventing the regulation. Storekeepers stocking stevia have been creative. For example, the sign in one store offered a suggestion to customers: DON'T SWEETEN YOUR COFFEE, SUPPLEMENT IT!

Ironically, the FDA's policy of classifying stevia as a nutritional supplement has some merit, but is unrecognized by the agency. Traditionally, stevia has been used as a digestive aid—a natural diuretic as a balancer of the blood sugar level, and as an aid in weight loss by decreasing the appetite for sweet foods.

STEVIA-SWEETENED COKE IN THE FUTURE?

Despite the FDA's adamant opposition to stevia, its policy may be challenged by powerful forces. For several years, the Coca-Cola Company has been working with Cargill to modify stevia so that the sweetener could be adapted to beverages and foods that appeal to health-minded consumers. The Coca-Cola Company has filed some two dozen patents to protect its formula for a modified version of stevia, which it has named rebiana. In anticipation of demand, Coca-Cola in a joint venture with Cargill has been developing stevia plantations in China, Paraguay, and Argentina. Cargill is conducting safety tests with rebiana to seek FDA approval by 2009. Coca-Cola could use the sweetener with some 400 brands of drinks in more than 200 countries, and Cargill could use it in numerous food-product applications. Can the FDA, with its long-time policy of placing obstacles in the path of stevia's approval as a sweetener, be expected to reverse policy? Perhaps.

According to an unnamed but prominent food lawyer quoted by *Functional Ingredients* in December 2007, "The FDA is twenty years behind the science with stevia, and knows it. They're just waiting for the right kind of application, and Cargill and Coca-Cola appear to have lodged just such an application. But it may be two years before GRAS [Generally Recognized As Safe] approval is forthcoming." Stay tuned.

Chapter 8

THAUMATIN: A VERY HIGH-INTENSITY PROTEIN SWEETENER

Today, commercial applications of thaumatin utilize the taste modifications, masking flavor enhancements, and synergistic properties to produce dramatic effects in food products.

—C.P. BOY, "THAUMATIN: A TASTE-MODIFYING PROTEIN." *INTERNATIONAL FOOD INGREDIENTS* (NO. 6, 1994)

Katemfe, an African fruit called "the miracle fruit of the Sudan" contains three large seeds surrounded by transparent jelly. The jelly is intensely sweet, with a slight licorice-menthol flavor, and causes other foods to taste sweet when used with it.

The katemfe fruit grows in the West African tropical rain forests from Sierra Leone to Zaire. For centuries local people have gathered this fruit and used the seeds to sweeten corn-based breads, sour fruit, and tea, as well as to make their palm wine more palatable. Records as early as 1837 show that the seeds were traded in West Africa.

In 1841 W. F. Daniell, a missionary stationed in West Africa, observed the uses of katemfe seeds. In 1855, he was the first individual to report on katemfe in a pharmacology journal. To honor him, katemfe was named botanically *Thaumatococcus daniellii*.

More than a century later, in 1972, H. Van der Wels and his colleagues isolated the protein in the katemfe fruit. By 1979, its structure was identified. The sweetness was found to be in a protein, named thaumatin, present in the seeds.

THE SWEETEST KNOWN NATURAL SUBSTANCE

Thaumatin is recorded in *The Guinness Book of World Records* as the sweetest known natural substance. Its sweetness is listed in several sources as having 100,000 times the sweetness of sucrose. However, most listings give lower estimates, such as 2,000 to 2,500 times as sweet as an 8 to 10 percent sucrose solution. Other estimates are from 1,500 to 2,500 times; 2,000 to 3,000 times or 3,000 to 5,000 times. Although the estimates vary, what is clear is that thaumatin is an extremely intense sweetener, and can be used at an exceedingly low level, in parts per million.

In the late 1970s, when thaumatin was being considered as a potential sweetener for commercial development, its attractive features were noted. It would be a natural, noncaloric, noncariogenic, high-intensity sweetener and flavor enhancer.

Shortly after identification of thaumatin's structure, commercial development was begun. The large protein responsible for the sweetness in the jelly was isolated, identified, and called thaumatin I and II. A process was developed to extract thaumatin from the katemfe fruit.

In 1977, Tate & Lyle, Ltd., in England, the world's largest independent sugar refiner, began to market thaumatin under the name Talin. Japanese companies purchased large quantities, and the sweetener become common in Japanese food products.

According to a present supplier of Talin, the Talin Food Company in Birkenhead, England, the katemfe fruit is collected from individual villages deep in the African rain forests. Then, it is shipped to the Ivory Coast and Ghana, where it is processed. The thaumatin is extracted from the fruit by purely physical methods, and remains unmodified. Then, it is shipped to England for final processing.

The Talin Food Company considers the thaumatin trade to be ecologically sound, and not destructive of the rain forests. The company's brochure, "Talin: The Natural Flavour Enhancer," claims to have "encouraged the maintenance of its natural forests, the katemfe fruit being harvested as an alternative to cocoa, coffee, or charcoal production, which destroy the forest environment."

APPROVAL FOR LIMITED USE

The European Economic Community (EEC), now known as the European Union (EU), approved thaumatin as a sweetener for applications including edible ices, some confectioneries, chewing gums with added sugar, dietary foods, and vitamin and mineral supplements. Thaumatin was approved as a flavor enhancer and taste modifier in water-based nonalcoholic beverages, dairy and nondairy desserts, and bakery products.

The Joint FAO/WHO Expert Committee on Food Additives (JECFA) and the European Commission's Scientific Committee for Food (SCF) regarded thaumatin as safe, and that no allowable daily intake (ADI) needed to be established. Because of the exceedingly low amount of thaumatin required to sweeten foods, it was exempt from any requirement to be listed on the label.

Thaumatin was approved for additional uses in some countries as a flavor adjunct in chewing gums, and for use in animal feed. Approved nonfood uses included cosmetics, toiletries, and oral care products such as toothpastes and mouthwashes.

In the United States, the Flavor and Extract Manufacturers Association (FEMA) organized an independent panel of expert toxicologists and pharmacologists to review the safety data on thaumatin. After deliberation the panel concluded that thaumatin was safe. The FDA approved the sweetener for general use in more than thirty different food categories.

THAUMATIN'S PROTEIN MOLECULE

In the early 1980s, Sung-Hou Kim and his colleagues at the University of California at Berkeley investigated the protein molecule of thaumatin. The National Institutes of Health supported more than five years of research. The findings of Kim and his colleagues, made available in March 1985 by the National Academy of Sciences (later renamed National Academies), found that the large thaumatin molecule consists of a polypeptide chain of 207 amino acids. The molecule contains two distinct structural regions. In one, the amino acids are arranged in slats (a structure common to many proteins). In the other, the amino acids form complex loops where the sweetness is present. Using x-ray crystallography Kim and his colleagues showed that these loops probably bind to taste bud receptors that recognize sweet substances. However, antibodies that bind to the looped regions can eliminate the protein's sweetness.

The unwieldy size and complexity of thaumatin's protein molecule discouraged attempts to synthesize thaumatin or to use genetic manipulation to overcome some drawbacks in the sweetener, such as the permanent loss of sweetness in heated thaumatin.

It was known that thaumatin produced in yeast cells lacked the folded molecular structure that gave thaumatin its sweetening properties. In the late 1980s, researchers at a California biotechnology company successfully inserted the gene for thaumatin expression into yeast cells. Later work showed that thaumatin would fold itself into a desired molecular structure when it penetrated yeast cell walls. This finding would make it possible to mass produce thaumatin more economically.

Different countries vary in their thaumatin regulations. Some permit its general use, in foodstuffs; others approve its general use as a flavor enhancer and sweetener in all foods; others limit its use as a flavor enhancer with flavors using no artificial sweeteners; others limit its use as a flavor enhancer in chewing gums. Some have specific product approval for its use in pharmaceuticals.

In Japan, where thaumatin is widely used, it is regarded as a natural food-component. Thaumatin has been approved for use in many countries, including Canada, Mexico, Brazil, Argentina, Paraguay, Uruguay, Korea, Indonesia, Taiwan, South Africa, Australia, New Zealand, and the United States.

VERSATILITY OF THAUMATIN

Food and beverage processors favor thaumatin because of its numerous attributes. At its lowest concentration, thaumatin potentiates other flavors such as peppermint, ginger, cinnamon, or coffee. In Japan, thaumatin has been used to enhance the aroma and boost the flavor of instant coffee. Thaumatin tames the taste of fiery and peppery flavors. It masks the bitterness or aftertaste in substances such as saccharin or salt substitutes and the metallic notes associated with synthetic high-intensity sweeteners. It is synergistic with flavor enhancers and increases the intensity of monosodium glutamate and 5'-nucleotides (both compounds are so-called flavor enhancers). Thaumatin masks acidity, and reduces the bitterness from caffeine or chocolate, and reduces the astringency in stocks and soups. It improves the mouthfeel in low-fat products and makes them seem creamier, and also gives a perception that the food has more fat than actually is present. Thaumatin reduces the perception of wateriness in diet beverages. It improves the viscosity and texture in yogurts and milk drinks. It gives a thicker texture to syrups and better mouthfeel in ready-to-eat meals. It reduces the powdery texture in reconstituted foods. The addition of thaumatin to mouthwashes gives the perception of increased viscosity and more body to the products.

Thaumatin is especially useful in chewing gums. It improves the gums' flavor impact and significantly increases their sweetness and prolonged perception of flavor. This makes it possible to decrease the amount of flavoring used, and thereby cuts production cost.

Blended with other sweeteners, thaumatin improves the sweetness profile of isomalt, sorbitol, and synthetic high-intensity sweeteners. It is synergistic with aspartame, acesulfame K, saccharin, and polyols.

The currently available thaumatin is heat stable, so it can be used in bakery products and in beverage formulations. It is stable, too, in a wide range of pH, from 2.0 to 8.0. Dry products containing thaumatin have a shelflife of more than two years.

Suppliers report that thaumatin may be used in products labeled "natural" claiming that the sweetener is a natural product, manufactured "by an ecologically sound production process."

Currently, Talin is available to food and beverage processors but not to the general public in retail markets. According to Michael Witty at the Imperial College of Science, Technology and Medicine in London, "one reason why thaumatin is not in more general use is its great expense and limited production. Modern methods of genetic engineering are now being used to develop rival methods to produce thaumatin and make it a more widely available food additive." (*Thaumatin*, CRC Press, 1994) If this sweetener is produced by means of genetic engineering, will it still be considered as a "natural" product?

This may not be welcomed news for consumers who seek "natural" sugars. Also, consumers should realize that thaumatin, used in products, is likely to be blended with other sweeteners that may be far less desirable.

Chapter 9

THE DIHYDROCHALCONES: BITTERNESS TURNED INTO SWEETNESS

One man's trash is another man's treasure.

—A YANKEE ADAGE

In 1958, researchers at the U.S. Department of Agriculture's (USDA) Fruit and Vegetable Chemical Laboratory in Pasadena, California, were searching for new uses for food industry wastes. They examined citrus peel, discarded from fruit processing, and commonly used in animal feed. Were there other possible uses? Indeed, yes. The investigators found that the bitter flavone glycosides from citrus fruit rind contained naringin, an intensely bitter substance. Even at low concentrations, naringin produces an extremely bitter taste, more bitter than quinine or caffeine that are used as bitter flavorings. However, naringin, converted to neohesperidin, becomes a substance that is at least 1,800 times as sweet as sucrose.

Unfortunately, the only food found to contain neohesperidin as a constituent is in the rind of one variety of orange, the Seville. This variety is common in Spain, but is not exported. The orange is prized as the main ingredient in the world-famous Seville marmalade.

The American scientists met the challenge. In several steps, they converted naringin, obtained from a plentiful supply of grapefruit rind, into neohesperidin. About a hundred pounds of grapefruit rind are needed to make one pound of naringin. But this small amount of naringin converts into about 13 pounds of neohesperidin, which has the sweetening power of about 450 pounds of sucrose.

CHARACTERISTICS OF NARINGIN

Naringin is from a group of substances known variously as dihydrochalcone (DHC), neohesperidin dihydrochalcone (NHDC), or neohesperidin (DC). They are regarded as a type of flavonoid.

In 1963, NHDC was discovered by two researchers who were studying bitter compounds in citrus fruits. After they hydrogenated a particular citrus phenolic glycoside, they noted that the resulting compound was intensely sweet—from about 1,500 times to 1,800 times sweeter than sucrose.

The intense sweetness of neohesperidin has certain drawbacks. The perceived sweetness lags somewhat in starting, but then lasts for a long time, with an even later effect described as a "menthol-cooling" or "licoricelike" sensation in the back of the mouth. These features might be problems for food and beverage use but possible assets for products such as chewing gums, candies, dentifrices, and mouthwashes.

Why the Sweetness of DHC Lingers

The slow onset and lingering aftertaste effect of DHC sweeteners may relate to the general property of phenols. They bind readily with proteins. DHCs, with their phenolic groups, may bind rapidly and indiscriminately with protein present in saliva. In that case, it would take time for the DHC activity to use up available saliva protein before binding to taste receptor sites. Three sites responsible for the sweetness have been located on DHC molecules and their analogs. They fit a model in which the surface configuration of a sweetener has three sites at specific angles to each other. This idea is reinforced by another observation: the DHC molecules have two phenol rings, with part of the three activating sites distributed between them. Saccharin and cyclamates have only one similar site per molecule. It is possible that both of these compounds pair up with a single receptor on the tongue to create the sensation of sweetness.

Investigations were extended to other members of DHC. For example, hesperidin dihydrochalcone glycoside was found to be present in sweet oranges. Variations exist among DHCs in terms of intensity, time lag, duration, mouth site affected, and background flavor. It is believed that DHCs have potential uses as sweeteners, flavorants, and flavor enhancers, but to date, only NHDCs have been developed commercially.

SAFETY TESTING

The DHCs have undergone extensive toxicologic tests by the USDA and commercial producers. Although most of the media reported that no harmful effects were observed, this is not accurate. Although long-term studies with rats fed high doses of DHC showed no increase in tumor incidence, an apparent interaction between the sweetener and the laboratory diet resulted in decreased growth of the animals. In tests with dogs, some animals showed mild thyroid hypertrophy, elevated liver weight, and testicular atrophy.

It may be argued that such adverse effects were observed at high feeding levels—unrealistic in terms of the levels likely to be consumed by humans. However, the use of high feeding levels is an accepted protocol in toxicologic studies to demonstrate safety of a substance. High feeding levels overcome the limitations of animal studies: using a relatively small number of animals tested compared with the human population, a range of individual responses, and the limited time span of the experiment. The use of high feeding levels provides a margin of safety.

In 1968, when the U.S. cyclamate ban went into effect and also attempts were being made to ban saccharin, scientists at the Weizmann Institute of Science in Rehovot, Israel, increased their work on naringin. Dan Amar and Yehuda Mazur reworked the chemistry of naringin, named neohesperidin dihydrochalcones, (Neo-DHC), and designed a process for its manufacture. Amar and Mazur conducted toxicologic tests with Neo-DHC, and did not observe any harmful effects.

In 1987, the European Union (EU) declared NHDC safe for human consumption. In 1990, the EU included the sweetener in its Proposal for the Council Directive on Sweeteners. The sweetener was considered safe for a wide range of food applications, including nonalcoholic beverages, beers, desserts, edible ices, confections, sauces, and feed supplements. However, it has not been widely approved by all EU countries. Elsewhere, it is available in Switzerland, the Czech Republic (not yet a member of EU at the time), and Turkey. Both Australia and New Zealand regulate it as an artificial flavor. The United States permits its use solely as a flavor ingredient for use in sixteen food categories at levels below its sweetness threshold. To date, no petition has been filed with the FDA for its use as a sweetener. In the late 1990s, companies from Spain and Israel had considered seeking regulatory approval in the United States but were dissuaded. According to a spokesman, Abraham Bakal, from ABIC International, a consulting firm to one of the interested companies, the petitioning process would have been lengthy and very costly. Easier approval might be gained with its use in animal feed. Bakal reported that such use would increase palatability of feed and result in weight gain for the animals.

Worldwide, NHDC is marketed as Citrosa by a Spanish-based company, Exquim, a subsidiary of a pharmaceutical group, Ferrer Internacional. Citrosa is marketed as a high-intensity sweetener and also as a flavor modifier.

The usefulness of naringin's bitter quality is being utilized as well. This flavonoid was found to be bitter even at concentrations of one part naringin to 50,000 parts water. Atomergic, the trade name of a commercial bitter flavor powder made from naringin, is produced by Atomergic Chemicals Corporation in Plainview, New York, and available to processors who can use it to replace quinine or caffeine as bitter agents in foods and beverages. The DHCs are used by processors, but currently are not sold at the retail level.

Chapter 10

PLANT-DERIVED SWEETENERS: USED TRADITIONALLY, BECOMING RECOGNIZED

Let not things, because they are common,
enjoy for that the less share of our consideration.
—PLINY, THE ELDER, *HISTORIA NATURALIS*, BOOK XIX, SECTION 59

Numerous plant-derived sweeteners are known and have been used traditionally in various regions of the world. To date, stevia is a notable exception. It is one that reached commercial developments, albeit by torturous means. Recently, lo han fruit has emerged as another available plant-derived sweetener. A number of other such sweeteners are known. Some actually reached some degree of development, only to have plans thwarted and abandoned. Others await future investigation and possible development. Meanwhile, the promoters of patentable synthetic high-intensity sweeteners have succeeded in quelling efforts to develop nonpatentable plant-derived sweeteners.

LO HAN FRUIT

Lo han fruit (*Momordica grosvenorii* or *Siraitia grosvenori*) is a wild vine indigenous to southern China where it is known as *lo han kuo*. The plant has a perennial tuberous root and gourdlike fruit. The Chinese have used lo han fruit widely in household medicine. They have cultivated the vine and trained it over trellises in special gardens created for it in forested mountainous areas.

Tons of green, unripe lo han fruit have been shipped yearly to drying sheds at Kweilin in Kwangsi Province. The dried fruits lose much weight, and then can be packed carefully in boxes, shipped to Canton and also exported to Chinese communities outside of China, including the United States. Traditionally, the dried fruit has been used to treat colds, sore throats, and minor stomach and intestinal problems.

Lo han fruit was first studied by botanists in the 1930s. Specimens were shipped to the United States through a grant of the National Geographic Society. The species name assigned to it honored Dr. Gilbert Grosvenor of the Society. He had encouraged botanical as well as geographic explorations in China.

One researcher, C. H. Lee, found that the sweet principle in lo han fruit could be extracted by water, either from the fibrous pulp or from the rind of the fruit. Also, a 50 percent alcohol extraction was satisfactory. The rind yields an extract that can be purified more readily than the pulp.

Structural studies of lo han indicate that the sweetener constituents are mogrosides, a group of triterpenoid glycosides that are present in the fruit. With recent interest in this sweetener, Q. Xiangyang and colleagues at Huazhong Agricultural University in China investigated the mogrosides in lo han. They examined the effects of lo han extracts on pancreatic islets in insulin-dependent mice and on normal healthy mice (the controls). Diabetes had been induced in the insulin-dependent mice by treating them with a drug (Alloxan), which is used to produce this disorder in experimental animals. The researchers found that when the lo han extract was used therapeutically it had no effect on the normal mice, but had beneficial antidiabetic effects, presumably from the mogrosides, on the insulin-dependent mice. The researchers suggested that, in addition to lo han's value as a low-glycemic sweetener, it might be an acceptable sweetener for diabetics.

The sweetness of commercially available lo han is estimated to range from 200 to 250 times the sweetness of sucrose. Other estimates are as high as 300 times the sweetness of sucrose. Lo han remains stable when it is heated in cooked foods.

Lo han is produced by Danisco Sweeteners in Ardsley, New York. Western Commerce Corporation in City of Industry, California, distributes a fruit concentrate Nu-Sweet and FrutSweet powder. Both products contain concentrates derived from lo han. The powder also contains chicory. Sometimes lo han is blended with xylitol. Other companies distribute products containing lo han concentrates. Wisdom Natural Brands in Gilbert, Arizona, offers Sweet & Slender, a product reported to curb cravings for sweets, and at the same time, promote fat burning. This product is promoted as being safe for diabetics and hypoglycemics. Lo han fruit extracts are SlimSweet and SugarNot. R. W. Knudsen uses a concentrate of lo han to sweeten its diet spritzers. Amax NutraSource, Inc., distributes products with lo han.

YACÓN

One plant that has become of interest for possible commercial development is yacón (*Polymnia sonchifolia*), a sweet root vegetable, purple on the outside, and orange on the inside. The pigmentation suggests that yacón is a rich source of carotenoids as well as being a sweetener. Yacón is indigenous to the Andean region of South America, where it has been cultivated before the arrival of the conquistadors.

In the 1930s, attempts to cultivate yacón in Europe were limited. Awareness of this vegetable increased dramatically after 1989, when it was described in *Lost Crops of the Incas* published by the National Research Council (NRC).

Presently, Peru is the largest producer of yacón. It is also cultivated widely from Venezuela to northeastern Argentina, and in lesser amounts, in Brazil, Japan, Thailand, United States, and New Zealand.

Sometimes yacón is called "leaf cup." Its high sugar content in the root consists mostly of oligofructose, a nonabsorbable dietary sugar. As a result, the vegetable is low in calories, and can lessen the peaking of blood sugar in diabetics. Also, as an oligofructose, yacón has probiotic properties. It promotes beneficial bacteria in the colon, and helps the body absorb some minerals, notably calcium. Yacón contributes a significant amount of dietary potassium. Also, it contributes some vitamins and antioxidants. This root vegetable can be eaten raw, or added to drinks, syrups, bakery products, or pickles. Although yacón holds promise as a source for a sweetener, to date, it remains undeveloped.

"MIRACLE BERRY"

The berry from the "miracle fruit" (*Synsepalum dulcificum*) makes sour foods taste sweet. Bushes bearing these red berries grow abundantly in the inland regions of the African Gold Coast. For centuries, the natives have been eating the berries to improve the taste of stale staple gruels turned sour, and to sweeten some palm wine.

From time to time during the last four centuries, explorers made references to this remarkable berry. In 1852, W. F. Daniell, who also had reported on katemfe (see Chapter 8), observed the berry's taste-altering effects and termed it a "miraculous berry." The term held, and the berry became known as the miracle berry. Daniell took samples back to England, where they were considered a curiosity.

A century later, with a serious quest for alternative sweeteners, this berry was no longer regarded as a mere curiosity. Researchers isolated a protein from the berry, and named the protein miraculin. The protein was found to be 2,500 times sweeter than sucrose, and was capable of altering taste perception for up to twelve hours.

Miraculin looked promising. In 1968, a small company with strong backing and funding was formed in the United States to develop miraculin. The company planted a million bushes, developed a process to isolate miraculin from the berry, and successfully completed test marketing. But they failed to anticipate the obstacles ahead.

CHANGING SOUR TO SWEET

The active principle in the miracle berry is a glycoprotein—a protein with sugar groups attached—which coats the tongue in a very thin but durable layer. It is thought that the sweet sensation is produced by the protein attaching itself to the receptors of the taste buds and modifying their function, somewhat like an anesthetic. This is analogous to the property of certain deodorizing preparations that function by anesthetizing the olfactory nerves temporarily and making it difficult to detect disagreeable odors. Others do not believe that miraculin acts in that manner, but rather that it influences the response to acid of the taste receptors on the palate in such a way that the recognition stimulation pattern is changed from sour to sweet. The glycoprotein contains 6.7 percent sugar (L-arabinose and D-xylose). The purified protein is tasteless. It is destroyed by boiling and by exposure to organic solvents.

In 1973, the company petitioned the FDA for Generally Recognized as Safe (GRAS) status for miraculin. The agency denied the petition, and classified the substance as a food additive. That classification signaled the cessation of all marketing. The company was unable to raise additional money to appeal, and was unable to fund the costly comprehensive tests necessary to prove miraculin's safety as a food additive.

In 1974, the company declared bankruptcy. Three years later, the FDA reviewed the case and concluded that the data did not "assure the safety of either general or limited use of the miracle fruit and its products for use in foods," stated in a press release, *Health, Education, and Welfare News*, May 23, 1977.

SERENDIPITY BERRY

Another red berry, also from West Africa, and known as the Nigerian berry *(Dioscoreophyllum cumminsii)*, has long been used to sweeten sour foods in that area. The sweet taste from the fresh berry, like miraculin, persists. It lingers for an hour or longer. The Nigerian berry contains a soluble low-calorie protein.

The Nigerian berry was rechristened the "Serendipity berry" because the fortunate discovery of the source of its sweetening characteristic was made only on the very last day of scheduled research. Robert H. Cagan, Ph.D., a biochemist, was the principal investigator of this berry, and his preliminary studies suggested that the sweet substance in the berry might be a large protein molecule. His investigation was advanced by James A. Morris, Ph.D., a postdoctoral student who spent a year purifying and identifying the molecule. The molecule was found to be about thirty times larger than a sucrose molecule. Cagan and Morris named the protein "monellin" after the Monell Chemical Senses Center, a research center devoted to basic multidisciplinary research in the field of the chemical senses. Work with monellin at the Monell Center in Philadelphia, Pennsylvania showed that the sweetener was up to 3,000 times sweeter than an equal weight of sucrose, and fifteen times sweeter than aspartame. At the time when Morris and Cagan were examining monellin, less than 50 milligrams of the substance was available to determine its composition, structure, and properties. A protein molecule of monellin's size held an interesting possibility for taste research in unraveling the chemical structure required for sweetness. They found that the purified fine, white, powdery monellin was a soluble, biodegradable protein. It contained almost no calories.

THE STRUCTURE OF MONELLIN

The large monellin molecule has ninety-two residues and an intact tertiary structure that is necessary to produce its sweetness. Monellin consists of two non-covalently bound chains of fifty and forty-two residues. When separated, neither shows sweetness. But the two chains, recombined partially, form a tertiary structure that again shows sweetness.

Further studies revealed that monellin is somewhat related to thaumatin. However, monellin proved to be more adaptable in its natural form.

In the late 1980s, Sung-Hou Kim and his colleagues at the University of California at Berkeley, California, researched monellin and thaumatin as high-intensity protein sweeteners that were potential candidates for commercial development. Kim and his associates identified the structures of both sweeteners (see Chapter 8). Although their sequences of amino acids differ, both sweeteners appear to possess many structural similarities. It is likely that both interact similarly with taste bud receptors to produce a sweet taste. However, they differ. Unlike thaumatin's characteristics as a taste modifier, monellin does not alter the taste of a bitter substance. Unlike thaumatin, monellin would not serve as a masking agent.

Kim and his colleagues found that monellin, in its natural form, loses sweetness when it is heated. Its two interlacing strings of amino acids are unbound by heat, and at high temperature they tend to separate. The researchers discovered that by inserting genes from a mutant version of monellin—in which the two adjacent loose ends are bound—a microbially-produced single-stranded monellin could be created. It has a three-dimensional structure that allows it to recover its shape and sweetness after having been exposed to heat.

By the late 1990s, there was interest in the commercial manufacture of monellin, as a potential competitor of synthetic high-intensity sweeteners. Keiji Kondo and his associates at the Kirin Brewery Company in Japan succeeded in producing a genetically-engineered yeast that could produce monellin in large quantities. The yeast selected was one approved in the United States as a regulated food additive. Results of the work were gratifying. Monellin accounted for up to 50 percent of the water-soluble proteins in the yeast concentration. This amount was approximately equivalent to the amount of the sweetener present in the serendipity berry. Also, Kondo and his associates developed a simple method to purify monellin's protein. This development was an important consideration for commercial production of the sweetener. Nonetheless, despite the high hopes of the researchers, monellin awaits future development. As noted in the journal *MD* (Jun 1979), the primary impediment in bringing monellin and other alternative sweeteners closer to the commercial stage "appears to be the regulatory climate that inhibits investment in the studies needed to establish required safety data." Also, the synthetic high-intensity sweeteners that came to dominate the market discourage investment for developing sweeteners from plant-based materials.

UNFULFILLED PLANS

In 1986, the NutraSweet Company, a subsidiary of the Monsanto Chemical Company, announced jointly with DNA Plant Technology (DNAP) an agreement to develop economic sources of naturally derived sweeteners. Under the agreement's terms, NutraSweet would support research and product development work conducted by DNAP, and would allow DNAP to share in resulting profits.

The DNAP program would utilize both traditional plant breeding methods and biotechnology to develop new plant varieties that could enhance greatly the specific desirable characteristics such as superior varieties of plants that would produce greater quantities of sweeteners.

This announcement was noted briefly in *Chemical & Engineering News*, Aug. 11, 1986.

HERNANDULCIN

A monograph titled "Natural History of New Spain" written between 1570 and 1576 by a Spanish physician, Francisco Hernández, led modern researchers to a remarkably sweet plant. Hernández had described a plant known to the Mexicans as *Tzonpelic xihuitl*, translated as "sweet plant,"

Hernández described the plant so accurately, and accompanied his text with a detailed drawing of the plant, that pharmacologists at the University of Illinois in Chicago could identify it in 1985. A team, consisting of Cesar M. Compadre, John M. Pezzuto, and A. Douglas Kinghorn, all at the Program for Collaborative Research in Pharmaceutical Sciences, along with Savitri K. Kamath, at the Department of Nutrition and Medical Dietetics, examined the plant, now renamed *Lippia dulcis Trev.*, collected in Central America. The researchers analyzed compounds in the plant and identified the chemical structure of a pure, colorless oil in the plant. The main component was found to exist mostly in the leaves and flowers, and to be about 1,000 times sweeter than sucrose. To honor Hernández, the sweet component was named hernandulcin.

The purified substance was taste-tested by a panel of seventeen trained volunteers. They found that the sweetener had some drawbacks. It was described as "somewhat less pleasant than sucrose" and it exhibited "perceptible off- and after-taste as well as some bitterness," the tasters reported to *Science* (Jan 25, 1985). Researchers hoped to modify hernandulcin to make it more palatable.

In testings, hernandulcin had some positive features. In mouse studies, the sweetener did not cause biochemical mutations in standard tests that indicate a cancer-causing potential. Even when the sweetener was administered at high dosage levels, the findings were negative. Other tests indicated that the sweetener was not cariogenic. This feature is found with all protein-based sweeteners, unlike carbohydrate-based sweeteners.

Although the researchers filed for a patent application for the sweetener in 1985, and had begun to negotiate with a food company, development of this sweetener appears to be in limbo.

BRAZZEIN

Brazzein is a high-intensity sweetener from a plant protein found in a vine fruit (*Pentadiplandra brazzeana*) in tropical West Africa. The fruit has been consumed by indigenous populations for centuries, and its reddish fruit, slightly larger than a grape, is sold presently in Nigerian markets.

In 1994, sensory scientists Ding Ming and Göran Hellekant, both at the University of Wisconsin in Madison, Wisconsin, working with brazzein, made interesting discoveries. They found that the fruit's sweetness resulted from a previously unidentified, relatively small protein in the plant. The protein is only fifty-four amino acids long. Its lysine-rich amino acid sequence bears little resemblance to those of other sweet proteins, which usually contain a far greater number of amino acids (for example, thaumatin has 227). Also, the protein is quite stable. It survives high heat for at least two hours, and retains its sweetness even when subjected to a wide range of acidic and alkaline solutions.

Brazzein is only one of six proteins thus far identified to taste sweet to humans and other primates. Among these proteins are thaumatin and monellin (already discussed). Yet, the structure of brazzein does not appear to resemble the structures of either thaumatin or monellin. Its structure has more in common with some plant-defense proteins and scorpion toxins. This similarity does not explain brazzein's sweetness. However, it may explain how the protein evolved. Brazzein's resemblance to proteins that plants use to defend themselves against microbes suggests that previously its precursor had a similar function in the fruit. Hellekant speculates that through mutations, the original protein may have lost its defense capacity and became sweet.

Joseph Brand, associate director of the Monell Chemical Senses Center, considers these findings important in the context of protein sweeteners. Comparing the structure of brazzein, which is smaller and more rigid than those of thaumatin and monellin, Brand suggests that researchers will better understand how all three of these sweeteners bind to sweet-taste receptors.

After brazzein was identified as providing the sweetness in the plant's protein, there was an obstacle for any practical application. It would be too costly to extract the protein from the native source. Then, a possible solution was found by means of genetic engineering. By inserting the gene for the brazzein protein into field corn, it might become commercially feasible to develop the sweetener.

In 1998, Nektar Worldwide, at the time located in College Station, Texas, was formed to develop a commercial production system for brazzein. A project was developed by the combined efforts of Nektar Worldwide (by then relocated in Fort Lauderdale, Florida) and ProdiGene, in College Station. ProdiGene provided the technical capabilities and enabling technology required to develop an efficient production system in corn.

Jim Eckles, president and CEO of Nektar Worldwide, reported that because this natural plant-based sweetener can be extracted from corn in a conventional milling operation while preserving the value of the other corn products, brazzein is expected to be extremely cost-effective to produce. The company expects to extract one kilogram of brazzein from a ton of corn. This equates in sweetness to at least 1,000 kilograms of sugar. Currently high-fructose corn syrup (HFCS) is the leading sweetener in the United States. The technology with brazzein could produce a new HFCS with twice the sweetness, without adding calories. Eckles expects full-scale brazzein production at some future time. Also, at that time, the company intends to submit a self-determination of GRAS status to the FDA. The product will be submitted as a flavor modifier in order to facilitate a prompt entry of brazzein into the marketplace, when the time is suitable.

ROSARY PEA

A weedy vine (*Abrus precatorius*), commonly known as the rosary pea, grows worldwide in tropical areas. It is especially abundant in the Caribbean region and in southeast Asia,

In Malaysia, traditionally tea was sweetened by using a 50:50 ratio of rosary pea leaves and tea leaves. In Indonesia, rosary pea leaves have been used to sweeten a stimulant called "betel quid," as well as used therapeutically for tropical sprue. Such widespread and long-time use of the rosary pea in these countries has not produced any reports of harm.

With funding from the National Institutes of Health (NIH), Dr. A. Douglas Kinghorn, a professor of pharmacognosy previously mentioned for his work with stevia and hernandulcin, and his graduate student, Dr. Young-Hee Choi, both at the College of Pharmacy, University of Illinois, in Chicago, conducted research on abrusosides, including rosary pea, as potential sweeteners. They gathered leaves from the rosary pea near Miami, Florida, where the vine is regarded as an invasive weed. They identified compound abrusosides A, B, C, D, and E as sweet saponins in the leaves. Abrusosides, the sweet components in rosary pea leaves, are triterpine glycosides that are chemically unique to these sweeteners.They are from 30 to 100 times sweeter than a 2 percent solution of sucrose. A derivative of one of the saponins was even sweeter—about 150 times sweeter than sucrose. Abrusoside E was only marginally sweet.

The sweet abrusosides are highly stable. Unlike many other sucrose substitutes, these compounds do not break down in cooking or baking. They are described as having highly pleasant taste qualities, with no disagreeable aftertaste.

Because *A. precatorius* grows abundantly, only its leaves need to be gathered to make the compounds. The plant, itself, remains intact. This feature would make its use as a sweetener ecologically sound, with no decimation or threatened extinction of a species.

Safety tests did not demonstrate any cariogenicity (ability to damage the teeth) or toxicity. The sweetener does not appear to cause water or sodium retention in the the human body, as does another plant-derived sweetener, licorice.

In order to obtain regulatory approval to market this sweetener, Kinghorn reported that it would be necessary to separate the sweet constituents from other constituents in the rosary pea leaves. The researchers found that they could do this by making the sweetener water soluble in the form of ammonium salts.

Kinghorn admitted to *Food Chemical News* (Sept 4, 1995) that regulatory acceptance of the sweeteners represents "a daunting hurdle." He estimated that it would cost some 200 million dollars to satisfy the toxicological testing requirements needed for FDA approval of the abrusoside sweeteners. Using the route of petitioning for GRAS approval as an additive would not be easy, either. Kinghorn expressed hope that the "years of apparently safe human exposure these applications represent will help convince U.S. regulators to accept sweeteners derived from the leaves." In view of the FDA's history of repudiating such proof, Kinghorn's hope seems overly optimistic.

Research Corporation Technologies (RCT) in Tucson, Arizona, is providing some "industrial leverage" in an attempt to gain commercial use of the sweetener. RCT received a patent for abrososides as sweeteners, and can make them available for licensing by commercializing them for the University of Illinois. Kinghorn also sought a patent in Japan. At present, the sweetener is unavailable.

SWEET LEAF TEA

The Chinese sweet leaf tea plant (*Pterocarya paliurus*) contains sweet saponins. Dr. Kinghorn, mentioned above and for his work with other plant-derived sweeteners, investigated this plant, too. He found that the plant was used in remote areas of Hubei Province, China, to sweeten foods in cooking. In examining this plant, Kinghorn and his colleagues isolated pterocaryosides in the plant, which are sweet saponins. Kinghorn reported to the American Chemical Society in 1995 that the compounds in this plant probably lacked a commercial value. However, he noted that "study of plant usage within a society can aid in the discovery of new useful compounds."

SWEET SHOOT

Sweet shoot (*Sauropus androgynous*) is a southeast Asian plant, also called chekkurmanis, katook, and katuk. Its sweet leaves are used to flavor soups and stews and are eaten as a vegetable, a green dye in pastry, and an ingredient in an alcoholic drink "brem bali." To date, it has never been developed for commercial sale.

OSLADIN

Osladin is derived from the rhizome of a fern that grows in many areas of the world called *Polypodium vulgare L.* It is a steroidal saponin, but lacks the bitterness of these substances. Yugoslavian researchers discovered a sweet glycoside extract in the plant, that bears a structural relationship to DHCs (discussed in Chapter 9). Osladin resembles saccharin in its level of sweetness, being about 300 times sweeter than sucrose.

The yield of osladin from the fern is so meager that its commercial development is doubtful. Nevertheless, the fern holds interest. Some compounds related to osladin were under investigation at the Northern Regional Research Laboratory, USDA, in attempts to relate the sweet-taste phenomenon to certain types of structures.

SWEET CICELY AND HYDRANGEA

Some commonly recognized garden plants contain sweet principles that have been used, but are not likely to be developed commercially. Among them is sweet cicely (*Myrrhis odorata*), sometimes called the "candy plant." This graceful fern, commonly grown in home gardens, has a sweet licoricelike flavor in its leaf. It is used as a sweetener and flavor enhancer in homemade conserves, but is not developed commercially.

The dried leaves of the hydrangea (*Hydrangea macrophylla*) contain a sweet principle named phyllodulcin. In Japan, this plant is known as *ama cha*, and used to sweeten tea served at a flower festival to honor Buddha. Phyllodulcin has not been developed commercially.

CHICORY ROOT FIBER AND OTHER FLAVORS

In the early 2000s, a blend named Just Like Sugar was introduced, consisting of chicory root fiber, maltodextrin, vitamin C, and flavors extracted from orange peel. According to the manufacturer, this product contains no calories, sugar, fat, cholesterol, sodium, carbohydrates, or protein. Its granular composition allows it to dissolve readily in hot and cold liquids. The manufacturer states that this product is as sweet as sucrose, gram for gram. The product was marketed through a distributor MG Europe in Hungary, Austria, Germany, France, Finland, Denmark, Norway, Sweden, the Netherlands, Switzerland, Italy, Spain, Portugal, Czech Republic, Slovakia, Croatia, Bosnia-Herzegovina, and Serbia-Montenegro. By 2006, the product was marketed in the United States and Canada in food stores and by mail orders.

Part Three

HIGH-INTENSITY
SYNTHETIC
SWEETENERS

Chapter 11

CYCLAMATE: APPROVED AS SAFE—LATER, BANNED

There is no theoretical reason to believe that the effect of cyclamate is proportionately less at lower doses; with many carcinogens, the observed rule is that lower doses simply take a longer time to take effect.

—DR. JOSHUA LEDERBERG (NOBEL RESEARCH SCIENTIST),
STANFORD UNIVERSITY SCHOOL OF MEDICINE, 1970

The story of cyclamates is inextricably intertwined with the story of saccharin. Some developments with both synthetic sweeteners are so strikingly parallel that one has a sense of déjà vu. Cyclamates, like saccharin, were discovered accidentally, and by current standards, also due to sloppy practices in a chemical laboratory.

The year was 1937. A young researcher, Dr. Michael Sveda at the University of Illinois, was studying various compounds as possible fever-reducing drugs. He isolated the barium salt of N-cyclohexylsulfamic acid. He smoked while working with this substance. Casually brushing off some tobacco shreds clinging to his lips, he noted that his finger tasted intensely sweet. Sveda knew that the barium salt of the acid was relatively toxic, so he prepared the sodium salt, which was to be called sodium cyclamate. Its potential uses to mask the taste of bitter pills, and to sweeten substances, were recognized.

By 1942, Sveda and his superior, Dr. Ludwig F. Audrieth, jointly patented cyclamate and its salts. Sveda also worked on the development of DDT. Ironically, both of these substances would be heralded as beneficial, only later to be condemned and banned.

Cyclamates were synthesized from sodium or calcium salts of cyclohexylsulfamic acid. Cyclamate is thirty times sweeter than sucrose, and has a sugarlike taste. Although cyclamate is not a high-intensity sweetener such as those developed later, it combined well with other sweeteners. It was stable. It was soluble in liquids. These features made it attractive for use in diet soft drinks. Cyclamate became the most popular synthetic sweetener in the 1950s and 1960s.

In 1950, Abbott Laboratories launched the first commercial production of sodium cyclamate. The following year, with approval by the FDA, the company also marketed calcium cyclamate. The DuPont Company, Monsanto Chemical Company, Pfizer, Pillsbury, and others soon followed.

AN EARLY SYNTHETIC SWEETENER

Dulcin, an early synthetic sweetener, was available in 1883. Dulcin was about 250 times sweeter than sucrose. (For the relative sweetness of sugar and sweeteners, see Appendix C.) It was used for more than fifty years in the United States and elsewhere.

In 1960, disquieting news concerning dulcin came from Japan. A woman and her infant were examined at the Department of Pediatrics at Iwate Medical Center, Japan. Both the mother and infant showed signs of malnourishment. In addition, the baby was malformed. The physicians ruled out malnutrition or radioactive exposure as likely causes of the malformation.

During questioning, the woman mentioned that early in her pregnancy she had eaten dulcin because it was cheaper than sugar. Her dulcin consumption was estimated to be about 0.3 grams daily. It was thought that the synthetic sweetener probably was responsible for the infant's malformation.

In tests, dulcin was found to cause liver cancer in rats. The United States had banned its use in 1950, but it had continued to be used in Japan (Information from *Fact*, Nov–Dec 1966).

FROM LIMITED TO GENERAL USE

At first, cyclamates were used for special dietary purposes, mainly for diabetics and persons who needed to restrict their weight. Cyclamate-containing products carried the same legend as saccharin: "Contains (brand name inserted) as a non-nutritive, artificial sweetener which should be used only by persons who must restrict their intake of ordinary sweets." This statement, devised by the Food and Drug Administration (FDA) in 1941, was intended to allow the marketing of saccharin-sweetened foods to meet special needs, but at the same time, to serve as a warning to sugar-rationed wartime consumers that the food value of sugar was not present in such products. The statement, originally devised for saccharin, also was applicable for cyclamates.

In time, however, cyclamates (like saccharin) extended into *general* use. No clear definition existed regarding what constituted a dietary food. Processors labeled food products containing synthetic sweeteners as dietary merely because the omission of sucrose spared some calories. The dietary tag was used by packers and retailers as a promotional gimmick. The FDA proposed a new labeling regulation that, if enacted, would have limited the dietary claim to those foods or beverages with significantly reduced calories. But the agency was deluged by industry protests, and the proposed regulations remained in limbo for decades. Meanwhile, by sly editing, processors transformed the term "non-nutritive" into "no calories!" and the phrase "should be used only by" into "recommended for" The cautionary warnings had been converted into selling points.

FIRST CYCLAMATE SAFETY REVIEW

In 1955, the FDA requested a cyclamate review by the Food Protection Committee of the National Academy of Sciences (NAS). The committee judged that cyclamate's limited use was not hazardous at a low daily intake level for special dietary purposes. Although not challenging cyclamate's safety, the committee noted that the available scientific data did not assure safe unrestricted use by children, pregnant women, or persons who suffered from lower bowel diseases or other conditions. Despite this concern, the FDA took no action to limit cyclamate's use.

Cyclamates, less intensely sweet than saccharin, were used to mask saccharin's bitter aftertaste, and were combined with saccharin in many low-calorie soft drinks, canned fruits, baked goods, soups, bacon, puddings, salad dressings, toppings, syrups, chewing gums, and toothpastes, in addition to many tabletop uses to sweeten coffee, tea, breakfast cereals, and other foods.

In 1957, F. J. Helgren was awarded a U.S. patent describing the synergism of combined sweeteners. He noted that a 0.2 percent solution of sodium cyclamate had an equivalency of 3.2 percent the sweetness of sucrose. By combining the two solutions at a 10:1 ratio of cyclamate to saccharin, the equivalency of sweetness to sucrose increased to 16 percent in the blend. The synergistic effect was dramatic. The higher the percentages of cyclamate and saccharin in solution, the greater became the increase in sweetness.

Processors used this finding of synergism to advantage. By combining two or more sweeteners, they could use less of the sweeteners and achieve a higher degree of sweetness at lower cost. In addition, processors reasoned that by using lower amounts of several sweeteners, any potential health risks from individual sweeteners would be lessened. The first practical application of this synergism was the joining of cyclamate with saccharin as a viable commercial combination, and it became popular with processors. The practice continues, often with more than two sweeteners in the mixes.

The combination was used mostly in diet soft drinks. Unfortunately, the combination of cyclamate with saccharin did not reduce health risks, but rather increased them. Combining these two synthetic sweeteners likely caused many of the problems noted in the tests conducted during the 1960s. It was found that in combination the two sweeteners form a weak carcinogenic effect, and was found to cause cancer in rats. (In 1978, the National Research Council (NRC) would deem saccharin to be a weak carcinogen.)

The dulcin case (see inset on page 184) led Professor Ryoza Tanaka of the Iwate Medical Center in Japan to study the effects of synthetic sweeteners in fetal mice. He found that cyclamates affected the fetus at an even lower level than thalidomide, the drug that had caused gross malformations in the human fetus. Tanaka's findings, extrapolated from mice to humans, had important implications. The data suggested that a pregnant woman, drinking as few as two bottles of cyclamate containing-diet soft drinks daily, might reduce by 50 percent her chance of having a normal live birth.

THE ESCALATING CONSUMPTION OF CYCLAMATES AND SACCHARIN

The greatly increased use of cyclamates and saccharin began in the 1960s. Remember that cyclamates are about 30 times sweeter than sucrose and saccharin is about 300 to 500 times sweeter than sucrose. Thus, for every pound of cyclamate used, it had 30 times the sweetening power of sucrose; and saccharin from 300 to 500 times the sweetening power of sucrose.

In 1960, the average U.S. annual consumption per person for saccharin was 1.9 pounds; for cyclamates, 0.3 pounds. By 1968, saccharin use had increased to 5.0 pounds; and cyclamates reached 2.2 pounds. After the cyclamate ban, saccharin use rose steadily. By 1980, saccharin consumption had risen to 7.1 pounds. These figures were released in the United States Department of Agriculture's (USDA) "Sugar and Sweetener Report," in December 1976, February 1979, and December 1980. The USDA arrives at such figures by dividing the total population by total consumption. The total population includes segments who are nonusers of synthetic sweeteners, so that the *actual consumption by users probably is higher than the statistical figures given in these reports.*

SECOND CYCLAMATE SAFETY REVIEW

In 1962, the FDA requested another cyclamate safety review. Once again, the Food Protection Committee recommended that cyclamate use be restricted to special dietary foods. The committee raised questions about cyclamate safety for broader use, and stated in its report that "the priority of public welfare over all other considerations precludes, therefore, the uncontrolled distribu-

tion of foodstuffs containing cyclamates." The committee noted that cyclamates consumed at high levels exerted a laxative effect, more pronounced in
children than in adults. Studies had been limited to adult males, yet data were
needed of the effects on women, as well as on the embryo, infant, and young
child, all being vulnerable groups needing lower tolerances than adults. Little
was known about the way the normal body metabolized cyclamates, nor the
body's ability to metabolize these sweeteners by persons with chronic diseases such as diabetes, or disorders of the kidney or large intestine. The committee cautioned that "it is not unlikely that the per capita consumption of
cyclamates will exceed 5 grams [daily] if the potential usages of this material
in foods and beverages is exploited."

The FDA took no action to limit cyclamate use. According to estimates, the
suggested 5 gram limit could be exceeded readily by persons who ate various
foods sweetened with cyclamates and drank several bottles of diet soft drinks
daily—a dietary pattern that was not uncommon. Cyclamates were being
used, increasingly, by individuals as well as by processors in a greater variety
of foods and beverages, and used at higher levels. Food and beverage processors found that they could replace six dollars' worth of sugar with about sixty-
four cents' worth of cyclamates and achieve a similar sweetness level.
According to a 1963 industry survey, 31 percent of all households used synthetic sweeteners; before long, it would reach 75 percent.

The Food Protection Committee's reviews consisted of evaluating reports.
They did not engage in any research. The reviews were notably lacking in any
sense of urgency. Critics noted that the committee, dominated by individuals
with limited toxicological knowledge, tended to ignore possible subtle, long-
term risks. Furthermore, the group was either unable or unwilling to prod the
FDA into action to curb cyclamate use.

Meanwhile, the medical community began to express concern about the
uncontrolled and indiscriminate use of cyclamates. Rightly, doctors regarded
the cyclamates as drugs.

The *Medical Letter* (Sept 11, 1964) noted that safety data for cyclamates
were incomplete. The *Medical Letter* is an independent, peer-reviewed, non-
profit publication that offers critical evaluations of drugs to health professionals. Many questions regarding the toxicity of cyclamates and saccharin were
unknown and needed to be resolved. Yet no research studies of these synthetic sweeteners had been published in those years. The *Medical Letter* recommended a toxicological reappraisal of synthetic sweeteners in pregnant
women and their breastmilk, as well as in healthy individuals. It was known
that cyclamates and saccharin, consumed by pregnant women, are carried
through the placenta and delivered to the developing fetus. Also, these synthetic sweeteners are transported from a lactating woman into breastmilk fed

to the infant. According to the *Medical Letter,* continued promotion and extended cylamate uses "are regarded as against the public interest, and action by the medical profession, health authorities, and federal agencies to inform, and protect consumers is in order."

The *Medical Letter* was critical of the claims for synthetic sweeteners' effectiveness for weight control and deemed them "of questionable value." Also, the *Journal of the American Dietetics Association* reported no significant differences between weight losses in users and nonusers of synthetic sweeteners.

The Abbott Company answered charges raised by the medical publications and claimed that the safety research had already be conducted for cyclamates and the results had been filed with the FDA. The *Medical Letter* responded by saying that unpublished evidence was inadmissible because the confidential data had not been reviewed by independent scientists.

Abbott released the data. One study with laboratory animals purportedly demonstrated cyclamate safety by the absence of adverse effects on fertility, pregnancy, the fetus, and offspring. Another study, of only two weeks' duration, was offered as proof of absence of adverse effects in patients with impaired kidney function. Another study presumably showed that a large number of children who had consumed cyclamate showed no ill effects attributable to the sweetener. But at the time, the study was still being analyzed. Other studies included one that allegedly demonstrated that the substitution of cyclamates for sucrose was beneficial for weight reduction, and another that cyclamates were excreted from the body without pharmacological effects. The last conclusion, the *Medical Letter* asserted, was refuted by Abbott's own data.

The FDA reviewed the studies as well as new experimental data. In May 1965, the agency concluded that there was no evidence that, at present use, cyclamate posed health risks.

Pandora's Box Opens

Shortly after this announcement, several reports from different sources, questioned both the effectiveness and safety of synthetic sweeteners. Pandora's box was opening.

In June 1965, the claim for cyclamates as weight reducers was shattered. Instead of keeping weight down, *synthetic sweeteners appeared to increase the craving for sweets.* For diabetics who departed from their customarily prescribed low-carbohydrate diet and became dependent on synthetically sweetened foods, grave health consequences could result. Researchers at the Frances Stern Food Clinic in Boston had conducted studies on a hundred diabetic women to learn whether the synthetic sweeteners helped them to adhere to a carbohydrate-restricted diet. The conclusion was reported in *Medical World News* (Feb 13, 1970): "There is little basis for implying that adherence or nonadherence to a carbohydrate-restricted diet is related to the use of a noncaloric sweetener."

Medical journals began to publish clinical reports about cyclamate's effects on humans, demonstrating a wide range of symptoms, ranging from dizziness, rash, itch, ear fluttering, and photosensitivity, to sleep interference. Some reports suggested possible links between cyclamate consumption and retardation and mental aberrations in children. Cyclamates were found to interfere with many types of drugs: reducing the effectiveness of an oral antidiabetic drug; increasing the hypoglycemic effects of chlorpropamide (a drug used by diabetics); potentiating the diuretic effects of thiazide with resulting excessive potassium loss; potentiating the anticoagulant effect of coumarin; binding strongly to plasma protein and resulting in displacement of other drugs similarly bound; and reducing absorption of lincomycin, an antibiotic used to fight bacterial infection. Ironically, cyclamates were used to flavor some antibiotics.

By September 1965, hard evidence abounded about cyclamate's health hazards. Results were announced from a nine-month study in which rats were fed cyclamate at various dietary levels. Cyclamate decreased conception ability, produced stunted offspring, and caused litter deaths. Rats on a diet containing 5 percent cyclamate for nine months suffered a 12 percent growth impairment; and at 10 percent cyclamate, a 50 percent growth impairment. The female rats appeared to bear normal offspring, but a few months after the young were weaned, their growth rates declined. Fifteen percent of the offspring of rats fed 5 percent of cyclamate in the diet had stunted growth; and 35 percent of the offspring of rats fed 10 percent of cyclamate in the diet had stunted growth.

This research had been conducted by the Wisconsin Alumni Research Foundation (WARF), funded by the Sugar Research Foundation, which develops and supports basic and applied scientific research. The Research Foundation became the World Sugar Research Organisation, Ltd., in 1968. The Sugar Association, its parent organization, is composed of members of the sugar industry. This group had voiced concern over the surging popularity of synthetic sweeteners, which obviously were cutting deeply into sugar sales. Data from these studies were not challenged, but motives were.

The Sugar Research Foundation continued its funding of WARF's studies. By 1967, rat studies yielded very damaging evidence. Among other effects, cyclamates were found to cause increased adrenal weight and structural changes in the adrenal glands, testes, kidneys, and pancreas; pituitary gland damage; a high incidence of kidney stones; fewer white cells in the blood of male rats fed 10 percent cyclamate in the diet; and a retarded growth rate. Adult rats on restricted food and 5 percent cyclamate in the diet, produced a first litter that died within five days; and the second litter, within seven days. Conception was totally suppressed in adult rats fed 10 percent cyclamate in the diet.

Charges and countercharges followed. Abbott scientists reported that no other researchers were able to duplicate WARF's results and that, to date, definitive independent research had not been conducted.

WARF then released Japanese studies, reported earlier in the year, which showed teratogenic effects (inducing birth defects) in rats fed cyclamate during the first two weeks of pregnancy. Abbott scientists and FDA pharmacologists responded by saying that the Japanese studies had not been duplicated either.

Pressured by the sugar interests and by congressmen who had been prodded by this group, the FDA issued a contract to help fund animal and human cyclamate studies, led by Dr. Frederick Coulston at Albany Medical College in Albany, New York. The studies would receive additional financial support from two cyclamate producers (Abbott Laboratories and E. R. Squibb), and the Sugar Research Foundation. This study could hardly be viewed as independent research, but nevertheless would extend understandings. Cyclamates were to be tested with rats and monkeys, as well as with prison volunteers, for possible effects on enzyme systems, liver tissue, and reproductive functions including sperm production.

As the studies progressed, Coulston admitted that, as yet, cyclamate could be neither exonerated nor condemned. But, as Coulston was quoted in *Science News* (Aug 26, 1967), "use should be restricted to persons who really need to cut out sugar." Otherwise, Coulston said, "it is possible their use will get out of hand." The greatest concern was the wellbeing of children, who might drink four or five bottles of diet cola daily, along with synthetically sweetened candies and cookies. Up to that period, only one study with children had been reported, and the results were inconclusive.

Cyclamate's Toxic Breakdown Compounds

Another issue was given attention. Cyclohexylamine (CHA) is the basic chemical from which cyclamates are manufactured. CHA, used in many manufacturing processes, including insecticides, is known to cause dermatitis in contact with the skin; or, if inhaled, can lead to convulsions. This toxic compound can be present as an impurity in cyclamates, or produced during food processing in cyclamate-containing products. But nobody had suspected that CHA might be produced within the body, human or animal, after cyclamate consumption.

Originally, Abbott scientists claimed that cyclamates are not metabolized by the body, but simply are excreted as cyclamates. However, Japanese researchers reported that some individuals excrete CHA, indicating that the body can break down cyclamate into at least one metabolite. Later work at Abbott Laboratories, as well as at the Albany Medical College, supported the Japanese finding. CHA was found in the urine of about 12 percent of all persons consuming cyclamates, even at low cyclamate consumption levels. In animal experiments, the metabolite was found in cyclamate-fed dogs and in a strain of rats. Later, it was discovered that CHA, itself, breaks down further to an even more toxic form, dicyclohexylamine.

Early cyclamate studies showed chromosomal damage caused by CHA. CHA was not found to be carcinogenic, and cyclamates were not likely to cause cancer by damaging a cell's DNA. But no studies had been performed on mammalian cells, and none were conducted using CHA.

Data from animal tests suggested that high doses of CHA, fed over extended periods of time, caused testicular atrophy in rats and reduced their body weight. Also, Dr. A. J. Collings, who had conducted cyclamate research while working for Unilever for several years, had found CHA to be active pharmacologically. Collings was concerned that children would be at greatest risk because they were likely to consume more synthetic sweeteners than adults. Because of CHA's testicular effects in rats, the substance might be active in boys and young men who convert cyclamate to CHA.

It was not known why cyclamate metabolism is variable among humans, or even variable within the same individual at different times. About 75 percent of the population convert less than one-tenth of 1 percent or less of cyclamate to CHA, by microbial organisms present in the colon and the cecum (a pouch at the entry to the large intestine). The degree of conversion depends on the individual, not on the amount of cyclamate consumed, nor the length of time of its consumption. At the other end of the continuum, however, 1 percent of the population converts 60 percent or more of cyclamate to CHA. Of the CHA formed in individuals, at least 90 percent is excreted in the urine within two to four days after the cyclamate has been consumed.

What is not excreted in the urine has been absorbed in the gut. Little of it builds up in the blood or tissues. What is excreted in the urine has been metabolized, variably, in the gut but not metabolized by the liver. It is excreted unchanged by the kidney.

In rat experiments, CHA ingestion led to hypertension, with a transient dose-dependent rise in arterial blood pressure. This finding was worrisome, if CHA also leads to hypertension in humans. An individual who already is at cardiovascular risk because of high blood pressure, could be at even greater risk if the individual also happens to be a high converter of cyclamate to CHA.

Additional breakdown products from cyclamates have been identified in humans: cyclohexanone, cyclohexanol, and cyclohexylhydroxylamine. They probably result from CHA metabolism, because they are found in the urine when CHA is present.

Additional disturbing news reported by Dr. Marvin Legator, chief of the FDA's Cell Biology Branch, was that in both test tube and in animal studies, even moderate amounts of CHA caused significant amounts of chromosome breakage. Thus, the metabolite was a suspected mutagen. Also, it was a suspected carcinogen. The incidence of chromosomal breakage both in sperm and bone-marrow cells was related directly to CHA levels. The breaks, occurring mostly in one section of the chromosome, were likely to have carcinogenic effects. Chromosome breaks occurred at relatively low CHA levels, comparable to CHA levels metabolized by humans.

Other studies showed that CHA and cyclamates were transported from the pregnant rhesus monkey through her placenta into the developing fetus. Cyclamates were transported only to a limited extent, but CHA crossed the placenta readily.

At Albany Medical College, tests with prison volunteers who consumed cyclamate showed that nine out of twenty-four individuals were plagued by severe and persistent diarrhea; the higher the dose, the worse the condition. Of the twenty-four men, seventeen converted cyclamate to CHA. In some, the metabolite was found to cause vascular constriction and increased blood pressure. This feature was regarded as a potential risk for cardiac patients with high blood pressure who might be using cyclamates for weight control. Also, noted was a marked increase in protein-bound iodine. Patients could be misdiagnosed and treated for hyperthyroidism, but in reality, they might be showing signs of high cyclamate consumption.

Some scientists began to voice nagging questions. Why were these findings not found when cyclamates were tested originally, before being given approval? Were the initial tests incomplete, slipshod, or both? The drug companies and the scientific investigators had complied with FDA standards, but newer findings illustrated gaps and inadequacies of the testing protocols.

THIRD CYCLAMATE SAFETY REVIEW

In 1967, the FDA requested a third cyclamate safety review by the Food Protection Committee. Newer toxicological findings and increased cyclamate usage made it urgent to reevaluate. In 1957, the annual sale of cyclamates was two million pounds; by 1967, the annual sales had reached 15 million pounds. It was anticipated that the volume would reach 21 million pounds annually by 1970. Three-fourths of the entire American population was consuming nonnutritive sweeteners. The FDA had tolerated uncontrolled usage, and clearly the situation was out of control.

In 1968, the Food Protection Committee released its new review, and repeated the mantra that "totally unrestricted use of cyclamates is not warranted at this time." The committee noted the lack of specific information about consumption patterns: the range of intake by different age groups; the extreme upper levels of these ranges; and the number of individuals consuming the extreme upper levels. The committee found it difficult to evaluate some of the ongoing, incomplete toxicological studies, and recommended additional research to clarify existing animal studies. The committee repeated its past position, and added that intake of 5 grams (5,000 milligrams) or less per day of cyclamates by adults should present no risk, but the daily intake should be based on body weight. The committee suggested that an adult should consume no more than 70 milligrams (mg) of cyclamates per kilogram (kg) of body weight daily. This recommended limit of 70 mg/kg was less stringent than the limit set by the Food and Agricultural Organization and World Health Organization (FAO/WHO) of the United Nations, of 50 mg/kg of body weight.

The FDA scrutinized the new report because it contained implications for regulatory policy. Also, tardily, the agency had begun systematically to build some expertise concerning synthetic sweeteners. The FDA requested Dr. John J. Schrogie of its Bureau of Medicine and Dr. Herman F. Kraybill, of its Bureau of Science, and formerly at the National Cancer Institute (NCI), to evaluate the latest safety reviews. After their reviews, Schrogie and Kraybill judged the new report to be superficial. They were quoted by Philip Boffey in *The Brain Bank of America: An Inquiry into the Politics of Science* (McGraw-Hill, 1975) by describing the report as:

> . . . a largely uncritical review of the available material. Conclusions of the studies are included without proper regard for the quality of methodology originally used. Studies lacking adequate statistical design are given equal weight with sounder studies; many clinical and epidemiological studies yielding questionable conclusions are included. Possibly erroneous results gain added stature and interpretive errors are perpetuated.

Schrogie and Kraybill suggested that the committee had placed undue reliance on usage figures supplied by an industry survey that was "fraught with great hazard of error," and they charged that the committee chose to ignore some pertinent teratogenic and mutagenic studies.

According to Boffey, who had made a detailed study of NAS's cyclamate reviews, the only geneticist serving on the Food Protection Committee's 1969 review was Dr. James F. Crow, who had concluded that the evidence added up to a "fairly strong case that cyclamates represent a mutagenic hazard to man."

Boffey reported that Crow asked that his name not be included in the report because he could not endorse it. No hint of Crow's input appeared in the report. His views were not afforded space as a minority report, and the committee never acknowledged his dissent. Crow was listed merely as a "consultant" on the report, a designation that conveniently allowed the committee to imply that he had contributed to the report, but without his signature.

As a result of the new review, the FDA lowered its previous recommended upper limit for cyclamate that had been 5 grams daily for an adult. In April 1969, the agency urged individuals using cyclamates to reduce their limit to 3.5 grams daily for adults, and 1.2 grams daily for children. These limits were applicable to a one hundred-fifty-four-pound adult or a fifty-four-pound child. Because some diet soft drinks contained up to a gram of cyclamate in one 12-ounce bottle, young children easily could exceed the recommended upper limit. These revisions and suggestions simply confused the public. Consumers found it impractical, if not impossible, to control cyclamate use on the basis of label information on synthetically sweetened foods and beverages.

The FDA proposed a new regulation to require that such products include a declaration of cyclamate content in milligrams, along with a statement specifying the upper limits recommended for adults and children. This labeling recommendation was never implemented.

Labeling was a minor issue in the cyclamate affair, as controversy continued to rage over the scientific issues. The sugar interests kept sounding alarms about cyclamate's dangers. The Abbott Laboratories appealed to processors using cyclamates to assist in a public relations campaign to defend cyclamate's safety.

Meanwhile, Dr. George T. Bryan, an oncologist (tumor expert) at the University of Wisconsin in Milwaukee, had been investigating cyclamates. Bryan had devised a technique that was capable of demonstrating the cancer-inducing potential of substances. By implanting pellets containing the tested substance into the bladders of mice, the substance's cancer-inducing potential could be identified. The technique was highly sensitive, reproducible, and accepted as valid.

Bryan recognized that no attention had been given to the urinary bladder as an organ susceptible to cyclamate's cancer-inducing potential. Bryan conducted tests, using surgically implanted pellets composed either of sodium cyclamate and cholesterol, or solely cholesterol as a control. The bladder exposure to cyclamate was very brief because half of the compound disappeared from the pellets within about an hour. The animals in each group were allowed to live for thirteen months, then sacrificed and examined. Bladders of any animals that had survived more than 175 days were examined microscopically. The cyclamate-treated mice developed seven times as many bladder tumors as the control group. Bryan claimed that the induction of tumors in the bladders of the mice by pellet implants predicted the cancer-inducing property of orally ingested cyclamates. The results suggested that cyclamate is a cocarcinogen.

Although many scientists supported Bryan by endorsing the validity of the pellet implant technique, the FDA rejected it as controversial and inappropriate. The FDA argued that other studies had shown that a broad range of foreign substances—including glass beads, paraffin, calcium oxalate concretions, or wood particles—with no further treatment, implanted in the bladders of mice, could induce tumors.

Another controversial study that played a role in the FDA's decision regarding cyclamate's regulatory fate was a study by Dr. R. M. Hicks and her colleagues at Middlesex Medical School in London, England. In a controlled group of female Wistar rats, they implanted a known direct-acting bladder carcinogen, (nitrosamide N-methyl-N-nitrosourea, with the acronym MNU), in the bladders of the rats, using presumably noncarcinogenic low doses. Another group of rats received similar doses of MNU, followed by dietary intake of sodium cyclamate. None of the control rats developed bladder tumors, but 50 percent of the rats implanted with MNU followed by cyclamate feeding developed bladder tumors. The results suggested that cyclamates are tumor promoters. This finding raised concern that humans, exposed to low levels of carcinogenic substances—in cigarette smoke, for example—could develop cancer if, at the same time, they were consuming cyclamate-containing foods and/or beverages. Some attempts to replicate the Hicks' studies failed, and other studies contradicted the findings.

Disquieting Data Mounts

Within the FDA, disquieting data mounted. In addition to Legator's findings, Jacqueline Verrett, Ph.D., a FDA biochemist research scientist, had been working with 10,000 eggs containing chicken embryos injected with cyclamate ninety-six hours after incubation—a period of time corresponding to the critical early months in human pregnancy. Many of the hatched chicks were deformed, with twisted spines, underdeveloped eyes, dwarfed and missing wings and legs, and most frightening, flipper arms and legs—the familiar characteristics of thalidomide babies.

Early in October 1969, in a dramatic presentation, Verrett displayed some of the deformed chicks before national television cameras. She implied that pregnant women should avoid cyclamate consumption.

Verrett's presentation was followed swiftly by FDA Commissioner Dr. Herbert L. Ley, Jr. requesting NAS to evaluate Legator's new data and Verrett's findings. One researcher in the Department of Health, Education and

Welfare (HEW, which was later renamed Health and Human Services, HHS), as reported in *Business Week* (Oct 18, 1969), expressed fear that "panic would force the federal government to make decisions based on practical necessity rather than scientific evidence. Not only the industry but millions of Americans could suffer."

Events moved rapidly. Ley's request for a new NAS review prompted HEW Secretary Robert Finch to assail the FDA's varying cyclamate assessments, and he accused the agency of "waffling." While the FDA was attempting to formulate official actions, Abbott Laboratories sent new data to the agency showing that rats fed high-cyclamate levels during most of their lifespan developed cancer. This information was reviewed promptly by the National Cancer Institute (NCI) and by NAS's Ad Hoc Subcommittee on Cyclamate Safety.

On October 18, 1969, in a move that surprised the general public but not the cyclamate industry, HEW Secretary Finch and Surgeon General Dr. Jesse Steinfeld called a press conference. They invoked the Delaney Clause, and ordered cyclamates removed from GRAS, and reported that they were initiating a banning procedure, with an orderly market phaseout of cyclamates by February 1, 1970. The United States ban was followed by similar bans in Great Britain, Canada, Sweden, and elsewhere.

Cyclamate was the first case for which the Delaney Clause was invoked. The Delaney Clause, included in the Food, Drug and Cosmetic Act as amended in 1958, provides that "no additive shall be deemed safe if it is found to induce cancer when ingested by man or animal, or if it is found, after tests which are appropriate for the evaluation of the safety of food additives, to induce cancer in man or animal."

The Delaney Clause was named after U.S. Representative James A. Delaney (D-NY) who had chaired a committee, Chemicals in Food Products, that held protracted hearings from 1950 to 1958. The committee's work culminated in the Delaney Clause being inserted into the 1958 amendment to the Food, Drug, and Cosmetic Act, and later into the Color Additive Act, amended in 1960.

When the committee proposed that the Delaney Clause be incorporated into the amended legislation, it was opposed both by the FDA and by industry groups, but supported by the scientific and medical communities. George P. Larrick, the commissioner of the FDA, opposed any mandatory carcinogenic testing and refused to admit that cancer causation should receive any special mention. Industry opposed the clause, which would necessitate costly testings, possible bannings, and loss of public trust.

The FDA reluctantly agreed to include the clause in the proposed 1958 amendment only after Delaney threatened to block the FDA's own bill from coming to a vote. Industry charged that the clause was "rigid" and "unscientific," and it "worked against the broad public interest." Industry falsely charged that the clause allowed for "no scientific judgment of the results of research." However, cancer experts contended that the clause allowed "much room for the exercise of scientific judgment" and that "no one at this time can tell how much or how little of a carcinogen will be required to produce cancer in any human being."

Originally, the FDA had been established to protect the public from harmful substances in consumer goofs. Yet the agency never supported the Delaney Clause, the purpose of which was similar to the agency's original purpose. Both the FDA and the industries likely to be affected by the Delaney Clause recognized that it would be difficult to get rid of the loathsome legislation. The public regarded the Delaney Clause as beneficial, and rightly so.

Reluctantly, the FDA invoked the Delaney Clause with cyclamates, and then with DES (diethylstibestrol). When saccharin qualified for being banned under the Delaney Clause, the FDA devised a clever means of circumventing the legislation (discussed in Chapter 12). The FDA's accommodation allowed industry to live with a defanged regulation.

Due to the FDA's spineless policy and inept fumblings with the cyclamate issue, Commissioner Ley was replaced. On his last day in office, Ley held a press conference. He was quoted in the *New York Times* (Dec 30, 1969) as saying candidly, "The thing that bugs me is that the people think the FDA is protecting them. It isn't. What the FDA is doing and what the public thinks it's doing are as different as night and day."

There was more fallout, Verrett, who had conducted the chick egg experiments, was chastised for "going public" with the findings. After working fifteen years for the FDA as a research scientist, she had to leave. Later, she would coauthor a book, *Eating May be Hazardous to Your Health: The Case Against Food Additives* (Simon & Schuster, 1974). Verrett claimed that, if anything, "the situation today is worse precisely because we now know much more about the dangers of food additives, and less protective action is being taken. It seems that our government protectors have simply dug in, hoping to weather out what an FDA official once called the 'dangers of rampant consumerism.'"

Verrett had contended that chick embryo studies, like other animal studies, although far from being foolproof, nevertheless were useful conducted along with mammalian tests. Verrett felt that chick embryo studies should not have been ignored, yet frequently they were.

The NAS-NRC cyclamate reviews came under sharp criticism. A "special interest" charge was made by author Philip M. Boffey in *The Brain Bank of America*. When asked to judge food additive safety, such as cyclamates, Boffey charged that NAS-NRC "continuously acted in the interests of the food industry," and "downplayed the likelihood of such long-term hazards as cancer, genetic defects, and birth defects." Boffey continued:

> No one has charged that committee members are guilty of blatant conflicts of interest in the sense that they profit directly from the recommendations they make. Rather, the complaint is that the committee members are just a bit too close to industry—too sympathetic to its problems—to permit objective judgment in a situation where the economic stakes are high and the scientific advice is subject to various interpretations.

Another reason for the Food Protection Committee's "leniency" Boffey explained, "is that it has long been dominated by scientists who tend to be more concerned about immediate acute effects than about long-term chronic effects." Also,

> The Committee's panels have seldom included anyone primarily expert in mutagenesis or teratogenesis, and the members expert in carcinogenesis have been a small minority. Yet in many cases the most alarming evidence of hazards associated with a particular chemical has involved precisely these long-term effects.

A BAN ON CYCLAMATES AND THE AFTERMATH

In retrospect, cyclamates should never have been granted GRAS status, which automatically bestowed the privilege of exemption from classification and regulation as a food additive. If cyclamates had been classified as a food additive, safety tests would have been mandatory. At an early stage, when questions had been raised concerning cyclamate safety, the FDA had an obligation to remove cyclamates promptly from GRAS. If the agency had acted properly, the ban would have been instituted decades earlier, because cyclamates lacked the necessary proof of safety. Countless numbers of people would have been spared from needless carcinogenic exposures as well as other damaging effects.

The cyclamate ban announcement resulted in wild stock market trading. Frantic speculators attempted to unload diet product stocks before prices dropped precipitously, and to buy sugar stocks before their prices soared. Heavy cyclamate consumers went on shopping sprees and hoarded cyclamate-sweetened foods and beverages.

Barron's newsweekly magazine, which typified most reactions from the business and financial communities, termed the federal actions as "arbitrary, unreasonable, and capricious" (Nov 23, 1969). *Barron's* found a few scientists who branded HEW's ban as a sweeping decree after a "hurried meeting" and "on the basis of experiments employing only twelve rats." These charges were patently untrue.

Earlier studies had suggested a link between cyclamates and cancer, but the warning signs had been ignored. At least twenty-one published cyclamate studies, mainly from 1951 to 1968 and reviewed by NAS's committee had revealed cancerous effects. However, the committee judged that the tumors formed not much more frequently in cyclamate-fed rats than in the controls, and on that basis, dismissed the findings as insignificant.

Among the twenty-one studies was a crucial one conducted by the FDA from 1948 to 1949. A large number of rats were fed a cyclamate-saccharin mixture over a two-year lifespan. When the 1969 bladder cancer report was received from Bryan, the FDA assigned two pathologists from its Bureau of Science to reexamine the earlier data and microscopic tissue slides. They had concluded that, indeed, there *had* been reason to suspect cyclamates of cancerous effects as early as the late 1940s. However, the warning signs were not shared with others. The NAS's committee had never been given specific data from these early studies regarding the incidence or variety of possible tumors in the rats. Thus, the committee's suspicions had not been aroused,

Another study, from 1951, demonstrated that cyclamates could induce ovarian tumors. This study was available to NAS's committee, but was not released publicly until after Finch's October 18, 1969 cyclamate ban order. Again, the warning sign had not been shared.

A month after Finch's actions, the economic blow was eased for industry. By legal legerdemain, the FDA would no longer classify cyclamates as food additives but would reclassify them as drugs. This deft maneuver skirted the Delaney Clause, which is applicable to foods but not to drugs. Cyclamates now would be considered as over-the-counter nonprescription drugs and labeled as drugs. Cyclamates could be used in foods and as sugar substitutes in liquid and tablet forms, with labels stating the cyclamate content of average servings. The ban against cyclamate use in diet soft drinks and other beverages would remain in effect.

This attempt at reclassification backfired. The FDA was willing to approve cyclamates and cyclamate-containing foods if companies filed "abbreviated" new drug applications, waiving safety and efficacy proof customarily required. Representative L. H. Fountain (D-NC), who chaired the congressional hearings on cyclamates, declared such approval as "ill advised" and illegal. Fountain demanded that such approval be rescinded promptly.

Safety had not been proven for cyclamates. On the contrary, by then, there was a sizable body of evidence demonstrating harmfulness. Efficacy had not been proven. Evidence showed that cyclamates lacked value in weight-control programs. Dieters depending on synthetic sweeteners tended to make up for the calories not present by consuming extra portions of foods and beverages. Such individuals lost weight no faster than those who used sugar in moderation.

Early in 1969, rat experiments in Holland demonstrated that cyclamates *stimulated* the appetite and led to weight *increase*. As reported in *Nature* (Jan 4, 1969), the researcher concluded, "if this is true for man, then weight reduction will be more difficult if the diet contains cyclamates."

With neither safety nor efficacy proven, the FDA was forced to reimpose a total cyclamate ban, issued on August 14, 1970, to become effective September 1, 1970. A nationwide survey conducted during the month after the cut-off date showed that half the stores were still selling foods and beverages containing the illegal cyclamates. The FDA took no vigorous action to enforce the order, and relied merely on voluntary compliance.

On October 8, 1970, the House Committee on Government Operations justifiably criticized sharply both the FDA and HEW for improper cyclamate regulation. The committee charged that by 1966 a genuine difference of opinion existed among qualified experts regarding cyclamate's safety, and by then, the FDA had the obligation to withdraw GRAS status for cyclamates and to ban them.

The committee charged that:

The FDA failed for several years to protect the public against possible health hazards associated with cyclamates despite a clear legal obligation to do so. The FDA aggravated the consequences of its inactions by permitting the use of cyclamates in food to reach massive proportions. The FDA attempted to permit the continued marketing of cyclamate-containing products through illegal regulations and procedures. The decision to permit the continued marketing of cyclamate-containing products was made by the Secretary of HEW, not by the FDA. The HEW used an outside advisory body to make recommendations on matters that had already been decided, involving a basic issue which the advisory body was not qualified to decide. NAS-NRC panels that considered the safety of cyclamates in food were not asked to provide the basic information necessary for determining if cyclamates should remain on the GRAS list.

For anyone not following the cyclamate developments closely, the committee had provided an excellent summary. After firing these volleys, the committee recommended that in the future, the FDA and the HEW should "take prompt and effective actions to guard against repetition of the mistakes made in the regulations of cyclamates." Perhaps the committee already had a premonition that the two agencies would repeat the same folly in their future handling of the saccharin issue.

The committee further recommended an immediate and objective review of any GRAS list substance whenever its safety was questioned, and its prompt removal from the list. The agencies were advised to confine their use of scientific advisory bodies to consideration of clearly defined issues that are within the competence of such bodies. Also, such groups should not be asked to advise on matters that the regulatory agency, the FDA, has the capacity to resolve. Food and drug safety questions should be decided "strictly in compliance with legal and scientific requirements and without regard to economics and other extraneous considerations." But economic considerations did continue to play a role.

Post-Ban Activities

Shortly after the total ban, producers of cyclamate-containing foods and beverages attempted to recoup their losses through different strategies. They dumped products for whatever prices they could get. Or, they donated them to charity and were rewarded with substantial tax savings. Throughout America, high mounds of diet soda were stacked in thrift shops, frequented mainly by the poor. In developing countries, the poor also became the recipients. One shipment of 60,000 cases of a low-calorie drink, intended for calorie-starved Laotian refugees, was stopped by the action of a U.S. congressman who considered the gesture to be "cheap and cruel." Taxpayers would have picked up the $42,000 shipping cost and the company would have enjoyed a tax break, according to the account in the *Wall Street Journal* (Aug 7, 1970).

By 1972, in response to activity described as "an enormous amount of lobbying," a bill was introduced in the U.S. House of Representatives to reimburse manufacturers and distributors who claimed economic losses caused by the cyclamate ban. The bill opened the way for claims estimated between $120 million and $500 million against the federal government. The bill proposed that the government should pay damages, even though no one charged the government with any wrongdoing. The premise posed by the processors, who had used cyclamates in their products, was that they had relied in good faith on cyclamate's safety because of GRAS status. The bill passed in the House, but was killed in committee hearings in the Senate. However, a decade later, in the summer of 1980, the California Canners and Growers (CCG), a farm cooperative of nearly two thousand members, filed suit seeking damages due to financial losses that they claimed to have suffered from the 1969 ban. The CCG won the first battle to obtain compensation. The U.S. Claims Court recommended that CCG be awarded $6.4 million because the FDA "misrepresented" scientific evidence in determining that cyclamates were carcinogenic. The amount could go as high as $8.2 million if an amount for interest or equity for loss of capital was included.

At the time of the ban, about 57 percent of CCG's inventory consisted of cyclamate-sweetened fruits. The Diet Delight line of products held the largest market share for sugar-free canned fruit—over half of CCG's inventory. In 1983, the company had filed for bankruptcy.

Bills introduced both in the Senate and the House permitted compensation to growers, manufacturers, packers, and distributors for damage suffered under the cyclamate ban. However, no money was paid. There would have been a long road ahead. The federal government could appeal the court's decision. If no appeal was filed, the ruling would revert to Congress, which might approve, reject, or modify it. In the case that the decision would be appealed, it would go to a review panel of three judges, and then back to Congress. Ultimate recompense appeared dim.

Attempts to Reinstate Cyclamates: Petitions and Rejections

After the cyclamate ban, studies were continued in various research laboratories, here and elsewhere. In newer tests, researchers used more animals, different species, higher cyclamate doses, and longer test periods than in the earlier studies. The newer tests failed to confirm earlier research implicating cyclamates as carcinogens, but other adverse effects were newly discovered.

By 1973, the Calorie Control Council (CCC) spearheaded a drive to lift the ban and put cyclamates back into production and marketing. The CCC is an international association representing the low-calorie and diet food and beverage industries, including American and Japanese saccharin manufacturers, soft drink companies, and pharmaceutical companies. The drug industry followed these activities with interest.

In November 1973, Abbott Laboratories petitioned the FDA to reinstate cyclamates as safe additives. By mid-February 1974, Abbott had complied with the FDA's request to submit data by dramatically placing into public view at the Hearing Clerk's office some 400 studies, bound in seventeen weighty volumes, along with supplementary binders. The FDA assigned a team of toxicologists, nutritionists, and chemists to review the voluminous data before passing them along to NAS's Food Protection Committee. Both Abbott and the FDA were smarting from the stings of earlier criticism. This time, they attempted to have thorough analysis and review.

By September 1974, the FDA rejected Abbott's petition, on grounds that the data were "inconclusive." The FDA reported that, as yet, questions about cyclamate's cancer-causing potential were still unresolved. The FDA requested further scientific studies.

By March 1975, the FDA reversed its position and told Abbott that it need not conduct additional time-consuming safety tests. The agency would make a decision based on the available evidence. At the same time, the FDA requested NCI to convene a blue-ribbon panel to conduct a fair evaluation of all evidence bearing on cyclamate's cancer-causing potential, and to make recommendations. Abbott interpreted this news as encouraging.

Ten days later, at a forum convened by NAS, and sponsored by the U.S. Public Health Service (PHS), the FDA, and the HEW, further heartening news followed. The NAS President, Dr. Philip Handler, charged that the experiments leading to the cyclamate ban were badly designed, inconclusive, and should not have warranted any action at that time.

Scientists selected to participate in the NAS forum were mostly proponents for cyclamate reinstatement, and the well-publicized meeting was hardly representative of a balanced view. Handler himself had served from 1964 to 1969 as a member of the board of directors of a company that used cyclamate in its brand of sweetening agents. Handler had told Boffey, who was critical of NAS's industry affiliations, that he had resigned his directorship and sold his company stock when he assumed presidency of NAS in 1969. Handler also said that the company had been marketing the sweetener before he joined the board, and his role was to maintain liaison with the research departments that were not involved with cyclamates. Nevertheless, Handler was associated with a company that had participated in the phenomenally increased cyclamate use, and Boffey had concluded that Handler presumably "retains the conditioning of a corporate director who would tend to regard the products of his industry as beneficial and efforts to ban them as unreasonable."

The NCI's panel could not reach a unanimous agreement in its review. By the middle of December 1975, in a preliminary conclusion, three of the five members agreed tentatively that cyclamate is not a *strong* carcinogen. The remaining two hedged, stating that cyclamate may be a *weak* carcinogen and there is no way to prove its absolute safety. What people do not realize is that weak carcinogens are not readily detected, and for this reason, long and widespread exposures to them are apt to occur. Strong carcinogens, being more readily identified, have a better chance of being withdrawn more promptly, and exposures to them are likely to be briefer and affect fewer people.

By January 1976, the panel report went to NCI's director, who, after reviewing it, sent it to the FDA by mid-March. After a nine-month review, the final report concluded that evidence from animal studies did not establish the carcinogenicity of cyclamates or CHA.

While the panel was deliberating, FDA scientists were reviewing other cyclamate studies. The agency concluded that large amounts of cyclamate in test animals can affect their growth and reproduction; cause testicular atrophy; and elevate blood pressure. Even if there is no cancer issue, based on these additional findings, any permissible safe level would be too low for practical use of cyclamate as a sweetener.

On May 11, 1976, the FDA advised Abbott to withdraw its petition to readmit cyclamates. Subsequent studies suggested that cyclamates, at doses approximating ordinary uses, caused human genetic damage.

Abbott informed the FDA that it would *not* withdraw its petition. This defiance forced the FDA to issue a formal denial of the petition, after which Abbott could request a public hearing. For the next two years, like a soap opera, protracted hearings were held. Repeatedly, Abbott petitioned, and repeatedly, the petitions were denied.

By 1978, an FDA administrative law judge, Daniel Davidson, reviewed the case and concluded that cyclamates had not been proven safe and therefore the ban could not be lifted. Nevertheless, Abbott continued to re-petition.

On February 4, 1980, Judge Davidson again rejected Abbott's petition, reiterating the statement that the data did not prove safety. Once more, Abbott re-petitioned, and again, the petition was denied. By then, newer evidence including mouse and rat studies showed increased numbers of tumors in the lung, liver, bladder, and lymph systems in cyclamate-fed animals. Other animal studies showed that cyclamate could affect chromosomes adversely, suggesting that the sweetener could cause inheritable genetic damage and could lead to Down's syndrome, mental retardation, and altered metabolism.

In 1982, during the Reagan Administration, Marian Burros, food writer for the *New York Times*, noted that the FDA would be more receptive than previous administrations to regulatory changes. In the altered political climate, once again, Abbott, accompanied by the CCC, petitioned the FDA for cyclamate approval. The petitioners submitted some seventy-five additional new studies that allegedly confirmed cyclamate's safety.

Examining Cyclamate's Carcinogenicity

In response to the third petition, the FDA's Center for Food Safety and Applied Nutrition (CFSAN) formed a Cancer Assessment Committee (CAC) specifically to address the carcinogenic aspect of cyclamates. The CAC was a twelve member panel, consisting mostly of individuals sympathetic to cyclamates. One panel member was Dr. Robert V. Morgan, of Environmental Health Associates in Oakland, California. Morgan described the company as a "contract research and consulting firm that accepts money from industry, government and unions." Another member was William Havender, Ph.D., at the University of California in Berkeley, who described himself as a "private consultant." He had served on the Board of Scientific Advisors of the American Council on Science and Health (ACSH), a group funded generously by food and chemical interests, including Abbott and other pharmaceutical companies manufacturing cyclamates. Havender had, in the past, been strongly critical of the cyclamate ban. The CCC, one of the petitioners for reinstating cyclamates, admitted to paying the travel expenses of Drs. Morgan and Havender to attend and participate as speakers at the CAC meeting.

Another panelist was Albert C. Kolbye, Jr., president of the Nutrition Foundation, an organization comprised of major food processors and refiners. The foundation's board of trustees read like a "Who's Who" of the food industry. Kolbye, both a physician and attorney, formerly had been at the FDA.

Other pro-cyclamate panelists included James L. Emerson, D.V.M., Ph.D., who was affiliated with the Coca-Cola Company and the International Life Sciences Institute (ILSI), an organization that represents concerns and interests of the food industry. Another was Robert H. Kellen, president of CCC, the co-petitioner in Abbott's request to reinstate cyclamates.

Chairman of the CAC panel, Dr. Richard J. Havel, was director of the Cardiovascular Research Institute of the University of California in San Francisco. His expertize was not carcinogenicity, the issue CAC had been asked to address. Havel also admitted that the panel lacked any expert in teratogenicity, an issue closely associated with carcinogenicity and mutagenicity.

Of the twelve member panel, Rodney E. Leonard was the sole consumer representative. Leonard, executive director of the Community Nutrition Institute (CNI), decried the attempt to "rehabilitate" cyclamates by focusing narrowly on carcinogenicity, but ignoring unresolved issues such as chromosomal damage and birth defects. According to Leonard, the abrupt banning of cyclamates effectively had foreclosed the needed continuing study of cyclamate's teratogenicity and mutagenicity, as well as the issue of CHA. Leonard charged that the ban was a deliberate move by the administration to avoid having to confront another thalidomide-like controversy. He called the proceedings "another case in which the FDA manipulates the scientist . . . this committee is told that it can examine only the question of carcinogenicity, and only after the FDA has decided cyclamate is not a carcinogen." Leonard claimed that the panel was being asked merely to rubber stamp a pro-cyclamate decision that the FDA already had made internally, and he added "that's as stacked a hearing as I've ever attended." Leonard reported that:

. . . apparently tumors do occur, and that fact alone suggests that at a minimum, perhaps we should take the time to perform a new array of tests . . . the major question about cyclamate was not whether it causes cancer, but whether it causes birth defects and whether it breaks down chromosomes. The question is whether the chemical is a teratogen and a mutagen. If the scientific community chooses to avoid these issues, then it condones an injustice and denies its responsibility to insure that science is a servant of the public interest and not a handmaiden of the regulatory politics.

The Committee on the Carcinogenicity of Cyclamates, formed by NAS, convened a "public meeting" for July 31, 1984. The meeting had been announced in the *Federal Register*, a daily publication more apt to be read by Washington, D.C. politicians and industry-affiliated lawyers than by scientists residing outside the Washington, D.C. beltway. Also, limited notification was given to selected organizations, but notably failed to reach individuals whose input would have been valuable.

Four former FDA Commissioners, Drs. Charles C. Edwards, Alexander M. Schmidt, Donald C. Kennedy, and Jere E. Goyan, were *not* informed about the public meeting, and learned about it only after it had taken place. Yet all four had served at the agency during cyclamate deliberations. None of the men had been afforded an opportunity to explain or defend their actions.

Dr. W. Gary Flamm, who had served as the FDA's Director of the Office of Technological Sciences during the time of cyclamate deliberations had *not* been notified about the public meeting. Nor had Marvin M. Legator, Ph.D., who had served as the FDA's Chief of Genetic Toxicology, been informed of the public meeting. Yet, during Legator's work at the FDA, he had conducted studies on cyclamate-induced chromosomal aberrations. After learning about the public meeting of which he had *not* been notified, Legator remarked that "no one I would have expected to have seen attend an impartial hearing was heard from." At the time, Legator was professor of the Division of Environmental Toxicology at the University of Texas in Galveston. In an interview with *Medical Tribune* (Sep 5,1984) Legator asked rhetorically, "why is there all this hullabaloo, when it was the industry's own studies and their own interpretations that led to taking it [cyclamate] off the market in the first place?"

Another scientist *not* informed about the public meeting was John H. Turner, Ph.D., professor of biostatistics and human genetics at the University of Pittsburgh, in Pittsburgh, Pennsylvania. Turner reported that in the last five years there had been an "explosion of efficiency" in the field of toxicology testing, and the ability to extrapolate human risk from animal systems. He and other laboratory researchers, who might have made valuable contributions at the meeting, had not been informed.

The CAC had not been asked to assess the safety of cyclamate; solely its carcinogenicity. In 1985, after CAC members had spent more than a year reviewing all the existing studies on cyclamates and carcinogenicity, the panel concluded that the collective weight of the numerous studies "does not indicate that cyclamate by itself is carcinogenic." However, CAC noted that one or two rodent studies suggested that cyclamate might be a tumor promoter or a cocarcinogen. The CAC recommended that these studies should be repeated and that additional research should be conducted to relate such studies to human health.

The CAC did not review data relating to CHA and testicular atrophy, claiming that the issue was outside its charge. But, CAC recommended that the issue "would need to be considered in detail" before cyclamates could be approved for broad use. The CAC noted that "there have been no assays for mammalian cell DNA damage and gene mutation for cyclamates and no DNA damage tests for cyclohexylamine." The CAC recommended that these and "more cytogenic studies should be carried out."

The CAC concluded that "even if cyclamate were to exert only a weak carcinogenic effect, its use would alter risk in millions of people." There had been no investigations of human cancer sites other than the urinary bladder. Research had been focused on the bladder because cyclamate is absorbed by the bladder and intestine. CAC was unable to estimate what effect cyclamate had on other parts of the human body.

The NRC repeated some of CAC's recommendations for further studies to detect possible mammalian cell DNA damage and gene mutation induced by cyclamates.

Both Drs. Turner and Legator suggested three areas that NAS should consider before considering any reintroduction of cyclamate:

1. The significance of variations in metabolism need to be studied. About 70 percent of humans excrete it unchanged, but, about 30 percent of humans metabolize it into CHA, which can be toxic.

2. The teratogenicity of cyclamates should be examined. This had been a major concern at the time of the ban, but subsequently ignored, due to the sole focus on carcinogenicity.

3. Mutagenicity should be assessed, especially because improved testing techniques, could yield better data.

Currently, cyclamate is being used in some fifty countries worldwide. In Canada, where cyclamate was never banned, it is used widely in candies and chewing gums, and as a tabletop sweetener. In Europe, except for the United Kingdom where cyclamate is not permitted, the sweetener is combined with saccharin in diet beverages and in tabletop sweeteners, despite the earlier evidence about the danger of combining these two sweeteners. Cyclamates have a strong market niche in developing Asian countries, with its cost lower than aspartame.

CYCLAMATE IN LEGAL LIMBO

As of 2008, the petition to reinstate cyclamate in the United States remains in legal limbo. Meanwhile, other sugar substitutes dominate the market. The competition is among pharmaceutical giants such as Monsanto, McNeil, Abbott, Johnson & Johnson, and others. The major sugar substitutes are far more intense in their sweetness than cyclamate, and they are popular with many processors and consumers. Although cyclamate remains unapproved for use in the United States, the ban has not prevented its production and exportation from the United States to foreign markets. Occasionally, the FDA seizes products sold in the United States illegally because they contain cyclamate.

Chapter 12

SACCHARIN: SWEET, CHEAP, AND DETRIMENTAL

Artificial sweeteners may be the nutritional disaster of our time.
—GEORGE V. MANN, SC.D., M.D. *POSTGRADUATE MEDICINE,* JULY 1977

Saccharin was the first notable synthesized sweetener. It was discovered accidentally, and by current standards, due to sloppy procedures in a chemical laboratory. In 1879, Dr. Constantin Fahlberg, a graduate of the University of Leipzig, worked in a Johns Hopkins research laboratory under Dr. Ira Remsen. During his work on oxidizing *o*-toluenesulfonamide, Fahlberg synthesized *o*-benzosulfimide. One day, working with this compound in the laboratory, he munched on bread that tasted incredibly sweet. Suspecting that he had contaminated the bread, he analyzed the compound. He found that it was 300 to 500 times sweeter then sucrose, and named it saccharin. In 1880, Fahlberg and Remsen reported their discovery in the *American Chemical Journal.*

Shortly after, Fahlberg returned to Germany and obtained patents for saccharin and its commercial production methods. He obtained a U.S. patent in 1895, Fahlberg and his German coworkers began commercial production of sodium and calcium salts of saccharin. In the United States, in 1901, John F. Queeny founded the Monsanto Chemical Company in St. Louis, Missouri for the express purpose of manufacturing saccharin. Its commercial production began in 1902. Soon after, other American companies entered the market.

SUGAR REPLACER OR DRUG?

From the beginning, saccharin was regarded as a drug, possibly of limited usefulness for certain dietary purposes such as for diabetics. As early as 1890, a decade after saccharin was synthesized, the French Commission of the Health Association had decreed that saccharin was harmful, and forbade its manufacture or import. This ban was followed by the German government's action to limit saccharin's use as a drug, and expressly to forbid its addition to any foods or beverages. Similar regulations were enacted in Spain, Portugal, Hungary, and elsewhere.

In the United States, however, attempts to keep saccharin out of the general food supply were unsuccessful. American food and beverage processors favored the use of saccharin because it was cheaper, sweeter, and easier to handle than table sugar. By 1907, the American marketplace was flooded with saccharin-sweetened canned fruits and vegetables, candies, soft drinks, and bakery products.

Harvey Washington Wiley, M.D., who had conducted the unsuccessful campaign against glucose discussed earlier, attempted to keep saccharin out of the food supply. Wiley warned that "saccharin is a noxious drug and even in comparatively small doses it is harmful to the human system." He regarded the use of saccharin as a sugar replacer to be an adulterant of food as well as a deceptive practice.

Wiley served as chief of the Bureau of Chemistry at the U.S. Department of Agriculture (USDA). The bureau would later become a new agency, the Food and Drug Administration (FDA), with Wiley as its first Commissioner. At the FDA, Wiley initiated numerous actions against the food adulterators. Wiley brought action against Monsanto and presented what he considered to be satisfactory evidence regarding saccharin's harmfulness. But twice the case resulted in a hung jury. The ban was appealed, and hearings were held in the presence of President Theodore Roosevelt. One corn processor boasted that his company saved $4,000 in one year by using saccharin as a sugar replacer. Wiley shot back, "Everyone who ate that corn was deceived. He thought he was eating sugar, when in point of fact he was eating a coal tar product totally devoid of the food value and extremely injurious to health" (recorded later in Wiley's autobiography).

What followed was a celebrated exchange between Wiley and Roosevelt:

Turning to me in sudden anger the President changed from Dr. Jekyll to Mr. Hyde, and said. "You tell me that saccharin is injurious to health?" I said, "Yes, Mr. President, I do tell you that." He replied, "Dr. Rixey [Roosevelt's personal physician] gives it to me every day." I answered, "Mr. President, he probably thinks you may be threatened with diabetes." To this he retorted, "Anybody who says saccharin is injurious to health is an idiot."

Roosevelt's remarks broke up the meeting. According to Wiley, the incident was "the basis for the complete paralysis" of consumer-protective food regulations.

THE EARLY POLITICS OF SACCHARIN

In 1912, the federal government declared saccharin to be a drug. As a legal drug, saccharin was limited for use by diabetics, but not for healthy people. Later, its legal use was extended for special dietary foods.

Monsanto ignored the governmental restrictions and continued to manufacture and sell saccharin for general use. In 1916, the government brought charges, but the case was struck from the docket in 1925. By then, it had become apparent that no jury in St. Louis, Missouri would convict Monsanto of wrongdoing. The company was a powerful force in the community.

In 1911, Roosevelt ordered the establishment of a referee board of consulting scientific experts to review saccharin's safety. A fair evaluation might have been possible with unbiased scientists. But none other than Dr. Ira Remsen, co-discoverer of saccharin, was chosen to head the board and to select other members. Despite the glaring conflict of interest, Remsen did not recuse himself. He served and packed the board with cronies. Wiley viewed the board's composition as "the worst crowd of adulterators that ever infested a republic" (recorded in his autobiography).

The Remsen Board not only exonerated saccharin but usurped the functions and powers of Wiley's department. The board continued to hand down decisions that unraveled Wiley's accomplishments in protecting consumers against hazardous substances. Instead of regulating an increasing number of chemical additives that were being introduced into the American food supply—some of which were of dubious safety—the board removed most constraints.

Saccharin was *in*, and before long, Wiley was *out*. The Remsen Board's decisions cast a long shadow and ultimately bore some responsibility for many crucial issues that inevitably developed into major crises several decades later. For example, during World War I, as sugar was rationed and became scarce, saccharin use increased.

Judged by present standards, early saccharin safety tests were crude, unsystematic, and lacked controls. Nevertheless, many reports supported Wiley's evaluation.

SACCHARIN SUSPECT AS A CARCINOGEN

The first suspicion raised about saccharin's possible carcinogenicity came in 1948, in an FDA chronic toxicity test. In 1951, three FDA scientists reported that at some levels saccharin induced a high incidence of unusual cancer combinations. Inexplicably, the FDA ignored its own data, and saccharin remained GRAS (Generally Recognized as Safe).

EARLY WARNINGS OF SACCHARIN'S EFFECTS OTHER THAN HUMAN CANCER

In early reports, many from European medical and scientific journals, there were disturbing findings. Among them:

• One experiment demonstrated that saccharin was a protoplasmic poison. (Protoplasm contains the substances that constitute the living matter of plant and animal cells, and reveals the essential life functions of the cells.) Peas, first placed in a saccharin solution, failed to sprout. (*Pharmaceutisch Weekblad,* vol. 59, 1915)

• Saccharin was reported to induce cell proliferation and predisposed cells to cancer. (*British Medical Journal,* Oct 9, 1915)

• One-cell animals died in solutions of 1 part saccharin to 400 parts water. The stronger the saccharin solution, the less protein was digested. Saccharin inhibited the fat-digesting action of the pancreatic juices and possibly had poisonous effects on cells in the bloodstream and in tissues. Saccharin was found to be 12 times more toxic to one-cell animals than carbolic acid. The researchers concluded that extensive, prolonged human use of saccharin was unwise and objectionable, and should be prohibited totally from the food supply, and restricted for drug use. (*Archiv für Hygiene und Bakteriologie,* vol. 92, 1923–1924)

• Saccharin's adverse chronic effects in mammals were reported. (*Bollettino della Societa Italiana di Biologia Sperimentale,* vol. 11, 1936)

• Saccharin was linked to goiter symptoms, both in human clinical cases and in animal experiments. (*Bratislavske Lekarske Listy,* May 1938)

• Symptoms from saccharin use, reported in numerous medical journals, include hives, itching, nausea, sweating, swelling and blistering of the tongue, fluttering in the ear, lowered blood sugar, irregular pulse, and heartbeat. (*Journal of the American Medical Association,* Nov 1, 1965, Sept 4, 1967; *American Journal of Obstetrics & Gynecology,* Sept 15, 1971, Aug 15, 1972; *Cutis,* Jul 1972)

In 1955, the National Academy of Sciences (NAS) conducted its first synthetic-sweetener review. Interest focused mainly on the more recent sweetener, cyclamate. Saccharin was less scrutinized because its long-time use was apparently without ill effect. Yet, the FDA repudiates such evidence with long-time use with plant-derived sweeteners. Saccharin did not concern the panel. Earlier studies and reports were either discredited or ignored. In NAS's later reviews, in 1962 and 1968, a similar attitude prevailed.

In 1957, using a bladder pellet implant technique in a single limited experiment with twelve mice, researchers found that saccharin-containing pellets induced a significant incidence of bladder tumors. Despite this finding, saccharin remained GRAS.

In October 1969, the FDA announced that saccharin would be "restudied." By then, its use spanned more then half a century, yet very little valid information existed regarding its safety. An agency spokesman announced that some further testing was necessary to ensure that saccharin merits its "present clean bill of health." The FDA proposed that its scientists review all the scientific literature to learn what gaps in knowledge might still exist. The Monsanto Company provided the requested data to the FDA.

Dr. George T. Bryan, who had devised and used the pellet implant technique with cyclamate (discussed in Chapter 11) investigated saccharin using the same technique. At the end of November 1969, Bryan notified the FDA that saccharin-treated mice developed a high incidence of bladder cancer. By mid-January 1970, an FDA team visited Bryan's laboratory, reviewed all the slides and data, and confirmed Bryan's findings. Viewed microscopically, the saccharin-induced bladder cancers were qualitatively more severe than the cyclamate-induced tumors in Bryan's earlier studies. The tumors induced by saccharin were larger, appeared deeper in the bladder tissues, and apparently were in a more advanced stage. The tumors induced by saccharin were as malignant in appearance as ones induced by well-recognized powerful urinary bladder carcinogens used in experiments with mice, rats, or dogs.

Bryan acknowledged that a direct saccharin-cancer risk for humans had not yet been established. But strong suspicions had been raised. In *Science* (Jun 5,1970) Bryan cautioned that, "It may take years before it is known exactly how dangerous the substance is, and until then, its use should be restricted to those who need it for medical reasons."

Mainly due to Bryan's findings, the FDA announced in March 1970 that the agency had requested the NAS to review saccharin. After deliberating, by late July 1970, NAS's committee released its conclusions. Although newspaper headlines proclaimed, NO HEALTH HAZARDS FOUND IN SACCHARIN AND PANEL FINDS SACCHARIN SAFE, closer reading of the articles revealed the opposite. Far from exonerating saccharin, NAS's committee acknowledged that available information was incomplete, and urged further laboratory experiments. Questions needed to be answered, especially because cyclamates were unavailable (having been banned in 1969). As a result, it was likely that former cyclamate users would switch to saccharin, and thus increase both the number of saccharin users, and its total usage. Also, testing for effects in saccharin users would be confounded if previously, they had been cyclamate users.

The NAS's committee also wanted information on saccharin's effects with other drugs. Animal studies had shown that saccharin could interact with certain medications, including insulin. Diabetics might be at special risk. Also, it was found that saccharin crossed the placenta in the rhesus monkey during the late period of pregnancy, and was distributed to many fetal tissues. In contrast to saccharin's rapid excretion from the maternal kidney, saccharin cleared very slowly from the fetal kidney.

Despite these concerns, NAS's committee conclusions gave bland reassurances, picked up by the media that all was well. As reported in the *Washington Post* (Jul 23, 1970), NAS's committee announced that "on the basis of available information the present and projected use of saccharin in the United States does not pose a hazard."

SACCHARIN LOSES GRAS STATUS

Despite this reassurance, FDA still faced unresolved safety issues. By mid-September 1970, the FDA announced a possible restriction on saccharin use. The agency hoped to hold saccharin consumption to then-current or perhaps lower levels as a precautionary measure, should human health hazards be demonstrated at a later time.

In retrospect, FDA officials recognized that many difficulties in the cyclamate affair could have been avoided if, early on, the agency had imposed restrictions on the sweetener's use. The agency wanted to avoid repetition of this mistake. As with cyclamate, saccharin was being added to foods and beverages in increased and unregulated quantities. After the cyclamate ban, it had been thought that saccharin's distinctly bitter aftertaste automatically would limit its use, but processors had found compounds to mask the bitterness, and more saccharin was being added to products.

Nine months elapsed before the FDA finally suggested some curbing actions. On June 25, 1971, the agency proposed to withdraw GRAS status for saccharin and to place specific limits on its use. The agency formulated an unprecedented plan to place saccharin in a newly created category "provisional food additive." The FDA would use this new category when the safety of a food additive, already in use, such as saccharin, is questioned and some mechanism is needed to allow the additive to remain in use for economic reasons, while further studies are being completed. Saccharin would be "frozen" to existing levels of use pending the outcome of more research. Because completion of some ongoing research was expected to take as long as *ten years*, the interim status could serve as a convenient delaying tactic. No safety assurance could be given for the existing high level use, but the freeze would prevent economic losses, a consideration forbidden by safety laws.

Despite the fact that no "safe" level had been established, the FDA recommended that saccharin use be limited to about 1 gram a day for an adult, and proportionately less for a child. The limit—coincidental or not—matched the 1 gram daily intake of a heavy-saccharin-consuming, 150-pound adult. Most 16-ounce bottles of diet soft drinks sold at the time contained nearly 0.1 of a gram of saccharin, and some as much as 0.2 of a gram. Heavy users of saccharin-containing foods and beverages, who also used tabletop saccharin packets to sweeten foods and beverages, could easily exceed the recommended limit.

Furthermore, the recommended limit was based on a mathematical error in NAS's calculations, with a misplaced decimal point. The committee had intended to use a time-honored hundredfold safety margin, one hundredth of the dose level at which no apparent harm is observed in animals fed the substance. The error resulted in only a thirtyfold safety margin, considered by toxicologists as uncommonly narrow, but by the FDA as reasonably safe. Seven months elapsed before the FDA removed saccharin from GRAS status, effective February 1, 1972. The agency issued an interim provisional regulation restricting saccharin use pending completion of safety reviews. The FDA's actions were part of a more comprehensive program, long overdue, and mandated by the U.S. Congress, to review more than 600 GRAS list substances.

The FDA's actions with saccharin were precipitated by the nearly completed two-year rat feeding studies, conducted by the Wisconsin Alumni Research Foundation (WARF), and funded by the Sugar Research Foundation (later renamed the World Sugar Research Organisation, Ltd.). Preliminary reports indicated that some male rats fed saccharin at a 5 percent level in the diet developed bladder tumors that appeared to be malignant. If malignancy was confirmed by the government scientists and NAS's committee, the FDA would be obliged to invoke the Delaney Clause and ban saccharin. (For more information on the Delaney Clause, see page 196.)

In addition to the WARF studies, eleven more studies were nearing completion in the United States at the FDA and National Cancer Insitute (NCI), as well as in West Germany, Holland, and Canada. The various studies were being conducted with different animal species, including rats, mice, hamsters, and rhesus monkeys. Also, epidemiological studies had been launched in England, Germany, and the United States.

If saccharin were to be banned, the economic stakes would be high. In the early 1950s, only about 20,000 pounds of saccharin were used yearly in the United States. By 1976, the amount had escalated to about 7,000,000 pounds for food use, produced here and supplemented with substantial amounts imported from Japan and Korea. Only 15 percent of that total was used for

special purpose dietetic foods—the original intended use. Contrary to popular belief, only about one-third of all diabetics were using saccharin regularly.
The general public was consuming 75 percent of saccharin in diet soft drinks
and 10 percent as tabletop sweeteners. In restaurants it became commonplace
to have saccharin packets available along with sugar packets. Trade journals
reported that food service operators could cut sweetening costs by offering
saccharin. Restaurateurs were urged to use saccharin. "Promote iced tea
sweetened with (brand name) as a perfect diet drink, all year round. Patrons
love fewer calories while you save from high cost of sugar." Magazines read
by homemakers carried advertisements featuring recipes using saccharin,
"Sinlessly sweet snackin' squares" sweetened with saccharin, were described
as "unique, low-calorie snacks in fabulous flavors. So delicious they taste like
no-nos." Nonfood uses of saccharin as a flavoring agent appeared in tobacco
and cigarette paper; toiletry articles such as dentifrice, mouthwash, lipstick,
and cosmetics; and medical preparations including cough syrup, children's
aspirin, and antibiotics for pediatric use. Saccharin was used even in animal
food. At no point did the FDA engage in any public education campaign to
lower or discourage general saccharin uses as the Department of Health and
Human Services (HHS), did with tobacco use.

FDA FACES A DILEMMA

On February 27, 1973, the FDA announced that in its own carefully controlled
studies, suspicious bladder tumors were found in rats fed saccharin at 7.5 percent of the diet. It was thought that the tumors might have been caused by
impurities in the saccharin, or by mechanical bladder irritation caused by the
high saccharin level. The FDA announced that it would take no action, pending NAS's planned review of the study.

The FDA researchers also were examining saccharin for its possible reproductive harmfulness, such as birth defects and genetic changes. On May 21,
1973, the FDA reported that the pathology review of its study showed "pre-
sumptive evidence" that saccharin caused cancerous bladders in rats, and
retarded their growth rate.

The FDA was required to act by June 30, 1973. The agency had three choices. It could end, extend, or modify saccharin's interim status. Clearly, NAS
would be unable to meet this deadline with its review, because a deluge of
data was accumulating from various studies. The FDA extended the deadline.

One report showed that high saccharin doses exerted a cocarcinogenic
effect: that is, although saccharin, itself, had not initiated cancer, it had promoted the action of other substances that resulted in cancer. The researchers
suggested that mixtures of saccharin and other substances, such as cyclamate,

would be undesirable. Although cyclamates were banned in the United States, they still were permitted elsewhere.

Another study, reported in late 1973, by chemists at the National Institutes of Environmental Health Sciences (NIEHS), was the first to test saccharin with animals at average human use levels likely to be consumed, such as two tablets of saccharin in a cup of coffee. Saccharin used over long periods of time accumulated in the animals' bladders. The researchers recommended that regular saccharin users should discontinue saccharin consumption occasionally for several days to allow for tissue clearance. The FDA made no follow-up to this suggestion.

Some studies appeared to incriminate saccharin; others appeared to exonerate cyclamates. Rumors spread that saccharin might be banned and cyclamates reinstated. The FDA faced a dilemma. On one hand, a mistrustful public viewed the agency's actions as overdue, indecisive, and lacking in safety assurance. On the other hand, affected economic interests and heavy saccharin users viewed the agency's actions as arbitrary, capricious, precipitous, and unscientific. Whatever the decision, the agency would be faulted.

The lessons from the cyclamate affair made everyone wary of making decisions that might be viewed as hasty or taking actions before incontrovertible evidence was available. In evaluating saccharin, one NAS reviewer remarked to the *New York Times* (Nov 5, 1973) that "this is a job for a philosopher, not a scientist." He described his efforts as "an education in obtuseness—poor data derived from poor experiments."

For the new saccharin review, NAS's principal task was to examine unpublished reports of research conducted subsequent to the Food Protection Committee's 1970 review. After two and one-half years of deliberation, on January 9, 1975, the committee handed the FDA the long-awaited report, "Safety of Saccharin and Sodium Saccharin in the Human Diet." The conclusions were inconclusive: "The results of toxicity studies thus far reported have not established conclusively whether saccharin is or is not carcinogenic when administered orally to test animals."

The committee admitted that the results of the studies by the FDA and WARF suggested that bladder tumors were related to saccharin consumption, but they could not be interpreted as showing that saccharin, by itself, caused the tumors. At the same time, poorly designed tests failed to prove that saccharin is *not* a bladder cancer-inducer. The committee recommended additional studies to resolve the carcinogenic question as well as other safety issues, including saccharin's ability to be transmitted by the pregnant woman through her placenta into the embryo. Other issues involved the toxicological significance of saccharin's impurities; changes in urine composition after consumption of high saccharin levels; the relationship to bladder stones or calculi; and epidemiological studies relating cancer incidence with long-term saccharin consumption.

The FDA expected to examine NAS's review in order to determine, in consultation with the committee, what further tests were needed, and how they should be conducted. Meanwhile, the FDA would continue to allow saccharin to be available under its interim status.

Safety Issued Unresolved

Various groups sharply criticized NAS's review. FDA's director of Scientific Liaison charged that the overall tenor of the report left the unmistakable impression that a group of saccharin defenders were out to beat back the saccharin accusers, no matter what the cost to logic and scientific impartiality would be. Also, he disputed the committee's contention that saccharin could not be judged unsafe for humans on the basis of tumors in rat bladders. Yet, this was precisely how the judgment on saccharin's use as a food additive would be determined.

WARF's director also was critical of NAS's review, noting discrepancies in the committee's interpretation of WARF's findings. Only half of the saccharin-related tumors noted in WARF's study were included in the committee's review. The FDA took no action to resolve this discrepancy.

Numerous studies reviewed by the NAS were unpublished and unavailable to the public. Anita Johnson, Ph.D., then staff attorney for the Council for Responsible Nutrition (CRN), a dietary supplement trade group, attempted to examine eight negative studies that NAS had reviewed that allegedly disproved saccharin's carcinogenicity. Johnson found that two of the studies were inaccessible and four were uninformative and essentially useless. In two other studies, animal examinations were judged to be grossly inadequate. One study involved as few as seven animals; another had no microscopic examination of the bladder, although bladder tumors are not always visible to the eye. In one study, the control animals had such a high incidence of pituitary tumors that, according to NCI analysts, no chemical could be proven carcinogenic with such controls.

Multi-sites, with various organs as targets for cancer, is a common occurrence. Saccharin may be responsible for cancer in sites other than the bladder. In a preliminary analysis, Johnson found four positive studies. In a mouse study, overall tumors, primarily in the lung, increased significantly in the saccharin-fed animals. The study corroborated earlier FDA findings. In a Japanese study, saccharin-fed animals showed a dramatically overall high tumor incidence. In a Canadian study, there was a twofold increase in leukemias and lymphomas.

By the mid-1970s, even persons who wished to shun saccharin consumption, were exposed. Saccharin was used illegally by some food and beverage processors as a partial sugar replacer to offset high sugar prices. The FDA and state regulatory agencies were finding bakery products, candies, chocolate milks, frozen desserts, and other products customarily containing high levels of sugar to be adulterated with saccharin. The presence of saccharin was undeclared on labels, or cleverly disguised under the deceptive phrases of "flavoring" or "flavor enhancer."

Saccharin continued to enjoy its privilege of interim status for about six years, during which time its safety questions remained unresolved. During that time, at least twenty-three new studies indicated that saccharin might be carcinogenic.

Senator Gaylord Nelson (D-WI) charged that the FDA was violating the law by allowing continued saccharin use without a final determination of safety. He requested the General Accounting Office (GAO, later renamed General Accountability Office) to review the case. On August 16, 1976, GAO issued a report, "Need to Resolve Safety Questions on Saccharin," and urged the FDA to make a final decision. The GAO stated that the continued interim status:

> . . . seems contrary to the Food and Drug Administration's intent of permitting use of such additives for a limited time. Extended use of a food additive, such as saccharin, whose safety has not been established and for which a question of carcinogenic potential has been raised could expose the public to unnecessary risk.

The GAO expressed concern that the narrow safety margin of only thirty-fold was questionable, in view of many doubts that had been raised about saccharin's cancer-causing potential. The GAO recommended that authorized levels for food use should be based on the higher, more generally accepted hundredfold safety margin.

The GAO found that the impurity in commercial saccharin, similar in chemical structure to acknowledged carcinogens, was being permitted at levels much higher than necessary. With good manufacturing practices, a lower level could be achieved. The FDA had set the impurity tolerance level at 100 parts per million (ppm) based on industry's capability. But newer technology made it possible to reduce the level lower than 50 ppm, even as low as 3 ppm to 1 ppm. The GAO recommended that the permitted impurity level be required to be reduced to the lowest achievable one.

The GAO recommended that FDA *promptly* reassess its justification for saccharin's continued use, terminate its interim status, and issue a final regulation that either would continue, or ban its use.

Despite the GAO's call for prompt action, the FDA decided to follow its original intention of holding off any final decision until the completion of more studies by 1977 or possibly 1978.

Meanwhile, preliminary results of a Canadian study showed that saccharin's impurity could cause an increased incidence of bladder stones, as well as an abnormal increase in cell numbers.

On January 6, 1977, the FDA took action to restrict the impurity in saccharin to 25 ppm. In setting this limit, the agency admitted that it lacked any method capable of detection at this level.

FDA PROPOSES BAN

Ultimately the smoking gun was produced, with the long-sought conclusive evidence. The Canadian Health Protection Branch had undertaken far-ranging saccharin studies that had begun in February 1974. By 1977, one study showed "unequivocal" proof of saccharin's cancer potential. Three out of 50 male rats fed saccharin at 5 percent of their diet developed malignant bladder tumors; the female rats did not. However, of the offspring of the female rats, also fed saccharin, twelve males and two females developed bladder tumors. The studies indicated that saccharin, not its impurity, was responsible for the malignant tumors.

On March 7, 1977, FDA obtained the preliminary results of the Canadian data. Two days later, the FDA and the Canadian agency jointly announced actions that would lead to saccharin bans in both countries. The FDA invoked the Delaney Clause.

The FDA announced that the Canadian data did not indicate "an immediate hazard to public health" and therefore the agency would not consider any recall of existing products to be necessary. However, the FDA encouraged saccharin manufacturers to discontinue production. The agency announced that it would prepare documents as soon as possible—in thirty days or less—to propose the ban, to be followed by the customary sixty-day period for public comment and reaction.

Reactions were immediate. The Calorie Control Council (CCC) called the FDA's action "an example of colossal government overregulation and disregard of science and the needs and wants of consumers."

A major packer of saccharin-containing tabletop packets called the proposed ban "an outrageous and harmful action based on flimsy scientific evidence that has no direct bearing on human health. To act on the basis of one questionable experiment creates senseless damage to the public and to a two-billion-dollars-a-year industry involving thousands of jobs." In addition, the FDA received countless telephone calls and communications from irate individuals who demanded that saccharin be kept on the market. A spokesman for the American Diabetes Association warned that the ban could have "very grave effects for the 10 million America diabetics" (even though as mentioned earlier, only about one-third of diabetics used saccharin).

Consumer organizations and activists, as well as many scientists and physicians, supported the FDA's actions. The Canadian Diabetes Association, the Canadian Medical Association, and surprisingly, even a spokesman for the Canadian soft drinks industry, supported the Canadian action.

"If society is to make progress in preventing cancer, then the Food and Drug Administration should be commended, not condemned, for banning saccharin," reported Dr. Charles F. Wurster, an environmental scientist, to the *New York Times* (Mar 20, 1977). Wurster noted that near hysterical criticism was directed, "not at the cancer hazard, but at those who would protect us from it and even at the law they upheld." He wrote that a misleading motion was being circulated that saccharin had been used safely for decades without inflicting human harm. Most cancers are caused by environmental factors, yet only few human carcinogens are identified. The exact cause of the overwhelming majority of cancers remains unknown. Developed tumors do not bear identification tags naming the substances that, decades earlier, induced their cancer development. Saccharin may cause many cases of cancer, yet we have no way to establish the fact with certainty. In the human population, very large numbers of people are exposed to low levels of chemicals, but the impact of seemingly low doses may not be low for a carcinogen.

Three misleading statements made by saccharin proponents were repeated endlessly. Even currently, these canards continue to be used, not only regarding saccharin, but applied to many other substances.

1. *Humans would need to drink about 875 diet soft drinks or chew 6,700 saccharin-containing bubble-gum sticks daily to equal the saccharin dose given to the test animals.*

The statement has no scientific credence. A review of ten rodent feeding studies by a NCI pathologist showed that doses as low as *one-hundredth of one percent* saccharin induced cancer in a wide range of experimental conditions. This amount corresponds to about one and a half cans daily, not 875. Also, as Dr. George T. Bryan remarked, "whether you drink one can of artificially sweetened pop or (many) cans, you're at risk from the first drink onward," quoted in *Capital Times* (Madison, Wisconsin, Mar 21, 1977). Bryan's statement was confirmed by Dr. Richard Bates, FDA's Commissioner for Science, who testified that as little saccharin as is contained in just one can of diet pop could induce cancer in rats. Bates statement was reported in the *New York Times* (Mar 22, 1977).

2. *Anything can cause cancer if given at sufficiently high levels.*

This statement is untrue. Chemicals generally safe at low levels may be toxic at high levels, but will not cause tumors. Relatively few chemicals have been shown to cause cancer, even when fed at the highest possible doses.

3. *Small amounts of a chemical are safe for people, even though large doses cause cancer in animals.*

This statement is unfounded. No safe threshold dose has been identified for any cancer-causing chemical. In some instances, humans are far more sensitive than test animals; in other cases, less sensitive. In the case of thalidomide, the drug that caused malformed human offspring, the human was found to be 10 times more sensitive than the baboon, 20 times more than the monkey, 60 times more than the rabbit, over 100 times more than the rat, and 200 times more than the cat. Therefore, it is dangerous to underestimate animal data, and argue that extrapolation of results to humans indicates exceedingly small risks. The risks may be great, and such faulty underestimations may affect many lives adversely.

Cancer causation by a chemical at *any* dosage in laboratory animals must always be regarded as a warning signal of potential harm for humans. Every human carcinogen is also carcinogenic in animals. Many well-known carcinogens, such as vinyl chloride and diethylstilbestrol (DES), were first shown as being carcinogenic in humans. These considerations underlie the scientific consensus that there is no way to establish a "safe" level for human exposures, using the results of animal carcinogenicity tests. Yet, vested interests constantly attempt to convince the public that "safe" levels are achievable.

Positive evidence does not nullify negative evidence. The absence of cancer signs in one strain of species of test animals does not prove automatically the substance's safety. For example, the fact that saccharin failed to induce cancer in monkeys did not eliminate the substance's potential harm to humans, as indicated by test results of saccharin-fed rats.

These misleading statements and their unscientific bases were exploited by saccharin proponents to topple the Delaney Clause. "We ignore cancer-causation of animals at our peril," warned Wurster. The Delaney Clause protects us from this folly, wisely allowing no human discretion based on dosage for carcinogens, because there is no valid scientific basis for such discretion. Exposure to any amount of a carcinogen, regardless of how low the level, is risky.

In issuing the press release concerning the proposed saccharin ban, the FDA misled the public. The agency implied that the banning action was forced upon the FDA by the Delaney Clause. In reality, the FDA had the power and responsibility to ban saccharin even without invoking the Delaney Clause, as did the Canadian government which has no regulation comparable to the Delaney Clause. Food additives, such as saccharin, no longer on the

GRAS list, are covered by general food additive regulations. Indeed, on a later occasion, the FDA chose to ban DES, another carcinogen, without ever invoking the Delaney Clause.

FDA'S MISLEADING PRESS RELEASE

The FDA's press release further misled the public by repeating the lie about the need for daily consumption of 875 diet soda drinks to induce cancer. The agency's scientists knew better. Furthermore, the press release falsely stated that the agency's actions were based on the Canadian study, which gave rise to the ridicule that the FDA's actions were based precipitously "at the drop of three rats." Actually, the FDA's actions were based on at least a dozen or more cancer-positive studies prior to the Canadian findings, including its own studies and one from WARF. Additionally, saccharin was related to a wide range of cancer sites other than the bladder, particularly the ovary and the breast; and to different cancer types, such as leukemias, lymphomas, and lymphosarcomas.

FDA'S PLAN TO RECLASSIFY

On March 11, 1977, the FDA announced plans to consider classifying saccharin as a drug so that physicians could prescribe its use for weight control and for diabetes and other disorders for which weight control is important. Canadian officials announced plans to make saccharin available in pharmacies as a drug as of September 1, 1977.

The FDA's plan to reclassify saccharin as a drug was made because of the prospect that a saccharin ban would result in having no sugar substitute available. Cyclamates had been banned.

Despite the concern to retain saccharin for weight control and diabetic use, the value of synthetic sweeteners and synthetic-sweetened foods and beverages has never been proven for these purposes. On the contrary, animal studies showed that saccharin was *an appetite stimulant* because of its ability to reduce blood sugar. (Later, similar claims for weight control would be made for other synthetic sweeteners. They too, would be shown to be appetite stimulants.)

In 1974, on behalf of the Institute of Medicine, Dr. Kenneth Melmon stated that "the data on the efficacy of saccharin and its salts for the treatment of patients with obesity, dental caries, coronary artery disease, or even diabetes has not so far produced a clear picture to us of the usefulness of the drug," as quoted in *Sweeteners: Issues and Uncertainties* (National Academy of Sciences, 1975). This viewpoint was confirmed after the proposed saccharin ban. Saccharin offered no health benefits for diabetics, reported Dr. Harold Rifkin, a diabetes specialist associated with the American Diabetes Association in New York. Nor did saccharin offer any health benefit for dieters, according to Norine Condon, a dietitian with the American Dietetics Association in Chicago. Condon reported in *The Journal of the American Dietetic Association* (vol. 32, 1976) that "It's very much a psychological thing. People are used to eating lots of sweet things. They don't want to give up that flavor."

SACCHARIN PROMOTES WEIGHT GAIN, NOT WEIGHT LOSS

Saccharin has been promoted as an aid for weight loss. Some studies have shown that not only is saccharin ineffective for this purpose, but actually, it can *promote weight gain.* (Similar claims have been made for high-intensity sweeteners, but as we shall see later, high-intensity sweeteners such as aspartame and sucralose, like sacharrin, can promote weight gain.) Here are some findings with sacharrin:

• Peter J. Rogers and John E. Blundell from the Biopsychology Group at Leeds University, Leeds, United Kingdom reported in 1989 that in humans, saccharin *stimulates* subjective hunger. A saccharin solution increases hunger, whereas a caloric sweetener solution (glucose) of the same level of sweetness, reduces hunger. The result confirmed and extended previous findings that showed a different satiety capacity between synthetic sweeteners such as saccharin and a caloric sweetener such as sucrose or glucose. The substitution of saccharin for glucose not only *failed to reduce overall food consumption but led to significant increases in hunger and food intake.*

• William Bennett, M.D., co-author of The Dieter's Dilemna (Basic Books, 1983) reported that the sweet taste in diet soda stimulates the nerves on the tongue to send a message to the pancreas, causing it to produce a small amount of insulin. In turn, this causes a drop in blood sugar level, making the dieter hungrier than before, and especially to crave something sweet.

• Similar findings about saccharin intake increasing food consumption was noted in rat studies. M. G. Tordett and M. I. Friedman conducted a series of four different types of tests with saccharin. They found that the substitution of saccharin for nutritive sweeteners was unsuccessful for any decrease or maintenance of weight. The body merely decreased the metabolic rate to compensate for decreased calorie intake. Also, the substitution of saccharin appeared to increase food consumption by the rats.

• At a conference held in Washington, D.C. as early as 1982, sponsored by the American Cancer Society in cooperation with the American Academy of Family Physicians, Dr. Guy R. Newell, director of Cancer Prevention at the M. D. Anderson Hospital and Tumor Institute in Houston, Texas, reported that there are no scientific data that "prove or disprove the widely perceived benefits of saccharin in the management of diabetes, weight reduction and control, preventing dental caries, or its use to improve the taste of drugs and oral products." Newell concluded by saying that the guiding principle should be that individuals "should not be exposed to a suspect carcinogen unless definite benefit is derived."

Despite the extensive use of synthetic sweeteners, including saccharin, they fail to control weight or prove useful for weight reduction. Instead, they probably play a crucial role in the alarming rise in obesity. Yet, they are not singled out as factors, along with portion sizes, lack of exercise, and other lifestyle factors. What saccharin and other synthetic sweeteners have achieved is a very profitable high-volume sale of diet soft drinks, bakery products, confections, and other low-nutrient products.

OUTCRY AGAINST THE BAN

As with the ban on cyclamates, news of the impending saccharin ban sent heavy saccharin users scurrying to stores and sweeping the shelves clean of the sweetener to hoard supplies as future hedges. Food and beverage manufacturers ignored the FDA's suggestion to discontinue saccharin uses in their products, and they continued to produce record-breaking volumes of saccharin-containing products (*Newsweek*, Mar 1977). The mood was one of defiance.

As mentioned earlier, food and food chemical interests had opposed the Delaney Clause since its inception. When minor substances were banned, opponents grumbled. When bans were of great economic significance, however, such as the 1969 cyclamate ban, and in 1973, the first DES ban, opponents mounted stronger and stronger attacks to rid the nation of the loathesome legislation. Prompted by the proposed saccharin ban in 1977, opponents declared a full-scale war in their efforts to topple the Delaney Clause.

The CCC had a multimillion-dollar war chest and was reported to have spent an estimated 2.5 million dollars in the saccharin battle. Within days of the proposed saccharin ban, the CCC had placed some thirty-two full two-page advertisements in major newspapers throughout the country. The advertisements questioned the scientific tests, attacked the FDA, and urged readers to protest the proposed ban to their congressmen. The CCC distributed materials nationwide to news media and retained a prominent public relations firm to present CCC's views. Within the first three weeks following the ban proposal, CCC had invested 1.14 million dollars on congressional lobbying efforts. "Our basic thrust used to be scientific in nature," the CCC chairman said when interviewed by the *Washington Post* on May 3, 1977, but "recently, we've had to change our arena of action. We've become political rather than scientific in nature."

Political action proved successful. Ten days after the ban proposal, the U.S.

House of Representatives held hearings on the issue. Sessions were stormy, with charges and counter-charges volleying between saccharin defenders and opponents. Throughout the hearings, the Delaney Clause loomed large as a pivotal issue.

Some Washington, D.C. observers believed that the saccharin issue was chosen deliberately as a major battleground, not only to discredit the FDA but for food interests to gain power in other disputes over even more economically important food additive issues, "This is the best issue that we've ever had to take the FDA to task," reported a vice-president of a leading soft drink company to *Snack Foods* (Jun 1977). "If we don't do it now, we never will," he added. "There are 1,800 flavors we use in foods and the FDA will try to attack each and every one . . . Industry cannot live with an FDA that cannot accept science and creates a science of [its] own . . ."

Continued pressure on the U.S. Congress, largely from the direct actions of the CCC, and indirectly from individuals energized by the CCC to take action, succeeded in making some legislators call for modification of the Delaney Clause to accommodate for saccharin's continued use. Dozens of bills were introduced in the House of Representatives to stop the proposed ban.

Meanwhile, saccharin studies were continued. The House of Representatives' Subcommittee on Health and the Environment, which had held the saccharin hearings, requested NAS and NCI to review the Canadian study so that the FDA's evaluation would be double-checked by independent assessment. Also, the U.S. Congress financed an additional saccharin assessment by its own Office of Technology Assessment (OTA, disbanded by the George W. Bush Administration in 2006) scheduled to do short-term testing for mutagenic or other genetic changes. These tests were intended to serve as a basis for evaluating a number of bills pending in Congress dealing with saccharin. Preliminary findings from OTA's panel showed that saccharin was a weak cancer-causing agent, and there was no indication that the substance could be presumed to be safe for human consumption. The media treated the term "weak carcinogen" as relatively good news. But, as explained on page 223, the reality is that a weak carcinogen is of great concern to scientists.

The public outcry against the saccharin ban continued. On April 14, 1977, the FDA issued a compromise plan, intended to ease the proposed outright ban. The agency proposed to permit the continued marketing of saccharin as an over-the-counter non-prescription drug, provided that manufacturers could prove its medical value. Saccharin would be withdrawn as a general purpose food additive as well as a nonmedical ingredient in drugs, and in consumer items likely to be ingested, such as lipsticks, toothpastes, and mouthwashes. Obviously, as with cyclamates, saccharin's medicinal value might be hard to prove because drugs need to be proven safe and effective for their purpose.

The new FDA proposal, instead of calming the controversy, seemed to rekindle the furor. In May 1977, the FDA held two days of public hearings. Nothing new was added to the body of scientific knowledge. In a circuslike atmosphere, some demonstrators waved pro-saccharin placards before TV cameras, while others wheeled shopping carts filled with saccharin-containing products as props. On June 3, 1977, Representative Paul G. Rogers (D-FL) announced that he would introduce a bill that would place an eighteen-month moratorium on any FDA action with saccharin.

On June 18, 1977, the FDA announced results of a new Canadian study that linked saccharin use to bladder cancer in men. The study reinforced the FDA's position, and the agency officials thought that release of news of this as-yet-unpublished study might win them more support, offering as it did, conclusive evidence linking saccharin to human cancer. The Canadian study showed that men who used saccharin (or cyclamates, which were still legal in Canada) had a 60 percent higher risk of cancer development than nonusers. The FDA considered the new study to be sufficiently important to merit scrutiny by the scientific community and the public. The agency extended the comment period, which had been due to expire, and announced that it would also delay its ruling beyond the projected midsummer target date. As events broke, the target date became irrelevant. Regulatory control was about to be snatched away from the FDA when some 315 congressmen agreed to sponsor legislation to head off the proposed saccharin ban.

By early July 1977, both houses of Congress worked on legislation. Shortly before the summer recess, the Senate Health Subcommitee approved a bill placing a moratorium on the FDA's ban, pending results of a study by NAS's Institute of Medicine. The House committee approved a similar bill and appropriated $1 million for the FDA to permit further tests with saccharin and cyclamates, and any other sweeteners that the FDA might judge to be in need of more definitive tests.

Shortly after Congress reconvened, on September 15, 1977, the Senate held a day-long debate on saccharin. Senator Gaylord Nelson described the Senate bill as "a fundamental attack on the best food and drug law in the world," as reported in *Food Processing* (Nov 1977). Hale Champion, undersecretary of the U.S. Department of Health, Education and Welfare (HEW) and the highest government health official involved in the saccharin issue, warned against any delaying legislation. Champion regarded the moratorium as a bad precedent of congressional interference in the regulatory process.

FIRST MORATORIUM ON SACCHARIN BAN

Over this opposition, the Senate voted for an eighteen-month moratorium on any saccharin ban. The legislation would require a warning label on saccha-

rin-sweetened products and on vending machines that dispensed such products. Shortly after, the House voted for similar legislation. On November 23,
1977, the moratorium, passed and signed by President Jimmy Carter, went
into effect.

By November 1977, the OTA review for Congress was completed. In
twelve short-term tests, three were positives and the OTA panel reported "a
clear suggestion" that saccharin was mutagenic. Also, saccharin was carcinogenic in rats and in mice. The panel concluded that saccharin was a weak
human carcinogen.

As followup to the moratorium, saccharin studies were planned to meet
the specific requirements of the legislation. Once more, the FDA requested
NAS to review the scientific literature and assess saccharin's so-called health
benefits and its risks, as well as the social and economic impacts of its regulations. Weighing the social and economic impacts were newly introduced features that were intended to weaken the scientific facts. These elements were
part of the "benefit versus risk" concept that would become a popular feature
of all controversial issues, and frequently espoused by those interested in
downplaying the scientific facts. Another ploy that became popular was to
hurl the epithet "junk science!" without any attempt to build a case against
solid scientific evidence.

The FDA's eleven-member Saccharin Working Group evaluated the available epidemiological data, and concluded that they were insufficient either to
accept or reject the idea that saccharin use increases the risk of human bladder cancer. The group proposed a new study that it hoped would avoid the
pitfalls of past epidemiological studies with saccharin. The study would
include sufficient numbers, have controls, choose people from the general
population rather than from hospitals, and from selected high- and low-risk
areas. Based on these suggestions, the FDA and the NCI jointly announced
on January 25, 1978, the launching of a nationwide study involving some
9,000 adults: 3,000 with identified bladder cancer, and 6,000 randomly chosen
healthy adults from the same areas. Scheduled to begin in March 1978, the
estimated cost of this eighteen-month study was $1.375 million; by comple-
tion, it reached $1.5 million.

On November 4, 1978, the NAS released the first half of its two-part
review. For the very first time, NAS's committee stated conclusively that saccharin "must be viewed as a potential cause of cancer in humans" not only
because it was a weak carcinogen, but also because it was a cocarcinogen. The
latter was possibly even more important than the former. The evidence linking saccharin to cancer in test animals was so strong that further testing was
not needed. There was no evidence that saccharin had any health benefits.
The committee expressed concern that based on intake per body weight, the

greatest saccharin consumers of any age group were children under ten, mainly from their consumption of diet drinks. Because cancer may take years to develop, high saccharin consumption over many years placed children at particular risk.

In March 1979, the NAS released the second half of its review. Saccharin was only part of the review, which dealt with the broad issue of revamping the food safety laws. The committee urged a more flexible food safety policy that would give the FDA options other than a complete ban of food additives suspected as carcinogen. However, the committee members were unable to agree about how saccharin should be handled, either under the proposed scheme, or by Congress. The committee suggested a plan to assign categories to food substances, such as high, moderate, or low risks. Some members disagreed as to whether saccharin was a high or moderate risk and questioned the appropriateness of categorizing carcinogens or other substances that inflict irreversible damage.

SECOND MORATORIUM ON SACCHARIN BAN

On May 9, 1979, the Senate held hearings to assess saccharin's risks in view of newer findings, and to hear arguments for and against extending the moratorium. Among the newer findings was a significant report, based on work conducted by the American Health Foundation in New York. At first, the study seemed to prove saccharin's safety, but by November 1977, results showed the opposite. Bladder cancer risk in men who were saccharin users was nearly twice that of nonusers. The findings, sent to the NCI at the time, had not been released publicly. The timing had coincided with the congressional moratorium.

A delegation from NAS's committee took the saccharin issue and its attendant questions—with which the group had been grappling long and hard—and handed them back to Congress. The delegation explained at the Senate hearings that the saccharin issue would not go away on its own, and that Congress needed to make some decisions.

This episode illustrates a disturbing pattern: scientific issues are not resolved by scientists, but rather on the basis of politics and economics. This pattern is repeated again and again, with more recently introduced sweeteners as well as with a wide array of other consumer goods. Decisions made on the basis of politics and economics, rather then science, create unnecessary health risks for consumers.

Congress, with three options, faced a no-win situation. It could extend the moratorium, leaving itself open to charges that the economic impact outweighed health risks. Congress could return the issue to the FDA, which would begin banning action. In this case, the saccharin proponents would mount another vigorous campaign to defeat the proposed ban. Or, Congress could attempt to modify the Delaney Clause, in which instance, saccharin opponents, joined by a broad spectrum of groups interested in public-safety issues, would coalesce and attempt to keep the Delaney Clause intact.

With the nearing of the moratorium expiration on May 23, 1979, congress introduced new legislation for extending the moratorium. No bill could pass before the imminent deadline, but Congress obtained a promise from the FDA that it would take no immediate action. The agency awaited an indication of congressional intentions. Even if the agency again proposed a saccharin ban, the process to allow time for comments and reviews would require a minimum of fifteen months before any final action. The head of NAS's committee studying saccharin's risks urged consideration of an orderly three-year phase-out of saccharin.

THIRD MORATORIUM ON SACCHARIN BAN

On the day when the moratorium was due to expire, the House of Representatives began saccharin hearings. Following the hearings, the House passed legislation to extend the moratorium. Later, the Senate followed suit. The moratorium was extended until June 30, 1981, a compromise between proposals to extend it for another eighteen months or for three years. The extension was intended to give both Congress and the scientific community more time to develop a reasonable national policy and to provide FDA with greater flexibility in regulating food additives such as saccharin. The agency planned, but failed to develop a consumer education program to encourage decreased use of saccharin, especially by pregnant women and children.

The American Medical Association (AMA) recommended that pregnant women and young children should not use saccharin. A similar recommendation was voiced by Dr. Guy R. Newell, director of Cancer Prevention at M. D. Anderson Cancer Center in Houston, Texas.

At a 1982 conference sponsored by the American Cancer Society, in cooperation with the American Academy of Family Physicians, Newell cautioned that: "Certainly pregnant women should not consume saccharin at any dose level, and children should not be exposed to saccharin from early youth over a lifetime in the doses currently used in soft drinks."

When the third moratorium expired, Congress extended it for another two years, to end on June 30, 1983.

FOURTH MORATORIUM ON SACCHARIN BAN

In late 1979 and early 1980, three epidemiological studies of saccharin's potential role in human bladder cancer were released. The manner in which the media presented these studies led the public to believe that the new evidence refuted the Canadian rat tests by which saccharin had been condemned. "Saccharin Scare Debunked" and "Cancer Risk Denied for Sweeteners" were typical newspaper headlines. The diet food and soft drink industries magnified the distortion and claimed that saccharin safety had been affirmed. Understandings of the issue by the public and by Congress were shaped by this false perception.

In reality, the three new epidemiological studies did *not* refute the earlier animal tests. In general, they were in harmony. The first study, released on December 20, 1979, was of eighteen-month duration, conducted by the FDA and the NCI. It confirmed earlier findings that saccharin posed a human cancer risk. Because patients were questioned about their past, as well as present, use of synthetic sweeteners, cyclamates were included along with saccharin. Other possible carcinogenic factors in lifestyle were included. Preliminary findings indicated that there was no increased risk of bladder cancer among synthetic sweetener users in the overall population. But, heavy users (six or more servings daily, or two or more diet drinks daily) showed a 60 percent increased risk of bladder cancer. Heavy cigarette smokers (two packs a day for men; more than one pack a day for women) who also were heavy synthetic sweetener users, had a higher risk of bladder cancer than heavy smokers who were not users of synthetic sweeteners. Women, who normally would be at low risk for bladder cancer, but who used synthetic sweeteners or diet drinks at least twice a day, were at 60 percent greater risk of cancer than a similar group of women who had never used synthetic sweeteners. The risk increased with the amount consumed. Although the study was important, it was unlikely to settle the saccharin controversy because the demonstrated risks appeared to be limited to certain types of saccharin users. Half of the subjects in the study were sixty-seven years of age or older, and in proportion to their body weight, consumed far less synthetic sweeteners than their children and grandchildren. The possible effects on young people who consumed large amounts over long periods of time, could be assessed only two or three decades later.

The study's prime purpose was to determine if the cancer rate was much higher than expected, as had been suggested by one earlier but questionable epidemiological survey. The present study showed that the cancer rate was not much higher than expected. *But this answer was entirely different from being proof of no effect*—the spin given by the media.

The second study, conducted by the American Health Foundation and published in March 1980, found no statistically significant differences in bladder cancer patients who were saccharin users or nonusers.

The third study, conducted by the Harvard School of Public Health and published in March 1980, found that men who consumed more than three synthetically sweetened soft drinks daily had a greater risk of developing urinary tract cancer than men who consumed less. Increasing the frequency or duration of the use of synthetic sweeteners was not associated consistently with increasing relative risk. Although the researchers concluded that users of synthetic sweeteners have little or no excess risk of lower urinary tract cancer, they admitted that more time might be necessary to accumulate a carcinogenic exposure level.

Congress viewed these three new epidemiological studies as confirmation of earlier negative results, and its own wisdom in staying the ban. A large segment of the public was relieved to learn that their saccharin consumption was not very risky. Most scientists came to opposite conclusions. The scientific community recognized that the new studies needed to be interpreted in conjunction with the well-conducted animal studies. As a group, the animal studies had suggested that saccharin exposure increased the human bladder cancer risk in a range centering around 4 percent. But even the most elaborate of the three new studies, conducted by the FDA/NCI, would detect no change in cancer incidence smaller than 15 percent. Even prior to the study, officials at the FDA and the NCI knew that positive bladder cancer detection would be highly unlikely. The American Health Foundation and the Harvard studies included far fewer patients, and the studies were even less likely to detect evidence of saccharin's carcinogenicity. Neither study did detect it.

The moratoria provided additional time to gather and study new evidence, but they did not resolve the dilemma. According to Dr. Jere Goyan, then FDA Commissioner, the agency's position had been, and continued to remain, that saccharin is a weak carcinogen.

In 1983, the CCC publicized twenty studies of human consuming saccharin. The studies presumably showed no overall association between saccharin use and bladder cancer. One weakness of the epidemiological studies was that their focus was solely on bladder cancer, and ignored other possible effects.

Some of the shortcomings of the epidemiological studies would be noted more than a decade later, at a saccharin workshop held in San Francisco in 1994. Geoffrey Howe, at the University of Toronto in Canada, reported that some subgroups have an elevated risk of bladder cancer. He was quoted in *Food Chemical News* (May 2, 1994), "No matter what we do, epidemiology will never be able to declare absolute safety . . . especially for small groups of . . . people such as those who consume more then ten servings [of saccharin] a day."

At the same meeting, Claudia Hopenhayn-Rich, a consultant to California's Office of Environmental Health Hazard Assessment, reported that consumption in excess of the ten helpings of tabletop sweeteners a day (equivalent to four diet drinks) produced an elevated bladder cancer risk.

At the same meeting, a representative from the California Department of Health Services suggested that an epidemiological study should be done of young children of diabetic women using saccharin. Based on the rat data, critical periods of exposure to saccharin occur neonatally (after-birth) or during the period of rapid growth in the first week after weaning. Such infants might be exposed to saccharin both in the fetal stage from the mother's diet, and as young infants from breastmilk—as mentioned earlier—and saccharin-containing cough syrups. Unfortunately, even a proper epidemiological study might not yield meaningful data for decades.

FIFTH MORATORIUM ON SACCHARIN BAN

The moratorium was due to expire in 1983. Bills were introduced in both houses of Congress to "allow time for completion and review . . . of research on the safety of saccharin." The new moratorium, the fifth one to be passed to stay the saccharin ban, was extended to 1985.

In 1983, the FDA convened a panel to review a two and a half year study of saccharin "sponsored" (in other words, funded) by the CCC, and performed by International Research and Development Corporation (IRDC), a group the CCC described as "an independent contract research laboratory."

The IRDC's study found a "statistically significant" dose-relationship between saccharin in the diet and bladder tumors in rats at a 3 percent level of saccharin, and an "equivocal" relationship at a 1 percent level. The study found that saccharin caused tumors at lower levels in the diet than previously had been documented. Other researchers found that a diet of 5 percent saccharin caused tumors in rats.

When diabetics chose to use synthetic sweeteners, they tended to be heavy users. The American Diabetes Association (ADA) cautioned diabetics to use synthetic sweeteners "in moderation." The ADA did not define limits, but recognized that synthetic sweetener use had been increasing.

By 1983, consumption of soft drinks continued to expand in the United States at a dizzying rate. Diet soft drinks accounted for 17 percent of the total beverage market. The annual per capita consumption reached more than 40 gallons. By then, aspartame had been approved. Processors still favored saccharin, costing about $4 a pound, compared to aspartame, costing about ninety dollars a pound. Because aspartame's sweetness was more intense, less could be used. Often, the two sweeteners were combined.

In 1984, the CCC estimated that more tham 68 million American adults—40 percent of the entire population—regularly used saccharin or aspartame. This was an increase of more than 60 percent over the previous six years. The annual per capita saccharin consumption had soared more than 40 percent from the previous decade.

SIXTH MORATORIUM ON SACCHARIN BAN

In 1985, for the sixth time, the moratorium on the saccharin ban was extended, to 1987. Once again, the rationale given was to allow the FDA more time to consider the issue, and to learn if any new health studies warranted action. By then, some 170 studies had been conducted with saccharin since the original 1978 moratorium. By then, it was known that saccharin affected different species of animals differently, and triggered different effects at different doses. The NAS had concluded that "saccharin is a carcinogen of low potency in rats and a potential carcinogen in humans."

For the first time, the moratorium included a provision that any further proposals to stay the ban on saccharin must be based on scientific evidence acquired after 1978. This effectively ruled out the use of the contentious 1977 Canadian rat study as a significant part of any future FDA actions on saccharin.

The FDA was attempting to determine whether saccharin acts as a cancer initiator and as a cancer promoter. Ronald Hart, Ph.D., director of the FDA's National Center for Toxicological Research, testified that the FDA studies showed that both in rats and in humans, saccharin does act as a cancer initiator and as a cancer promoter. Hart reported that when human skin cells are subjected to a "safe" dose of a known carcinogen, and at the same time to a low dose of saccharin, the sweetener is "very effective in enhancing the transformation of the cells into malignant cancer cells." Also, Dr. Frank E. Young, then commissioner of the FDA, told U.S. Senators that studies conducted jointly by his agency and NCI produced evidence that synthetic sweeteners were cancer promoters. Their studies showed that heavy smokers who also used synthetic sweeteners had an increased cancer risk.

Another health concern about saccharin was its ability to cross the human placenta. Formerly, it had been thought that the placenta acted as a barrier to keep harmful things out. This was proven wrong. A study, reported in 1986, examined six women who had used saccharin during pregnancy. Five of the women were diabetics. Saccharin was identified in all samples of their urine and blood. Among the offspring, three had trace concentrations of less than 50 nanograms per milliliter (ng/ml) of saccharin, and three had concentrations ranging from 110 ng/ml to 160 ng/ml. Saccharin concentration in the cord blood samples in two infants was even higher than in the matching concentrations found in their mothers. Although this study used a very small sampling of women, the findings were important.

By now, groups such as the FDA, AMA, and ADA, as well as individual health professionals, were cautioning pregnant women to limit or avoid saccharin consumption. In 1986, the U.S. Department of the Treasury's Bureau of Alcohol, Tobacco and Firearms (BATF) ruled that any alcoholic beverage containing saccharin must carry a warning label "Use of this product may be hazardous to your health. This product contains saccharin which has been determined to cause cancer in laboratory rats." Among the affected beverages subject to such labeling were the popular low-calorie wine coolers.

SEVENTH MORATORIUM ON SACCHARIN BAN

As the end of the 1987 moratorium loomed, members of both houses of Congress introduced bills to extend the Saccharin Study and Labeling Act to allow continued use of the sweetener. A vigorous campaign "Save Saccharin" succeeded in having a five-year extension of the moratorium—the seventh extension since the original 1977 moratorium and the first time that the extension was made for a period longer then two years. This extension, to 1992, provided that justification of the ban need to be based on scientific evidence, counsel of qualified professionals, *and the support of the public* (emphasis added). Of course, the public support of saccharin users had nothing to do with scientific findings, and actually were diametrically opposite to the scientific findings. Campaigns to "educate" and 'inform" the public were launched by self-serving groups, interested in promoting saccharin sales both to processors and to consumers.

The campaign to promote saccharin use and to prevent it from being banned proved highly effective. The FDA received thousands of letters in support of saccharin and in opposition to any future ban. The saccharin products were promoted in advertisements targeted at the public. Different suppliers of saccharin competed for market shares, and one advertisement was challenged. The Cumberland Packing Corporation, in Brooklyn, New York, claimed for their product in an advertisement, "It's a fact, 30 million people prefer Sweet'n Low. That's 40 percent more than Equal." (Equal is a brand name for aspartame.) When challenged, Cumberland reported that its source for the statement was supplied by a leading national research company. Sugar Foods Corporation, a saccharin competitor, challenged the claim. The taste preference claim was based solely on market share data. The National Advertising Division of the Council of Better Business Bureaus, Inc., agreed that accepted industry practice substantiates a comparative taste claim by means of a taste test, not by market share data. As a result, Cumberland withdrew its misleading advertisement.

Later, Cumberland was in more serious trouble. The Internal Revenue Service (IRS) charged that between 1985 and 1994, Cumberland's president, vice president, some employees, and contractors "conspired to defraud" the IRS by submitting fraudulent invoices for services falsely represented to have been rendered to Cumberland, and paid the fake invoices and then deducted the payments as legitimate expenses on its tax returns. The funds were used, in part, to reimburse political campaigns in an attempt to obtain the support for the continuation of the Congressional moratorium on the banning of saccharin, the main ingredient in Cumberland's product, Sweet'n Low. This illegal political campaign reimbursement scheme was devised to evade the legal limits of contributions to federal and local political campaigns. Some $224,000 had been funneled to presidential campaigns and to various campaign committees of both major parties, as well as to individual members of the U.S. Congress of both major parties. The recipients were unaware that the contributions had been made in violation of the federal campaign contribution law. After pleading guilty, as part of the plea arrangement in 1990, Cumberland agreed to pay a fine of $2 million.

Steady pressure continued to be exerted to save saccharin and to remove any ban threat. On December 30, 1991, with little fanfare, the FDA published in the *Federal Register* its decision to withdraw the original 1977 proposal to remove saccharin from the U.S. food supply. This action would terminate the unprecedented series of repeated moratoria, and negate the one that was due to expire in 2002.

Due to the increased numbers of safety tests, by 1992 WHO/FAO's Joint Expert Committee on Food Additives (JECFA) listed saccharin as a substance that needed reevaluation. In the same year, the European Commission's Scientific Committee on Food retained a temporary average daily intake (ADI) for saccharin pending more information. Also, in 1991, a medical journal had appealed for safety reports of saccharin that were not based on research sponsored by industry.

The Canadian government was subjected to similar pressures as in the United States. In 1993, Canada's Health Protection Branch was petitioned to reinstate saccharin approval for use in cosmetics and pharmaceuticals. The CCC and the Canadian Soft Drinks Association petitioned for a Canadian reapproval of saccharin's use in foods and beverages.

DRUG INTERACTIONS

One aspect of saccharin that had been ignored was its ability to interact with some medication. For example, it cross-reacts with sulfa drugs.

Many pharmaceutical companies were adding saccharin to newly formulated medications. This use was questioned by Howard Frankel, M.D., Ph.D., who found the practice "both inappropriate and unnecessary, and makes no scientific sense." Frankel charged that government regulatory agencies failed in their responsibility to advise the public that saccharin had been added to some drugs, including non-prescription over-the-counter medications.

It had been assumed that saccharin did not alter liver function. However, a case reported by Drs. Francesco Negro, Alessandra Mondardini, and Franco Palmas, physicians in Turin, Italy, found that saccharin-containing drugs elevated the serum concentration of liver enzymes in a patient. Her level of enzymes returned to normal after discontinuation of the drugs, but rose again when the use of saccharin-containing drugs was resumed. To confirm their suspicions that saccharin was the culprit, they administered 12.5 milligrams (mg) of pure sodium saccharin to the patient daily for five days. Her serum liver enzymes rose. The doctors suggested that over time saccharin consumption could be a factor in the pathogenesis of liver damage for some individuals.

ATTEMPTS TO DELIST SACCHARIN
AS A PROBABLE CARCINOGEN

The National Toxicology Program (NTP), begun in 1978, coordinated the toxicology activities of the National Institutes of Health's National Institute of Health Sciences (NIHS), the Center for Disease Control's National Institute for Occupational Safety and Health (NIOSH), and the FDA's National Center for Toxicological Research (NCTR). The director of NTP is also the director of the National Institute of Environmental Health Sciences (NIEHS).

Since 1980, the U.S. Congress has mandated NTP to publish annual reports on carcinogens, listing all substances "(i) known to be carcinogens or which may reasonably anticipated to be carcinogens, and (ii) to which a significant number of persons residing in the United States are exposed." It was appropriate to list saccharin on both counts, and since 1981 saccharin has been listed in the Annual Report on Carcinogens.

One study, highly publicized by groups eager to have saccharin delisted and deleted from the Annual Report an Carcinogens, was based on tests with monkeys. Although this report has been cited frequently as exonerating saccharin as a carcinogen, careful reading of the study does not absolve saccharin. Three monkeys out of twenty in the group, given a high saccharin level, showed gross evidence of tumors.

Dr. Michael Jacobson, executive director of the Center for Science in the Public Interest (CSPI), one of the study's critics, claimed that the study offered a "largely one-sided review of the evidence" and that the review of epidemiological evidence by the study's authors "is even worse." Jacobson also charged a conflict of interest. One of the authors had served as a CCC consultant. Jacobson noted that this trade association had "lobbied for years to have the 'cancer' label taken off of saccharin" (reported in *Food Chemical News*, Feb 16, 1998).

Michael Jacobson also appealed to the U.S. Congress to enforce the requirement that products containing synthetic sweeteners be labeled adequately. From time to time, the FDA has seized saccharin-containing food products that had no label declaration of the presence of saccharin in the product.

An advisory panel of NTP met to consider a petition from the CCC to remove saccharin from the forthcoming Annual Report on Carcinogens, due in 1999. The NTP planned to review a new study submitted that allegedly demonstrated the safety of saccharin.

The study suggested that male rats fed saccharin developed bladder tumors only under "rat-specific" urinary conditions that induced high pH and crystal formation. The NTP panel had divided opinions about the study. Two members of the NTP Scientific Committee were critical. The panelists who favored delisting were criticized by epidemiologists who regarded the data as "flawed." Among these critics were Dr. Devra Davis, an epidemiologist at World Resources Institute in Washington, D.C. and Dr. Emmanuel Farber, a pathologist at Jefferson Medical College in Philadelphia. Farber had chaired the 1978 panel that had established saccharin as a weak carcinogen. The critics noted that cancers other than bladder cancers increased in some rodent studies with saccharin. Certain subgroups of people using synthetic sweeteners did appear to be at risk of bladder cancer. Farber reported "my concern is children, because they could consume lots of saccharin in soft drinks. That makes me nervous" (quoted in *Food Chemical News*, Nov 3, 1997).

Farber's concerns were strengthened by findings in a British study reported by C. A. Lawrie, of the Additives and Novel Foods Division of Food Science and Safety Group, Ministry of Agriculture, Fisheries, and Food. National surveys of food consumption showed that exposure to food additives on a body weight basis is likely to be higher in children aged one and a half years to four and a half years than in adults. National diet surveys showed that young British children in this age range consumed almost five times the equivalent amount as adults—taking body weight into account—of dairy products, puddings, and confectionery. They obtained more than 80 percent of their fluid intake (excluding milk) from soft drinks, or sixteen times the equivalent amount consumed by adults. Some of the puddings and confectionery, and many of the soft drinks, were sweetened with saccharin. As a result, the authors estimated that some children were receiving saccharin in quantities exceeding the ADI. In the case of soft drinks and saccharin, consumers had been advised to add extra water to saccharin-containing soft drink concentrate to reduce children's intakes of the sweetener. In the United Kingdom, manufacturers voluntarily added this warning to product labels, and reinforced it in nutrition leaflets.

On October 31,1997, the NTP scientific subcommittee decided in a split vote of four to three that saccharin should continue to be listed as "reasonably anticipated to be a human carcinogen" in its ninth edition of the NTP's Annual Report on Carcinogens to be issued in 1999.

The decision was a blow to the CCC which had submitted a petition to delist saccharin. The CCC issued a statement calling the action "extremely unfortunate and contrary to science."

The four subcommittee members who voted to retain saccharin on the list of carcinogens were:

- Dr. Eula Bingham, professor of environmental health, and former assistant administrator of the federal Occupational Safety and Health Administration (OSHA);

- Dr. George Friedman-Jimenez, director of Occupational and Environmental Medicine Clinic at Bellevue Hospital in New York City;

- Dr. Nicholas Hooper, a toxicologist with the California Department of Health Services; and

- Dr. Franklin Mirer, director of Health and Safety for the United Auto Workers.

The three subcommittee members who voted for delisting were:

- Dr. John Bailer, professor of biostatistics at Miami University, Miami, Florida;

- Dr. Steven Belinsky, an inhalation toxicologist at Kirkland Air Force Base in Albuquerque, New Mexico; and

- Dr. Clay Frederick, a senior toxicologist at the chemical company, Rohm and Haas.

Various epidemiological tests that had been performed (some sponsored by industry) came under critical analysis. Dr. Bingham said that she was "troubled by the generalization that you can dismiss higher risks in certain groups . . . You need to look at 'pockets' that show excess risks" (quoted in *Food Chemical News*, Nov 10, 1997).

Dr. Mirer added that he had been inclined to delist saccharin until he had reviewed the epidemiological studies. He said that "We can rule out particular risk rates, but not risks below the limits of detection."

Dr. Friedman-Jimenez said, "Subgroup analysis is important, and you want to avoid 'dredging the data' to create subgroups. But these subgroups were determined in advance. The epidemiological studies are not entirely reassuring. I don't feel comfortable with delisting."

Another reviewer, Dr. Sheila Zahm, an occupational epidemiologist at NCI, who also served as a consultant to the subcommittee, lamented the lack of two-generational bioassays, because saccharin is consumed heavily by women of childbearing age. She voiced her concerns to *Food Chemical News* (Nov 10, 1997) along with the other scientists, about increased sweetener use since 1970: "What was considered a 'high dose' then isn't any longer. I'm worried that exposure will increase still further if we delist saccharin."

Reviewers of the data expressed concerns about high saccharin intake by consumers, and that doses were closer to those of the test rats than originally thought. Harm from saccharin use may not be discerned in epidemiological studies except in highly exposed groups, and these groups did show signs of harm.

During a time for public comments related to the advisory panel meeting organized by the NTP, Jacobson, of CSPI, stressed the importance of studies suggesting that saccharin may cause tumors at sites other than the bladder. He said that "delisting saccharin would ignore the many indications of carcinogenicity and result in greater exposure of both children and adults to this probable carcinogen." He warned that "Delisting saccharin would be throwing all caution to the wind," and commended the subcommittee vote to continue listing saccharin in the forthcoming NTP's Annual Report on Carcinogens. He applauded the majority of the subcommittee's recognition that the scientific evidence did not justify saccharin's removal from the list of carcinogens. "Those scientists were not persuaded by industry's research on male rats that saccharin is safe for humans. However, we can expect the Calorie Control Council to lobby fiercely over the next year to delist saccharin," Jacobson predicted in *Food Chemical News* (Nov 10, 1997).

In a letter directed to the NTP, eight scientists urged that saccharin be retained on the list of carcinogens. They said that declaring saccharin safe:

> . . . would give the public a false sense of security, remove any incentive for further testing, and result in greater exposure to this probable carcinogen in tens of millions of people including children (indeed, fetuses). If saccharin is a weak carcinogen, this 'unnecessary additive' would pose an intolerable risk to the public.

These scientists stated that although the argument has been made that urinary bladder tumors in male rats caused by sodium saccharin are irrelevant to humans:

> . . . such arguments are flawed. Although the causation of tumors in male rats cannot be proven relevant to humans, neither can it be assumed to be irrelevant.

The letter was signed by:

- Dr. Samuel S. Epstein, professor of environmental and occupational medicine at the School of Public Health, University of Illinois in Chicago;

- Dr. Richard Clapp, Department of Environmental Health, Boston University in Boston;

- Dr. Devra Davis, Health, Environment and Development Program, World Resources Institute, Washington, D.C.;

- Dr. Emmanuel Farber, pathologist, Jefferson Medical College in Philadelphia;

- Dr. William Lijinsky, formerly with the Chemical Carcinogenesis Program, the Frederick Cancer Research Center in Frederick, Maryland;

- Dr. Erik Millstone, Science Policy Research Unit, University of Sussex, in Sussex, United Kingdom;

- Dr. Melvin Reuber, consultant on oncology and pathology, formerly at NCI; and

- Dr. Michael Jacobson, executive director of CSPI.

THE CLOSED DOOR MEETING THAT SAVED SACCHARIN

Despite the majority of the scientific counselors of NTP voting against the delisting of saccharin, by the end of 1998, NTP's executive committee, in a meeting closed to the public, voted six to three to delist saccharin from the forthcoming ninth Annual Report on Carcinogens, due to be issued the following year. The action was the fourth and final NTP saccharin evaluation. Jacobson called the vote "despicable, but not surprising" (*Food Chemical News*, Feb 16, 1998).

In anticipation of the NTP executive committee meeting, a saccharin review by the International Agency for Research on Cancer (IARC), a unit of WHO and partly funded by NCI, also concluded that saccharin does not pose a cancer risk. Jacobson charged that the conclusion was virtually predetermined by the composition of the twenty-six person group, "dominated by industry representatives and industry consultants." By Jacobson's count, "fully half of the people on the committee are affiliated with the food and chemical industries and/or had previously concluded that saccharin does not pose a cancer risk." Jacobson added that the review was "carefully rigged to exonerate saccharin." He noted "extraordinary conflicts of interest" and that the IARC evaluation was "completely inadequate from a scientific standpoint." Jacobson then cited a litany of specifics:

- IARC summarily dismissed the evidence from an NCI study—the largest and most sensitive human study ever done—that found links between artificial sweetener consumption and bladder cancer;

- IARC dismissed evidence from animal studies that showed saccharin to increase the potency of chemical carcinogens;

- IARC accepted completely industry's theory that saccharin caused cancer in the urinary bladders of male rats by a mechanism and only by that one mechanism, and that it is irrelevant to humans; and

- IARC ignored evidence that saccharin caused tumors in animals at sites other than the urinary bladder.

In view of IARC's biases, Jacobson recommended that HHS should demand that IARC withdraw its report; WHO should appoint a new director of its chemical evaluation process; and a new and balanced committee of individuals with impeccable integrity should reevaluate saccharin. If WHO should fail to take these actions, HHS should stop funding IARC. None of these recommendations, suggested by Jacobson and reported in *Food Chemical News* (Feb 16, 1998) were pursued.

DELISTING LEADS TO WEAKENED REGULATIONS

Saccharin, delisted as a substance "reasonably anticipated to be a human carcinogen" by the NTP, allowed the FDA on December 31, 1991 to drop its last proposed ban on the sweetener. The agency announced that "the safety of saccharin is no longer of concern and that these 1977 proposals [the bans] have become outdated."

After saccharin was delisted, regulatory control was relaxed. The U.S. House Commerce Committee amended the Food, Drug and Cosmetic Act to repeal the saccharin notice requirement that retail stores selling saccharin-containing products, to alert consumers about the health risks associated with use of the sweetener. Also, delisting allowed industry to drop the warning label requirement on saccharin-containing products.

In a 1998 survey conducted by the CCC, synthetically sweetened sodas and desserts were consumed regularly by 144 million American adults. Saccharin accounted for about one-third of all synthetic sweeteners sold in the United States.

If saccharin had been classified as a drug—Dr. Wiley's intention—it would not be available today. Drugs must be proven safe and effective. Saccharin is neither. As demonstrated in this chapter, saccharin is hazardous to health. Nor is it useful for its alleged benefits in weight reduction.

Chapter 13

ASPARTAME: A BREAKTHROUGH HIGH-INTENSITY SWEETENER

Any new substance, despite all the safety tests,
is surrounded by question marks.
—STANLEY GLASSNER, FDA FOOD AND COLOR ADDITIVES DIVISION,
THE NATIONAL OBSERVER, JANUARY 4, 1975

As with other synthesized sweeteners, the discovery of aspartame was by chance. In December 1965, James Schlatter, M.S., a scientist working at the G. D. Searle & Company, was researching peptides, involving amino acids, in an attempt to develop new drugs to treat ulcers. He noticed a white powder on his hand and brushed it off. Later, he wet his fingertips with his tongue in order to turn the pages of his research notebook. He experienced an extremely sweet taste from his fingertips. In testing, he discovered that the white powder was a combination of two amino acids, aspartic acid and phenylalanine. By themselves, neither was sweet. Combined, however, they became extremely sweet. He tried various combinations of other amino acids, but failed to produce the intense sweetness of aspartic acid combined with phenylalanine. A 4 percent solution of the compound in water was from 180 times to 200 times as sweet as a comparable sucrose solution. The sweetness of the compound had an even broader range, from 160 times to 220 times as sweet as sucrose, depending on the length of time the compound was in solution, the temperature, pH, and available moisture.

The taste of the sweetener was almost identical to sucrose, and it lacked saccharin's bitter aftertaste. However, unlike sucrose or saccharin, it lost its sweetness upon being heated.

Beginning in March 1966, the Searle Food Resources division, in Skokie, Illinois, began two years of extensive research with the compound, attempting to develop a viable commercial product. By January 1969, Searle began safety tests in order to submit data to the Food and Drug Administration (FDA). The company designated the compound as aspartame.

ASPARTAME'S PROBLEMATIC CHARACTERISTICS

Aspartame (1-methyl-N-L-alpha aspartyl-L-phenylalanine) is composed of commercially produced L-aspartic acid and L-phenylalanine. As amino acids, isolated from foods, both are problematic. Phenylalanine needs to be limited in the diet by women of childbearing years who are phenylketonuric and are unable to metabolize phenylalanine. Women may not know that they have phenylketonuria (PKU). High levels of phenylalanine in their diets can result in offspring with severe health problems, including mental retardation. Phenylalanine is a component of all proteins, but isolated phenylalanine, separated from protein foods, acts differently than when it is one of a number of amino acids present in protein foods. The other amino acids present impede its uptake by the brain. In isolation, without this impediment, excessive phenylalanine may reach the brain.

BLACK HUMOR

The safety concerns posed by all three synthesized sweeteners—cyclamate, saccharin, and aspartame—provided material for the cartoonist, Schochet. He drew two women seated in a cafe, who have been served hot beverages. One woman offers the other the bowl containing packets of sweeteners, and asks, "Cancer, diabetes, or phenylketonuria?"

Aspartic acid, the other amino acid, is well recognized as a neuroexcitor (an overstimulator of the brain). At a high level, it becomes a neurotoxin (a substance capable of producing brain damage). Aspartame is hydrolyzed in the intestinal lumen to phenylalanine, aspartic acid, and methanol (wood alcohol), which at a certain level becomes a toxin that can cause severe health problems, including blindness.

In metabolism, the phenylalanine breaks down, in sequence, from tyrosine to dopamine, to norepinephrine, and ultimately, to adrenalin. Aspartic acid breaks down to carbon dioxide and water. Methanol breaks down to formaldehyde, formic acid, and ultimately, to carbon dioxide. Both formaldehyde and formic acid are well recognized toxins. In addition, when aspartame breaks down, with heat, acidity, or over time, it forms metabolites (breakdown products). One is diketopiperazine (DKP) which has the potential to form carcinogenic nitrosamines. All these features, which would be recognized by chemists and biochemists, should have been early warning signals about the characteristics of the sweetener under development.

In February 1973, Searle filed a petition for approval of aspartame. Its uses would be limited to dry-based foods and beverages in the United States. Searle also petitioned for approval in Canada. In July 1974, the FDA approved these uses. Searle named the product NutraSweet.

FIRST SPECIAL TASK FORCE INVESTIGATION

The following month, August 1974, John W. Olney, M.D., and Attorney James S. Turner filed formal objections to the approval based on safety concerns. Olney, professor of psychiatry and neuropathology at Washington University School of Medicine in St. Louis, Missouri, expressed concern that aspartame might cause brain damage in young children. Earlier, Olney researched another neuroexcitive amino acid, glutamate, used in the flavor enhancer, monosodium glutamate (MSG). He had found that glutamate, at a level similar to what was being used as MSG added to baby foods, produced damage to the brains of laboratory mice. Olney was especially concerned that a meal containing both aspartame and glutamate—a common combination—posed an even greater threat of brain damage, especially to young children.

Turner, a consumer advocate attorney, had authored *The Chemical Feast* (Grossman Publishers, 1970), Ralph Nader's Study Group Report on the FDA. Turner filed formal objections to aspartame on behalf of the Community Nutrition Institute, an independent public service organization interested in consumer issues. Both Olney and Turner requested a hearing before a judge. The FDA denied the request.

Safety Tests Found Flawed

In response, however, the FDA commissioner was obligated to stay approval for aspartame in December 1974, pending validation of certain research studies conducted by Searle.

Ninety of the 113 tests had been submitted in the early 1970s to the mid-1970s. All of the aspartame tests submitted during that time by Searle and its major contractor, Hazleton Laboratories, were called into question, along with drugs tested, by a 1975 special task force investigation convened by the FDA. The findings were so serious that they led to the FDA's general counsel to request a grand jury investigation of Searle.

All of the aspartame tests that the FDA had considered "pivotal" (that is, critical key tests to establish safety) had been conducted during that time period. Eighty-eight percent of the tests had been conducted by Searle or Hazleton. The testing was described as "incredibly sloppy science" by Dr. Alexander Schmidt, interviewed later by *Common Cause Magazine* (Jul–Aug 1984). Schmidt had been FDA Commissioner at the time of the 1975 special task force investigation. He recalled, "What was discovered was reprehensible." Schmidt said that a pivotal test is of such importance that it needs to be repeated if it is found wanting. Yet only one pivotal test had been repeated after the 1975 investigation, and it was not even considered in the agency's safety assessment. Later, when the FDA's Bureau of Foods and the new FDA Commissioner Arthur Hull Hayes, who replaced Schmidt, decided that aspartame was safe, they relied on some or all of the early flawed tests. There was no evidence in the public record that Hayes or the Bureau of Foods ever explained how their decisions were reconciled with the questions raised by the task force about Searle's early flawed tests. Three pivotal tests used to determine whether aspartame might cause serious cancerous brain tumors had been brought to Hayes' attention by FDA scientists, during his deliberations, but not considered in his decision.

Problems with Laboratory Practices and Personnel

The 1975 task force investigations had revealed serious problems with laboratory practices at Searle and other companies. As a result, the FDA developed detailed regulations on good laboratory practices, which subsequently, all laboratories submitting test data needed to follow.

The 1975 task force raised concerns about the quality and training of personnel. Studies in reproduction and teratology (fetal damage) were judged "an extremely important phase in safety evaluation." Yet, the task force found that "the person responsible for most of the reproduction studies reviewed was apparently inexperienced in conducting studies of this nature and yet given full responsibility at Searle with a title of senior research assistant in teratology. His prior experience was one year's employment with the Illinois Wildlife Service where his work involved population dynamics of the cottontail rabbit." When asked by the task force investigator about his qualifications or training he had to conduct reproduction and teratology studies, he said that after his employment with Searle he attended one meeting of the Teratology Society, and Searle provided him with books on the subject. This man was responsible, also, to train and supervise a research assistant and two technicians. In this setting by the end of 1975, Searle had submitted eighteen studies related to reproduction and teratology.

The 1975 task force had no way to evaluate the quality of animal care facilities in the laboratory studies when the tests had been conducted, but in October 1975 they found "poor practices" at Searle. For example, an exterminator sprayed insecticides twice monthly with a fogging machine, without removing the animals from the room. The practice had been in effect at least since 1970. The investigators found no evidence that the treatment feed used in studies had been tested for pesticide content.

The 1975 task force reported that in studies conducted by Searle and by its major contractor, Hazleton, "little concern was evidenced for the need of proper quality control of homogeneity, concentration, or stability of the active ingredient-diet," and because of laxity, "there is *no* way in which it can be assured that animals received the intended dosages" (emphasis supplied).

The 1975 task force had examined a number of the pivotal tests and had raised questions about all of Searle's tests including the vast majority of the aspartame tests conducted between 1967 and 1975. The lead investigator, Philip Brodsky described as "one of the FDA's most experienced drug investigators," recalled in an interview with *Common Cause Magazine* (Jul–Aug 1984) that he had "never seen anything" as "bad" as Searle's testing. Brodsky said, "I wouldn't want to rely" on those tests "for making a decision about the products . . . There were too many errors."

The 1975 task force submitted its report in March 1976, and questioned all of Searle's tests between 1967 and 1975. Among its conclusions:

> At the heart of the FDA's regulatory process is its ability to rely upon the integrity of the basic safety data submitted by sponsors of regulated products. Our investigation clearly demonstrates that, in the G. D. Searle & Company, we have no basis for such reliance now.
>
> We have uncovered serious deficiencies in Searle's operations and practices which undermine the basis for reliance on Searle's integrity in conducting high-quality animal research to accurately determine or characterize the toxic potential of its products.
>
> We have noted that Searle has now submitted all the facts of experiments to [the] FDA retaining unto itself the unpermitted option of filtering, interpreting, and not submitting information which we would consider material to the safety evaluation of the product.
>
> Finally, we have found instances of irrelevant or unproductive animal research where experiments have been poorly conceived, carelessly executed, or inaccurately analyzed or reported.
>
> While a single discrepancy, error, or inconsistency in any given study may not be significant in and of itself, the cumulative findings of problems within and across the studies we investigated reveal a pattern of conduct which compromises the scientific integrity of the studies. We have attempted to analyze and characterize the problems and to determine why they are so pervasive in the studies we investigated.

These conclusions were made part of the public record at a later time, at the U.S. Senate hearings on aspartame.

SECOND TASK FORCE INVESTIGATION

In 1977, the FDA convened another task force to evaluate one of the pivotal brain tumor tests used to determine that aspartame was safe. This task force was headed by Jerome Bressler. The team found evidence—including a photo-graph—that the experimental rats may not have eaten the intended doses of the test substance, the aspartame breakdown product, DKP. There were indi-cations that the animals found DKP distasteful and may have avoided eating it, thus skewing the results of the tests. Bressler told *Common Cause* (Jul–Aug 1984) that "it was a lousy study; it was a sloppy study."

Searle submitted thirteen tests in an attempt to demonstrate that aspar-tame would not cause genetic damage. Memos in the public record show that FDA scientists who initially reviewed these tests found serious deficiencies in all of them. They described three of these studies as "incomplete individually and collectively."

After having stayed the approval of aspartame earlier, the FDA had con-vened a Public Board of Inquiry (PBI), and appointed three expert panelists outside of the agency. The panelists were Dr. Walle Nauta, a neuroanatomist at the Massachusetts Institute of Technology (MIT) in Cambridge; Dr. Peter Lampert, a neuropathologist at the University of California at San Diego; and Dr. Vernon Young, a nutritional biochemist at MIT. Nauta felt that "extensive testing" was needed to confirm charges that consumption of large amounts of aspartame, especially with carbohydrates, might affect brain chemistry.

During protracted PBI deliberations, the FDA, in addition to its two spe-cial task forces, also had requested a review by the Universities Associated for Research and Education in Pathology (UAREP) of fifteen pivotal toxicity studies of aspartame. As the review continued, the FDA decided that the agency itself would review three of the fifteen pivotal studies being examined by the UAREP in order to speed validation. After three months, the FDA vali-dated the accuracy of all three studies it had examined, and the UAREP vali-dated the remainder.

ASPARTAME APPROVED FOR USE AS A TABLETOP SWEETENER

In April 1979, Searle requested that FDA lift its stay on aspartame approval. The FDA denied the request, pending the results of PBI's recommendations. By January 1980, the PBI had examined two contested safety issues, and con-cluded that one of the issues was resolved adequately, but recommended additional scientific testing in the other. Also, the PBI recommended that all aspartame-containing products carry a warning label for individuals who had PKU and needed to restrict their diets.

The FDA commissioner disagreed that additional testing was needed. He contended that *additional evidence, unavailable to the PBI,* made additional test-ing unnecessary.

On July 15, 1981, the FDA announced approval for aspartame use as a tabletop sweetener, and with dry mixes and foods not heat processed. Searle would name the tabletop sweetener, available to the public, Equal.

Searle's long-range strategy was to petition for limited uses of aspartame, incrementally. At this point, Searle had not requested approval for the sweetener's use in soft drinks, so the 1981 approval did not include aspartame use for such purpose.

RUMSFELD RESCUES SEARLE

In 1977, the G. D. Searle & Company was regarded as an ailing drug and health-care company. Donald H. Rumsfeld became its president and CEO, and intended to rescue it. Rumsfeld had scant business experience. Searle had debts and was losing its edge in drug research (*Business Week*, Feb 8, 1982).

Five years later, Rumsfeld began to rebuild a nearly moribund research and development effort that had been discredited by the FDA with charges that Searle had falsified research data. Under Rumsfeld's management, earnings climbed. But the short-term gains in the drug market were dwarfed by its sales of aspartame, marketed as the tabletop sweetener, Equal.

Meanwhile, aspartame approval was being granted in other countries: 1979, in France; September 1979, in Canada; and February 1980, in Belgium and Luxembourg. In European countries it was sold with a brand name Canderel. By 1980, aspartame was approved in the Philippines; in September 1980, in Brazil; in February, in Mexico; and in June 1981, in Switzerland. In rapid succession, from December 1981 through September 1982, a number of countries worldwide followed suit: in Singapore, West Germany, Norway, Peru, Sweden, Australia, Venezuela, South Africa, Indonesia, Denmark, and Portugal. By 1983, aspartame was approved in twenty-two countries; by 1992, it was approved in more than ninety countries. Approval became virtually global. It is worth noting that many countries do not conduct their own safety tests, but depend on countries such as the United States for assurances. For this reason, it is vital not only to Americans, but also to people everywhere, that our testing is accurate and complete.

BREAKDOWN PROBLEMS

Among many safety issues that remained unresolved, one was DKP, the breakdown product of aspartame mentioned earlier. DKP is formed when aspartame is heated, or when aspartame is added to liquids (such as soft drinks) that may be stored for months. DKP, a secondary amine, might result in the formation of cancer-causing nitrosamines in the body. This unresolved issue concerned many scientists and researchers, especially after the FDA extended aspartame approval for use in soft drinks, in 1983.

Dr. Woodrow C. Monte, director of the Food Science and Nutrition Laboratory at Arizona State University, expressed concern about the breakdown of aspartame in products such as soft drinks, stored in hot climates such as the southwest. Monte found that after only six or seven weeks of storage at 86°F aspartame-containing soft drinks could produce over 3.9 parts per million (ppm) methanol (wood alcohol), and three times the upper limit tolerated by the Environmental Protection Agency in drinking water. Also, Monte noted that a disproportionately large share of soft drink consumption is in the southwest. Monte joined Olney and Turner in 1983 to urge the FDA to deny the approval of apsartame in soft drinks.

Aspartame proponents, as well as the FDA, had dismissed the problem of methanol. They were quick to point out that the amount of methanol in soft drinks was less than the amount of methanol contained in canned fruit juice. This argument was specious. There is a distinct difference between ingesting methanol by itself, and ingesting it along with food such as fruit juice. Real food provides two protective buffers against methanol toxicity. If the fruit juice breaks down in the can and forms methanol, at the same time it produces ethanol, which *protects* against methanol toxicity. Also, the ethanol slows the rate of conversion from methanol to formaldehyde, and allows time for some of the methanol to be eliminated from the breath and the urine. Actually, ethanol is administered as an antidote for methanol poisoning. The second protective buffer is folic acid, which helps break down methanol. Most foods contain folic acid; diet soft drinks do not.

The bottlers of diet soft drinks need many months to distribute their products. They recognized the breakdown problem. They found only about 65 percent of its starting sweetness in soft drinks after six months of storage under typical conditions (68°F).

AND THE LITTLE CHILD SHALL LEAD

As a school project, Jennifer Cohen, an eleven-year-old sixth grade student in Oradell, New Jersey, kept seven cans of diet Coca-Cola in the refrigerator, seven cans in an incubator at 104°F, and seven cans at room temperature (between 68°F and 70°F). After ten weeks, she found that the incubated soda contained 0.026 percent aspartame, and the two breakdown products, 0.002 percent DKP and 231 parts per billion (ppb) formaldehyde. The measurements were made at the Winston Laboratory, a testing laboratory in Ridgefield, New Jersey. The laboratory found that all of the drinks, including the refrigerated ones, had broken down to formaldehyde and DKP.

Jennifer paid for the expenses of her experiment with money she had earned baby sitting the previous year. A summary of her work, posted on www.dorway.com/jcohen.html (no longer an active web page) chided the FDA for failing to admit to the common scientific knowledge of aspartame's properties. "Can young Jennifer Cohen and her piggy-bank budget *shame* the FDA into doing its job?" She asked, "Will they *now* divorce the drug companies, reclassify aspartame as a cumulative toxic poison, and then mandate its removal from over 9,000 items in the human diet?" (*Food Chemical News,* May 5, 1997)

Bottlers of soft drinks were concerned, too, but for a different reason. The breakdown of aspartame, from some hydrolysis and cyclization (the formation of rings in a hydrocarbon), converts the sweetener to the dipeptides without the methyl ester, and results in a loss of some sweetness in the product, especially in very acidic drinks. This loss of sweetness would lower the quality of the drinks and reduce sales. The bottlers found that sugar and high-fructose corn syrup (HFCS) used in regular soft drinks helped maintain the sweetness of the product for six months or longer; aspartame in diet soft drinks degraded as quickly as two to three months.

In late June 1983, a week before the FDA approval, the National Soft Drinks Association (NSDA) requested the FDA to stay its approval until concerns over the stability of aspartame-containing soft drinks could be resolved. In Canada, aspartame had been in use with soft drinks, and apparently without problems. However, NSDA pointed out that storage conditions in cooler climates in Canada were not comparable to warmer climates elsewhere, such as the south and southwestern areas in the United States.

The NSDA sought to prevent marketing of aspartame for soft drinks because of "serious and unresolved questions about the public health." The NSDA declared aspartame to be "inherently, markedly, and uniquely unstable in aqueous media" and that the sweetener decomposes into unidentified compounds of unknown safety (*Congressional Record,* U.S. Senate, May 7, 1985).

The NSDA also charged that Searle "chose to use a semi-quantitative analytical method to analyze for numerous major [aspartame] breakdown products close to the limits of detection when that method is not the best method available . . . Searle itself has acknowledged the inadequacy of the analytical method that it chose."

Earlier, the NSDA had encouraged FDA approval. This last-minute reversal puzzled many people. *Business Week* (Jul 18, 1983) offered an explanation. The article cited unidentified industry sources who "suspect" that the Coca-

Cola Company and the Pepsi Company were behind the NSDA's sudden change of heart because "a delay would have given Coke and Pepsi time to absorb their heavy new-product marketing costs . . . and allow them to continue negotiating with Searle on a favorable supply contract."

ASPARTAME APPROVED FOR USE IN SOFT DRINKS

The FDA advised NSDA that the agency could not, in good faith, delay approval. Promptly after approval, both the Coca-Cola Company and Royal Crown Cola Company announced plans to use aspartame in their products. Widespread use of the sweetener would be stymied by its high cost. It was estimated that aspartame-sweetened diet soft drinks would cost bottlers about twenty-five cents per six pack; for saccharin equivalency, less than one cent. Later, some producers used some saccharin or sucrose along with the aspartame in soft drink products to stabilize the aspartame and to retain sweetness. Another approach was to add more aspartame to the products to make up for lost sweetness.

Some scientists and researchers expressed concerns about the FDA's approval of aspartame in soft drinks, which would lead to far greater consumption of the sweetener than had been anticipated when the acceptable daily intake (ADI) had been set.

Approval for Soft Drinks Questioned

Dr. Paul A. Lachance, a prominent and respected professor of food science and nutrition at Rutgers University in Rutgers, New Jersey, had urged the FDA to deny the petition for use of aspartame in soft drinks. He said that the existing data did not establish "reasonable certainty" that the proposed use would not be harmful. The questions of DKP formation and the release of free amino acids must be addressed. Lachance noted that although the FDA had concluded that neither aspartame nor DKP caused brain tumors in laboratory rats, the agency acknowledged "that high amounts of aspartame component amino acids may cause brain damage" (*Food Chemical News*, Mar 14, 1983). He said that aspartame was approved only because the available data established that the maximum projected consumption of aspartame for current approved uses was still far below any level even suspected of being toxic. But, the additional uses "reduce this implied margin of safety . . . the FDA must consider not only toxicity, but the fact that both phenylalanine and aspartic acid are recognized as exerting neurotransmitter activity considerably below the concentrations and durations of exposure involving the classical toxicological testing." The narrowed margin of safety must be recognized "between what could be labeled physiological levels with the possibility of exerting excitatory [effects] and over time, possible brain lesions." Lachance added that the FDA acknowledged that "it is believed that the (brain) lesion can be produced by a single surge of plasma GL/ASP [glutamic acid/aspartic acid] above some toxic threshold." Lachance said that there should be concern about the effects of repeated sub-toxic surges "because of the known actions of such compounds in the brain." Lachance's warnings reinforced the earlier ones of Olney.

Richard J. Wurtman, M.D., a neuroendocrinologist and director of the Clinical Research Center at MIT said that the use of aspartame in soft drinks may cause brain chemistry changes that can affect mood or behavior in some individuals. Wurtman cited rat studies. Replacing glucose in food by aspartame *doubled* the brain levels of phenylalanine in the animals. When the rats consumed carbohydrates along with the glucose or aspartame, the brain phenylalanine *doubled again.* The combination also *tripled* brain tyrosine (an amino acid) and blocked the normal rise in other chemical messengers. Wurtman noted that the amount of aspartame used in the rat studies was comparable to what an eight-year-old child might consume on a hot afternoon. Individuals most likely to experience behavioral changes after aspartame consumption were persons suffering from insomnia, Parkinson's disease, hyperkinesis, and persons using drugs that interact with plasma phenylalaline or tyrosine (such as levadopa or monoamine oxidase inhibitors). Phenylalanine is toxic to neurons at certain levels. With PKU, brain damage can be caused by high levels of phenylalanine. People who carry the gene for PKU are *twice* as sensitive to aspartame as others. Wurtman reported that the minimum level at which phenylalanine is toxic is unknown. He recommended that human behavioral studies be conducted to learn if the same effects of aspartame in the rat studies are duplicated when humans consume aspartame-sweetened soft drinks along with carbohydrate-rich foods.

On the very day when Wurtman issued his warnings, the Coca-Cola Company rolled out the nation's first aspartame-sweetened soft drinks. Later in the same week, the Royal Crown Company introduced its aspartame-containing soft drink.

The FDA rejected Wurtman's warnings. The agency claimed that all the issues raised by Wurtman had been reviewed thoroughly by FDA scientists, and they had not found any safety problems.

In addition to the problems of breakdown to methanol, formaldehyde, and DKP, problems were discovered in aspartame's ability to interact with other substances. In the presence of ascorbic acid (vitamin C) and a transitional metal catalyst, aspartame can produce benzaldehyde via a free-radical attack on aspartame. This finding was reported by Glen Lawrence and Dongmal Tuan, both from the chemistry department at Long Island University in Brooklyn, New York. The researchers noted that there was scant investigation of aspartame's interactions with other food components such as naturally present nutrients, or with other food additives.

Another unconsidered interaction was raised by the Coalition in Engle-wood Cliffs, New Jersey. In a letter dated February 24, 1999, to the FDA, the coalition reported that aspartame in milk and other dairy products does not break down in the stomach because these foods lower the stomach's acidity level and allow aspartame to survive much longer in exerting its effect. The coalition cited a study in which rhesus monkeys developed epileptic seizures after being fed aspartame in a milk-based formula. Seizures developed on day 200 of a year-long study. When the aspartame-containing formula feedings were discontinued, the seizure activity ended promptly. The coalition request-ed the FDA to require the manufacturer to perform a series of tests in which aspartame is delivered in a milk-based formula.

POSTMARKET MONITORING

Due to the contentious reactions that aspartame had provoked with its origi-nal approval in 1981, the FDA had established a plan for a postmarketing sur-vey. This is common procedure with drugs, but aspartame was the first newly introduced food additive to require formal postmarket monitoring of adverse reactions. The FDA's survey had two components. Manufacturers would sup-ply a poundage survey of aspartame sales made to the food and pharmaceuti-cal industries and a dietary survey, in which actual ingestion by a sample of the population would be reported.

In addition to these monitorings, the FDA furthered research on aspartame safety by contracting with Battelle Memorial Institute, a science and technolo-gy enterprise that develops and commercializes technology and manages lab-oratories for customers worldwide, to evaluate the effects of altered amino acid balance on rodent brain function, with an emphasis on neurotransmit-ters. Also in February 1987, the FDA funded the National Institute of Envi-ronmental Health Sciences (NIEHS) to study the impact of amino acid imbalances on seizure thresholds, and neurobehavioral functions in rodents. Another interagency agreement funded the Federal Aviation Administration (FAA), to study the effects of aspartame on the performance of airplane pilots on a number of complex laboratory-based tests of physical and mental func-tions. This study was devised after there were reported cases of airplane pilots who lost their licenses to fly due to eyesight problems that allegedly were caused by aspartame consumption.

The FDA established a passive system of review for consumer complaints about aspartame. The weakness of voluntary compliance caused the acting director of the FDA's Bureau of Drugs to recommend that aspartame be regarded as a drug, and that "safety evaluation of proposed new sugar substitutes be conducted as phase I studies under the Investigational New Drug (IND) Regulations." This recommendation was made in an FDA memorandum and released publicly by the late U.S. Senator Howard M. Metzenbaum (D-OH) during the U.S. Senate Hearings, NutraSweet—Health and Safety Concerns (Nov 3, 1987).

Inadequate Labeling

Metzenbaum recommended new regulations to make the reporting of adverse reactions to additives *mandatory*, not *voluntary*. Metzenbaum also wanted the FDA to require clinical testing for the approval of additives with potential behavioral or neurological effects.

The issue of adequate labeling of aspartame-containing products was discussed at the Senate hearings as well by others, including Dr. Wurtman and Dr. Reuben Matalon, director of Biochemical Genetics and Metabolism, and director of the PKU Clinic at the College of Medicine at the University of Illinois in Chicago. Although there was a warning statement on labels about PKU, there were additional needs not being met. The American Diabetes Association, in its "Position Statement on the Use of Sugar Replacers" (*Diabetes Care*, Jul–Aug 1987) encouraged the food industry to label the *amount* of aspartame in any given product in milligrams (mg) per serving. Dr. Matalon suggested that the problems of behavioral disturbances and birth defects in offspring of heavy aspartame users with PKU may be aggravated because the government did not require labeling to show how much aspartame is contained in each sweetened product. Dr. Wurtman told the FDA that, in addition to cautioning PKU individuals about products containing aspartame, the warning should extend to individuals with hypertension, Parkinson's disease, hyperkinesis (hyperactivity), and those on certain types of drugs.

After aspartame approval for use in foods, a bill was introduced that, if passed, would have required manufacturers to state on labels how much aspartame was in each serving. The bill was defeated in the Senate by a sixty-eight to twenty-seven vote. As a result, the presence of aspartame is declared on the label of soft drinks, but the amount used is not listed. (By 2006, labeling of aspartame was weakened further. The FDA considered allowing aspartame to be added to products such as ice cream, and merely to be listed as an "artificial flavoring," and not to require the sweetener to be listed specifically by the word aspartame.)

Valid findings from postmarket monitoring is nearly impossible unless the presence of additives is noted clearly on food packages, identifying both the substance and its quantity. Clearly, consumers cannot report any adverse effects if they are unaware of what they have consumed, and in what quantities they have consumed the substance.

After aspartame approval in soft drinks, and with greatly expanded uses of aspartame in soft drinks as well as in a greater number of food products, some scientists expressed concerns. They found that the daily intake by some individuals, especially children, was exceeding the established ADI level.

On October 18, 1983, at a meeting of the FDA with the National Consumer Exchange, the agency promised to continue monitoring a usage level via its postmarket survey to ease the accuracy for estimates of daily intake. The FDA assured the group that clinically, no subpopulation group, except persons with PKU or other individuals who needed to control phenylalanine intake, "have been identified who can suffer ill effects from longterm or excessive aspartame ingestion" (*Food Chemical News*, Oct 23, 1983).

COMMON ADVERSE REACTIONS

This reassurance did not match the facts. The FDA continued to receive, in ever-increasing numbers, reports from individuals who claimed that they were suffering ill health from aspartame consumption. The agency monitors complaints as part of its Adverse Reaction Monitoring System (ARMS) which tracks voluntary reporting from consumers and health professionals on adverse effects experienced from food products and food additives. The purpose of ARMS is to identify potential problems that require clinical investigation.

Voluntary reports of epileptic seizures linked to aspartame ingestion were investigated by FDA field personnel using interviews, questionnaires, and medical records. The results of these investigations, conducted from January 1986 through December 1990, involved 261 cases of reported seizures grouped by strength of linkage:

- Group A: 41 cases of reported seizures that recurred when a person ate different products containing aspartame.

- Group B: 35 cases of reported seizures that recurred each time the person ate one specific aspartame-containing product type.

- Group C: 51 cases of reported single seizure temporarily associated with the consumption of aspartame after which the person avoided aspartame.

- Group D: 124 cases of reported single or multiple seizure(s) that probably were unrelated to aspartame ingestion. Within this group, physicians' statements in patients' medical records indicated that seizures were not linked to aspartame, or that another condition likely caused the seizures (examples: brain tumors, brain damage, or congenital defects). Also, within this group were other reasons to reject aspartame's role in seizures: seizures occurring before aspartame intake; seizure(s) occurring months or years following aspartame intake; or absence of aspartame in the offending food or beverage.

Of the reports examined, thirteen individuals failed to provide adequate information and refused access to their medical records. Of Groups A, B, and C, 88 out of 127 cases of seizures were women. The peak incidence for them was thirty-one to thirty-five years of age. Of the 127 cases, 45 were considered ineligible for a potential causal link because the seizures occurred thirteen hours or longer after consumption of aspartame. (This was faulty reasoning, because monosodium glutamate, another compound that contains an amino acid that affects the central nervous system including the brain, has been linked to adverse reactions even twenty-four hours after ingestion.) The rationale given was that aspartame is hydrolyzed rapidly during digestion to phenylalanine and aspartic acid, and the half lives of these two amino acids are four to six hours following absorption into the portal vein, so it is unlikely that aspartame seizures occur more then twelve hours after ingestion. Of the 127 reports in Groups A, B, and C, data on the amount of aspartame consumed by 82 individuals was *below* the ADI limit. Only two individuals consumed unusually large amounts above the ADI level.

By January 1987, the FDA had received more than 3,000 adverse reaction reports for aspartame. Of these, there were multiple symptoms, but the major problem was headaches, accounting for about 600 of the reports. About 500 reports involved seizures after eating or drinking aspartame-containing products. About one-fourth of all the adverse reactions reported involved neurological and behavioral symptoms, allergic reactions, menstrual irregularities, and miscellaneous problems.

By July 1991, the FDA had received a total of nearly 5,000 complaints. Headaches remained the major symptom, followed in frequency by dizziness, mood changes, vomiting, nausea, abdominal cramps, and other discomforts. Almost 40 percent of all complaints cited diet soft drinks as the source of the problem.

By 1992, the FDA had received a total of 5,831 complaints. Headaches remained the most common feature. Use of diet soft drinks and aspartame tabletop sweetener were mentioned most frequently in the reports. Seizures were listed in 251 reports, but the FDA denied that most cases demonstrated any linkage to aspartame.

By 1994, the FDA had received a total of 7,232 complaints. Some of them were rejected and eliminated from the official summaries. Thus, only 6,583 complaints were directed to the FDA's Center for Food Safety and Applied Nutrition (CFSAN), or received from the NutraSweet Company, the Aspartame Consumer Safety Network, the 700 Club, as well as from individual health professionals and other interested parties. Headaches remained the commonest complaint, and other complaints were similar to those in previous reports. By then, reports received by the FDA about adverse reactions to aspartame comprised three-fourths of all reports about adverse reactions to substances in the food supply received by the agency.

MAJOR SELF-REPORTED SIDE EFFECTS IN 496 ASPARTAME REACTORS

H. J. Roberts, M.D., has studied aspartame more extensively, with patients perhaps, than any other physician. Known for his concerns and interest in aspartame and human health, he attracted many patients who ascribed many of their ailments to aspartame intake. With nearly 500 of his patients who claimed to suffer adverse effects from the sweetener, Roberts recorded and classified the various symptoms. Many patients suffered from multiple symptoms.

- Eye: decreased vision and/or other eye problems (blurring, bright flashes, tunnel vision)

- Ear: tinnitus (ringing or buzzing), severe intolerance to noise; marked impairment of hearing

- Neurological: headaches, dizziness, unsteadiness, or both; confusion, memory loss, or both; convulsions (grand mal epileptic attacks); petit mal attacks and absences (disorientation); severe drowsiness and sleepiness; paresthesias (pins and needles, tingling), or numbness of the limbs; severe slurring of speech; severe hyperactivity and restless legs; atypical facial pain; severe tremors

- Psychological/psychiatric: severe depression; extreme irritability, severe anxiety attacks; marked personality changes; recent severe insomnia; severe aggravation of phobias

- Chest: palpitations, tachycardia (rapid heart action) or both; shortness of breath; atypical chest pain; recently developed hypertension (high blood pressure)

- Gastrointestinal: nausea; diarrhea; associated gross blood in the stools; abdominal pain, pain on swallowing

- Skin and allergies: severe itching without a rash; severe lip and mouth reactions; urticaria (hives); other eruptions; aggravation of respiratory allergies

- Endocrine and metabolic: menstrual changes; severe reduction or cessation of periods; marked thinning or loss of hair; marked weight loss; paradoxical weight gain; aggravated hypoglycemia (low blood sugar); less control of diabetes

- Other: frequency of voiding (day and night); burning on urination (dysuria) or both; excessive thirst; 'bloat;" severe joint pains; fluid retention and leg swellings; increased susceptibility to infection

The FDA admitted that the passive surveillance program was not a controlled scientific study. However, the agency did not believe that the evidence warranted such a study.

The adverse reaction reports had peaked earlier, after which there had been a gradual decrease in the number of reports that the agency received. By 1994, there were 198 reports during the year, and the symptoms were similar to these noted earlier, and similar in demographic distribution, severity, and strength of association with the product. By the end of 1994, the NutraSweet Company informed the FDA that it planned to discontinue aspartame consumption surveys, but would continue to submit quarterly reports on the amount of aspartame sold to industrial customers in the United States.

The CFSAN policy did not *require* reporting on the use of any approved food additive. Reporting was voluntary. After the aspartame experience, CFSAN *requested* physicians and other health professionals to inform the center about any well-documented, severe reactions associated with foods, food additives, or dietary practices. Many health professionals cooperated. Because headaches seemed to play such a prominent role in the reports of adverse reactions to aspartame—nearly 20 percent—many health professionals responded on this subject.

Aspartame-Related Headaches

In a letter to the *New England Journal of Medicine* (Aug 14, 1986), Donald R. Johns, M.D., at Massachusetts General Hospital in Boston, noted the marked rise in aspartame-related complaints to the FDA after its approval of the sweetener in soft drinks. Johns noted that the most common cause of complaints were neurologic and behavioral symptoms, including headaches. Johns noted that dietary substances, including phenylalanine, tyramine, and nitrites are known to play a role in migraine headaches.

Johns reported a clinical case of a heavy user of aspartame-sweetened soft drinks and headache induction, and advised other health professionals that:

> Considering the widespread distribution of aspartame in food products and the relatively high prevalence of migraine and seizures, it is prudent to include inquiries about aspartame consumption in the evaluation of patients with these disorders. Future clinical observation of the possible role of aspartame as an inciting or provocative factor in migraine and other neurologic illnesses are obviously needed.

Richard B. Lipton, M.D., at the Department of Neurology at Albert Einstein College of Medicine and at the Headache Unit at Montefiore Medical

Center in Bronx, New York, along with his colleagues surveyed 190 patients with headache disorders at the Montefiore Hospital. The study was supported by a grant from the National Headache Foundation. The patients were asked to complete a questionnaire regarding the role of several dietary factors associated with their headaches. Of the 190 questionnaires distributed, 171 were completed fully, and analyzed. Compared with other headache sufferers, migraineurs were three times more likely to report aspartame as a definite headache trigger.

Shirley M. Koehler, M.S., and Alan Glaros, Ph.D., both at the Department of Clinical and Health Psychology at the University of Florida in Gainsville, found that the addition of products containing aspartame to the diet of migraineurs could produce a significant increase in the frequency of migraine episodes. Koehler and Glaros conducted a thirteen-week, double-blind, randomized, cross-over study with twenty-five migraineurs. Results indicated a significant increase in headache episodes for some subjects. Although the study was well designed, the number of participants was modest. The aspartame did not increase the intensity, but did increase the length of the migraine duration compared to the placebo. Also, the subjects experienced an increase in unusual symptoms during their headache episodes, such as dizziness, inability to see well, and a feeling described as "shaky." The researchers recommended future research to examine the amino acid content of subjects' diets to determine the amount of amino acids such as phenylalanine, L-tryptophan, and tyrosine present, as well as other triggering agents such as tyramine (another amino acid).

Another study of aspartame and headaches, conducted by S. S. Schiffman, was published in the *New England Journal of Medicine* (Nov 5, 1987). The study, conducted at Duke University in Durham, North Carolina, was double-blind. The number of subjects was still modest, but slightly larger than the Koehler and Glaros study. Twelve men and twenty-eight women were studied who had reported vascular headaches occurring within twenty-four hours of ingesting aspartame-containing products. All were given challenge doses of aspartame or a placebo in capsule form, followed by a washout period (time for the body to be cleared of the challenge dose), and then a cross-over challenge, followed by allergy testing a day later. The incidence of headaches after ingesting aspartame was 35 percent; after the placebo, 45 percent. Results of this short-term challenge failed to confirm consumer complaints that aspartame causes headaches in sensitive individuals. However, the study was criticized. The aspartame in capsules contained only traces of aspartame's breakdown products. In real-life settings, much aspartame is consumed in beverages in which, as mentioned earlier, some of the sweetener degrades. If the breakdown products, rather than the intact sweetener associated with headaches had been used, the study might have produced different results. The NutraSweet Company funded this study.

Even aspartame-containing chewing gums were found to induce headaches, as reported by Dr. Harvey J. Blumenthal and Dwight A. Vance, in *Headache* (Nov–Dec 1997). The cases reported involved three young women who were migraineurs. All three developed headaches after using aspartame-containing chewing gums. One woman was a forty-year-old homemaker who had suffered from migraine since she was twenty-five years of age. She observed that aspartame-containing chewing gum was a strong trigger of her typical migraine episodes. Another woman was a thirty-two-year-old executive assistant with a six-year history of migraine. She observed that whenever she chewed aspartame-containing gum, she had an inter-menstrual period migraine episode. She experienced a throbbing, bitemporal headache within forty-five minutes, which lasted for approximately ten hours, compared with her usual menstrually-related migraine episodes which lasted four to five days. The third woman was a twenty-five-year-old laboratory technician who had suffered from mild headaches for twelve years. She sought medical help when the headaches worsened. She was urged to stop smoking and to chew gum instead. She found that the use of aspartame-containing chewing gum produced her typical headaches.

A different problem induced by aspartame-containing chewing gum was reported in the *Australian Dental Journal* (Aug 1993) from New South Wales, Australia. A forty-seven-year-old man suffered from recurrent swellings (granulomatitis) in his upper lip from frequent use of an aspartame-sweetened chewing gum. The symptoms disapppeared when he stopped using the chewing gum as well as other aspartame-containing products.

Aspartame's Effects on Brain Functioning

Although headaches accounted for a large number of adverse reaction reports ascribed to aspartame, headaches are only one manifestation of neurological problems, ranging from brain dysfunction such as behavioral changes and panic attacks, all the way to brain tumors and brain cancers.

In a clinical update on aspartame, Daniel P. Potenza, M.D., and Rif S. El-Mallackh, noted in *Connecticut Medicine* (Jul 1989) the mounting number of reports, both published and unpublished, of aspartame as a factor in headaches, seizures, blindness, and cognitive and behavioral changes. They noted the serious lack of reliable epidemiological data. Also, they noted that pertinent data remained unpublished, and consequently, not subject to peer review. Despite these shortcomings, there appeared to be "sufficient data to indicate that a sector of the population may be susceptible to a variety of complications with long-term high-dose aspartame ingestion."

In May 1987, several clinical investigators presented their findings regarding the effects of aspartame on brain chemistry before federal government officials and industry executives in Washington, D.C. The meeting was organized by Dr. Wurtman.

One study, presented by Paul A. Spiers at Beth Israel Hospital in Boston, was about aspartame and brain functioning. Spiers's preliminary findings indicated that normal volunteers on a high aspartame diet (equivalent to the amount of the sweetener in about twelve cans of diet soda consumed in twenty-four hours by someone weighing 110 pounds) do worse than matched controls on standard tests of higher brain function. Unlike the controls, the performance of the high aspartame users worsened on each successive test. They also complained more of headaches and dizziness when they consumed aspartame. (Consumption of twelve cans of diet soda with a twenty-four hour period may seem unrealistic, but idiocyncratic use does occur.)

Louis J. Elsas, II, director of the Division of Medical Genetics at Emory University School of Medicine in Atlanta, Georgia, presented his study. He found that in individuals who have only one effective phenylalanine hydroxylase gene, phenylalanine slows brain waves at a dosage equivalent to only 34 mg/kilogram/bodyweight/day. Yet the ADI level established by the FDA is 50 mg/kg/bw/dy.

Reuben K. Matalon, mentioned earlier as a critic of inadequate labeling of aspartame, found that human consumption of aspartame at levels from 50 mg/kg/dy to 100 mg/kg/dy were not uncommon. Matalon found that when a high dose is continued over a period of a week, the phenylalanine level in 14 percent of normal subjects, and in 15 percent of those with only one functional phenylalanine hydroxylase gene exceeds the level considered as excessive for pregnant women.

Matthew J. During at MIT reported on tests conducted to observe behavioral effects of aspartame on rats. He found that high doses of phenylalanine inhibit synthesis of the neurotransmitter dopamine. Several other laboratory studies found that high doses of aspartame can increase the frequency of seizures, or lower the stimulation level necessary to induce them in laboratory animals.

At the previously mentioned U.S. Senate hearings on aspartame (Nov 3, 1987) several doctors gave statements regarding aspartame's neurological effects. Dr. Michael Mahlik at the Philadelphia College of Osteopathic Medicine cautioned about aspartame's possible inducement of brain dysfunction. Dr. Jeffrey Bada, professor of marine chemistry at the University of California at San Diego, cautioned that aspartame's degraded products had not been studied adequately. Dr. Roger Coulombe at Utah State University at Logan, expressed concern about aspartame's possible behavioral and neurological effects.

OPENING STATEMENT AT SENATE HEARINGS ON ASPARTAME (1987)

"If a food additive has potential neurological or behavioral effects, it should undergo human clinical testing, similar to the process a drug must undergo before it is put on the market. Only animal tests were required of NutraSweet, though at one point in the approval process FDA scientists had recommended that NutraSweet be tested like a drug. They were overruled. I wish they hadn't been—maybe a number of questions . . . would have already been answered."

—U.S. Senator Howard M. Metzenbaum (D-OH)

Dr. Wurtman, whose work was mentioned earlier, provided the FDA with records of eighty-six people who suffered brain seizures after consuming aspartame. None had brain abnormalities that could have caused the problem. The FDA remained unconvinced. Wurtman accused the NutraSweet Company of failing to refer seizure complaints to the FDA. A NutraSweet spokesman denied the charge and reported that the company referred all medical complaints to the FDA monthly.

Drs. Phillip C. Jobe and John V. Dailey, epilepsy researchers, conducted animal studies at the College of Medicine at the University of Illinois, in Chicago, financed with a $343,000 grant from the NutraSweet Company. Jobe and Dailey reported that aspartame did not bring on seizures in the tested rats.

Another manifestation of neurological problems related to high aspartame intake is panic attack. In correspondence to the *Lancet II* (Sep 13, 1986) Miles E. Drake at the Department of Neurology at the College of Medicine, Ohio State University in Columbus, reported a case of a woman cook who consumed from six to twelve cans of aspartame-sweetened cola daily. After a job transfer to a very hot kitchen, she increased her consumption of the drinks to about twenty cans daily. Within a week, she experienced panic attacks. She reduced her cigarette and coffee use, but the panic attacks failed to subside. Then, she reduced her diet cola consumption to two to three cans daily and the panic attacks subsided. When she increased her intake of the drinks to her former high consumption level, the panic attacks returned.

Retinal detachment in the eye was related to patients with depression and who consumed aspartame. Ralph G. Walton, Chairman of the Center for Behavioral Medicine and chairman of the Department of Psychiatry at Northeastern Ohio Universities College of Medicine conducted a double-blind study with forty depressed patients and forty people without depression. Each group consumed daily rations of aspartame equal to that in ten to twelve cans of aspartame-sweetened soft drinks. The depressed patients showed significantly more side effects than the controls, and they were especially vulnerable to severe effects such as retinal detachment. (*Biological Psychiatry*, 1993)

ASPARTAME AND LEARNING

A high school junior, Susie Morris, in Price, Utah won a first prize in the National Science Fair in 1998 for her three-year research study on the effects of aspartame on the learning ability of rats. Morris chose twenty-seven-month-old rats (equivalent to seventy-nine-year-old humans). She found that when rats were fed aspartame, the sweetener "destroyed the elderly rats' ability to learn." Two groups of rats were fed the same diet, but aspartame was added to the feed of one group. All of the animals were tested for their ability to find their way through a maze. The control group mastered the maze by the thirty-fourth trial. Morris reported that the aspartame-fed group "never mastered the maze and showed no sign of learning whatsoever." Instead, they engaged in "repetition of a meaningless behavior." (*Pure Facts*, Sept 1998)

Aspartame and Increases in Cancer

By the 1990s, aspartame's neurological effects continued to be publicized. Dr. John W. Olney, mentioned earlier, wrote a paper "Increasing Brain Tumor Rates: Is There a Link to Aspartame?" that was published in the *Journal of Neuropathology and Experimental Neurology* (1996). Olney noted the dramatic rise of brain tumors from 1975 to 1992 in several industrialized countries, including the United States. During this time period, brain tumor data were gathered by the National Cancer Institute (NCI) from catchment areas (surrounding areas served by an institution such as a hospital or school), representing 10 percent of the U.S. population. Olney analyzed the data and found that the increase in brain tumor rates in the United States occurred in two distinct phases: an early modest increase that perhaps reflected improved diagnostic technology; and later, a sustained increase in the incidence, and shift toward greater malignancy that needed to be explained by other factors. Olney wrote:

> Compared to other environmental factors putatively linked to brain tumors, the artificial sweetener aspartame is a promising candidate to explain the recent increase in incidence and degree of malignancy of brain tumors. Evidence potentially implicating aspartame includes an early animal study revealing an exceedingly high incidence of brain tumors in aspartame-fed rats compared to no brain tumors in concurrent controls. The recent finding is that the aspartame molecule has

mutagenic potential . . . (aspartame was introduced into the U.S. food and beverage markets several years prior to the sharp increase in brain tumor incidence and malignancy). We conclude that there is need for reassessing the carcinogenic potential of aspartame.

Olney conceded that numerous environmental factors in industrialized societies have been studied in relation to the increased brain tumor rates, yet aspartame has barely been mentioned as a candidate.

H. J. Roberts, M.D., director of the Palm Beach Institute for Medical Research in West Palm Beach, Florida, and a longtime critic of aspartame, wrote "Does Aspartame Cause Human Cancer?" in the *Journal of Advancement in Medicine* (1991). Roberts charged that aspartame's potential for cancer induction had never been evaluated seriously, but merely dismissed as a possibility. Roberts, as had Olney, noted the sharp rise in brain tumor rates in the United States following the approval of aspartame. Also, the two panelists on the FDA's PBI, Drs. Walle Nauta and Peter W. Lampert, were prominent neuroscientists. They were asked to evaluate evidence from two animal studies that potentially linked aspartame to malignant astrocytic (star-shaped cells especially neuroglial cells of nervous tissue) brain tumor. Nauta and Lampert had concluded that evidence from one study they examined was "bizarre" and totally unreliable, but that evidence from the other study appeared to show that "aspartame may contribute to the development of brain tumors." The two experts recommended additional research to rule out brain tumor risk, and also recommended that aspartame approval be withheld pending the outcome of such studies. Other expert FDA consultants had concurred with the panelists. However, in 1981, the newly appointed FDA Commissioner Arthur Hull Hayes judged that the brain tumor risk was minimal, and that no further research was necessary. He promptly approved aspartame after being in office for a few days. As a consequence, the specific studies recommended by the panelists were never conducted.

WORDS, BUT NO ACTIONS

"Within the general field of toxicological testing, the FDA Bureau of Foods views the development of behavioral teratological or neurotoxicological testing as one of the most important and urgent areas for future improvement. We await with keen interest the creation of testing paradigms that can be recommended for routine measurements of the neurotoxic potential of food additive substances."

—D.G. Hattan et al., "Role of the Food and Drug Administration in Regulation of Neuroeffective Food Additives." In *Nutrition and the Brain* edited by Richard J. Wurtman and Judith J. Wurtman (Lippincott Williams and Wilkins, 1985).

In 2005, results of an impressively large and well-designed long-range study of the carcinogenicity of aspartame were announced by the European Ramazzini Foundation, a non-profit private institution with official government recognition, located in Bentivoglio, Italy. The Foundation has conducted research in environmental health sciences, oncology, and toxicology for more than twenty-five years. The aspartame study was conducted on 1,800 rats (900 males and 900 females) from a colony used for more than thirty years by the Foundation. In order to simulate daily human intake, aspartame was added to the standard rat diet in quantities that ranged from 5,000 to 2,500, 500, 100, 20, 4, and 0 mg/kg/bw/dy. The diet began by feeding eight-week-old rats, and continued until spontaneous death occurred with the animals. A complete necropsy and histopathological evaluation of tissues and organs was performed on each deceased animal (to note any changes in the tissues and organs due to disease), with a total of more than 30,000 slides for microscopic examination.

Results of the experiment showed a dose-related statistically significant increase of lymphomas and leukemias in female rats. This statistically significant increase was observed at a dose level of 20 mg/kg/bw/dy—a dose that is lower than the ADI suggested by current regulations. The addition of aspartame to the diet induced a dose-related reduction in food consumption, but without causing a difference in body weight between the treated and untreated animals. The results demonstrated that aspartame is a carcinogenic agent, even when administered at dose levels very close to the acceptable one for humans. The data demonstrated that aspartame in the diet is not effective for weight loss. The International Agency for Research on Cancer (IARC) of WHO recognizes that long-term bioassays conducted on rats or mice are highly predictive of carcinogenic risk for humans. In view of the findings from this large-scale, long-range study, the Foundation called for "urgent reconsideration of regulations governing the use of an artificial sweetener in order to better protect public health, in particular that of children" (www.dorway.com or *Environmental Health Perspectives*, Mar 2006).

Other Health Problems Ascribed to Aspartame

In addition to the numerous problems ascribed to aspartame, are its effects on organs such as the liver, skin conditions, and carpel tunnel syndrome.

Misael Uribe, M.D., at the National Institute of Nutrition in Mexico City, wrote in a letter to the *New England Journal of Medicine* (Jan 21, 1982) that aspartame was potentially toxic in patients with liver disease. Uribe reported that the FDA had not considered this possibility. He felt that until controlled tests are conducted to assess this problem, it would be prudent to issue a warning to patients with advanced liver disease that they should avoid using aspartame.

Daniel P. McCauliffe, M.D., in the Department of Dermatology at the University of Texas in Dallas, and Kevin Poitras, M.D., at the Scott Air Force Base in Illinois, reported a case of a fifty-seven-year-old diabetic man who consumed about six or seven packets of aspartame-containing Equal and 36 to 48 ounces of aspartame-sweetened soft drinks daily. On occasion, he used other aspartame-containing products. He developed a lobular panniculitis (an inflammation of the skin and fat nodules, especially in the abdominal area). The man was advised to discontinue use of aspartame-containing products. Within twelve days, the nodules were gone, and there was no recurrence of the skin disorder.

McCauliffe and Poitras obtained pure aspartame from Searle and conducted double-blind studies. There were no lesions in subjects given the placebo, but lesions developed in subjects within five days of ingesting 300 mg of aspartame twice daily—equivalent to four 12-ounce cans of aspartame-sweetened soft drinks (*Journal of the American Academy of Dermatology*, Feb 1991).

Aspartame-induced hives was reported by Anthony Kulczycki, Jr., M.D., an allergist and immunologist, and professor of medicine at Washington University School of Medicine in St. Louis, Missouri, in the *Journal of Allergy and Clinical Immunology* (Feb 1995). He recruited seventy-five individuals who suspected that their chronic urticaria (hives) or angioedema (swelling) might be due to aspartame use. Of this group, fifty individuals experienced total relief from their symptoms after they avoided aspartame for two weeks. Some of them were willing to rechallenge themselves with aspartame, and they experienced skin reactions again. Some of the reactions were immediate; others, delayed; and some, chronic.

Kulczycki criticized an earlier study, sponsored by the NutraSweet Company, which had found no association of aspartame with hives. He identified flaws in the study, and suggested that confounding medications such as astemizole (a nonsedating antihistamine) should have been avoided for six weeks instead of only three weeks prior to the study (*Journal of Allergy and Clinical Immunology*, Feb 1995).

Kulczycki also identified aspartame allergy in six patients, and studied an additional forty-four potential patients. All suffered severe reactions. One patient experienced such throat swelling that she needed emergency treatment.

Earlier, in 1985, Nelson L. Novick, M.D., at Mount Sinai Medical Center in New York City had reported a patient who developed inflammatory nodules in the fatty tissues of her legs after aspartame ingestion. The inflammation developed on three occasions after aspartame ingestion.

Kulczycki contacted the FDA, because out of some 700 complaints ascribed to aspartame, at least sixty-two appeared to be very similar to the cases observed earlier by Novick, and later by himself. After Kulczycki's article appeared in the *Annals of Medicine* (Feb 1986), a number of individuals in the St. Louis area contacted Kulczycki to relate similar complaints.

Researchers Paula Robbins and Lawrence Raymond reported of a possible link between aspartame use and carpel tunnel syndrome in the *Journal of Environmental and Occupational Medicine* (1999). In North Carolina, three computer workers, all heavy aspartame consumers, experienced carpel tunnel syndrome symptoms of pain, tingling, and numbness in their hands and wrists. All three had been consuming from 6 to 15 grams of aspartame daily. All three stopped consuming aspartame-containing foods and beverages and all symptoms abated totally within two weeks, despite having made no other changes in their keyboarding work.

As noted in many of these reports, health problems developed with high aspartame use. In establishing the ADI for aspartame, the FDA failed to take into account the future greatly expanded uses of aspartame, especially with soft drinks. Obviously, some people exceeded the ADI. Dr. William M. Pardridge, professor of medicine at the Division of Endocrinology and Brain Research Institute, Blood-Brain Barrier Laboratory at the University of California in Los Angeles was concerned about the inadequacy of the ADI. In November 1983, Pardridge wrote to the FDA that its ADI was far too low. An eight-year-old child easily might consume far more by the time he or she finished an afternoon snack.

SUPPLY AND DEMAND FOR ASPARTAME CONTINUES TO SKYROCKET

The expanded consumption of aspartame by Americans is reflected by the statistics gathered by the Economic Research Service (ERS) of the U.S. Department of Agriculture (USDA) in the Sugar and Sweeteners Outlook report. In 1981, the consumption of aspartame in the United States was 0.2 pounds per person annually; by 1982, 1.0 pounds; by 1983, 3.5 pounds; by 1984, 15.8 pounds; by 1986, 18.0 pounds; and by 1986, 18.5 pounds.

It is not easy to appreciate the staggering amounts represented, until one extrapolates. With these figures, the USDA estimated that the sugar-sweetness equivalency of aspartame was 200 times that of sucrose. With increased aspartame use, saccharin use declined slightly, from 6.0 pounds per person annually in 1985 to 5.8, in 1986. The USDA estimated that the sugar-sweetness equivalency of saccharin was 300 times that of sucrose.

The total amounts of synthesized sweeteners (cyclamates and saccharin) used in 1970 was 6.0 pounds per person. By 1985, the amount (saccharin and aspartame) had risen to 16.0 pounds; by 1986, to 18.5 pounds; and by 1991, to 24.3 pounds. The year 1991 appears to be the last year the USDA tracked these sweeteners. After 1991, amounts were not included in subsequent issues of

Sugar and Sweeteners Outlook report, nor were they available from the USDA. However, the ever-escalating use of aspartame continued, and can be inferred in several ways.

By 1992, it was estimated that some 200 million people worldwise were using more than 5,000 different types of food and beverage products sweetened with aspartame. American consumption accounted for about 80 percent of the world's market of aspartame. The prediction was that consumption would more than double by the year 2000.

Soft drink consumption soared. In 1970, on average, the per capita consumption of soft drinks was 22.7 gallons a year in the United States. By 1992, consumption had risen to 48.0 gallons. The total soft drink consumption was estimated at 12.4 billion gallons, of which diet soft drinks accounted for 3.6 billion gallons—about 29 percent of the total.

The Marketing Research Corporation of America, an independent research group, was hired by Searle to monitor aspartame intake. The group collected data through June 1985. All age groups were consuming aspartame below the level of 34 mg/kg/bw/dy. This included data on high users and children of very low body weight. However, some individuals, notably Drs. Reuben Matalon and William M. Pardridge (both mentioned earlier) disputed these findings. They said that doses as high as 50 mg/kg/bw/dy actually were not uncommon.

Small children are most likely to consume the largest amounts, in proportion to their body weight, according to Deborah Thomas-Dobersen, senior clinical dietitian at the Health Sciences Center of the University of Colorado in Denver. Writing in the *Journal of the American Dietetic Association* (Jun 1989), she found that two- to five-year-old children had a mean potential exposure as high as 50 mg/kg/bw/dy, an amount that matched Matalon and Pardridge's estimates.

Another way to appreciate the growth of aspartame consumption is to examine the steady expansion of manufacturing plants. The demand for NutraSweet was so great that the Searle Company converted its Chicago area plant in mid-1982, spending $35 million for expansion. Meanwhile, the Ajinomoto Company continued to produce NutraSweet for Searle in Japan, to meet demands for the sweetener in the United States.

Searle, in a joint venture with Ajinomoto, announced in 1990 that U.S. plants would be enlarged, and new facilities would be opened in San Paulo, Brazil. Ajinomoto announced that it would increase its capacity substantially. In 1991, NutraSweet announced opening a new manufacturing facility at its August, Georgia location, at a cost of $100 million as well as investigating manufacturing site possibilities in Europe.

With aspartame patents due to expire in December 1992, the Holland

Sweetener Company planned to gear up to increase its share of the nearly $1 billion annual aspartame market. It planned to expand its existing plant in Geleen, the Netherlands, and to invest more than $60 million to increase its annual production capacity *fourfold*, to 4.5 million pounds of aspartame production by the end of 1993.

By 2005, Ajinimoto increased aspartame production, and announced that it would invest $58 million to expand existing manufacturing plants in Yokkaichi, Japan and in Gravelines, France, in order to meet the growing demands by food and beverage manufacturers. Completion was expected by 2006. The global capacity of aspartame was projected to reach 10,000 metric tons a year, to supply more than half of the world market.

The steady increases in production and sales of aspartame were attributable to large outlays for promotional blitzes. In 1983, Searle announced that it would spend more on advertising Equal, its aspartame-containing tabletop sweetener, than was spent in the entire sweetener substitute category the previous year. The two leading sellers of saccharin and aspartame had spent an estimated combined total of more than $3 million in 1982 on advertising.

Prior to Equal's market release, ads for the sweetener began to appear in medical journals such as the *Journal of the American Medical Association (JAMA)*; trade magazines such as *Restaurants & Institutions*; and popular magazines read by the general public such as *Womans' Day* and *TV Guide*. Two-page spreads were intended to whet the appetite, before the product was launched. In *JAMA* (Apr 15, 1983) doctors were told, "Your patients can't buy it, but they're gonna love it." The advertisement was accompanied by an offer for a free sample of chewing gum sweetened with aspartame.

In *Restaurants & Institutions* specific groups were targeted in different issues. In the February 1984 issue, a registered dietitian at the Dana-Farber Cancer Institute offers a testimonial that the "Dana-Farber Cancer Institute is keenly aware of the safety of the foods they provide, as well as the requirements of good taste." Another ad, in the same issue, featured the owner of a world-famous five-star Michelin restaurant in San Francisco, willing to attest to his enthusiasm about using Equal in his restaurant. *Womans' Day* carried a recipe with aspartame as an ingredient in an unheated food dish, and misled readers by stating that "unlike saccharin, it's made of two of the building blocks of protein. So your body treats NutraSweet as naturally as it treats any food you consume." Aimed at restaurateurs, another misleading ad announced that NutraSweet is "made from ingredients like those found naturally in many foods."

Later, the misleading information continued in advertisements. In several magazines, including *Better Homes and Gardens* (May 1988) and *Newsweek* (May 9, 1988), the text accompanying a picture of various fruits, read:

"In your eyes, NutraSweet doesn't have very much in common with all these different kinds of fruit.

"But the rest of your body will detect a rather remarkable similarity.

"NutraSweet, you see, is made of two building blocks of protein, like those found in foods that we eat every day.

"Including every one of the fruits that you see pictured here.

"Your body, of course, doesn't require such a long explanation.

"Because it understands these things naturally, and the way your body sees it, a juicy piece of fruit and NutraSweet have quite a bit in common."

"They both look good enough to eat."

Misleading statements continued to an even greater extent with aspartame advertisements by Ajinomoto. In *Food Product Design* (Jul 2001), a picture of two bees in a hive is accompanied by the caption; "The new choice for sweetness experts." The implication is, that like honey, consumers should regard aspartame as a "natural" sweetener.

SUGAR INTERESTS VS. SWEETENER INTERESTS

Declining sugar sales prompted the sugar interests to launch a nationwide campaign, begun on radio and in print in the mid-1980s, to remind consumers that sugar is "natural" and has been in long-time use. A trim woman in a bathing suit in a print advertisement emphasized that sugar does not make one obese. The campaign was reported to have been developed to counter the G. D. Searle & Company's advertisements for NutraSweet.

On August 15, 1984, the Sugar Association petitioned the Federal Trade Commission (FTC) to prohibit alleged deceptive advertising practices by Searle. The petition requested immediate action to prevent the practices that were contained in Searle's advertisements for aspartame. The claims that NutraSweet and Equal are useful for weight control, and for prevention of tooth decay were not substantiated adequately.

The petitioner requested that NutraSweet and Equal advertisements for health and safety claims be banned unless they disclose that:

- Most foods containing NutraSweet also contain carbohydrates and this combination has never been shown to be effective in weight control and/or caries reduction.

- Claims regarding no-cariogenicity of NutraSweet and other aspartame-containing products are based solely on animal studies.

- NutraSweet is aspartame, and health risks, including the possibility of mental retardation in children with PKU, may result from the use of aspartame.

Another Ajinomoto advertisement in *Functional Foods and Nutraceuticals* (Nov 2004) shows a picture of a human infant being breastfed. The accompanying text reads:

"Remember your first taste of aspartame? (in bold lettering) Mother's milk doesn't contain aspartame but it might as well. Aspartame is made from things which (sic) occur in larger quantities in other parts of our diet, and our bodies digest it completely naturally. The principal components of aspartame are the two building blocks of protein, just like those found in eggs, fruit, cheese, or fish—or even in mother's milk.

"A natural part of life."

A 2005 AD FOR ASPARTAME

"Currently, more than 200 million people around the world regularly consume aspartame-containing products. Aspartame is now approved in 134 countries . . . "With the World Health Organization asking what food and drink companies are doing to help children avoid the perils of being overweight, Ajinomoto Aspartame provides an important part of the answer . . . "Thanks to aspartame, beverage manufacturers are leading the food industry by providing excellent low calorie products which children all over the world enjoy . . ."

From a two-page Ajinomoto ad for aspartame in *Food Product Design*, May 2005.

In July 1987, the National Advertising Division (NAD) of the Council of Better Business Bureaus took action when it found a misleading NutraSweet advertisement. The text read, "If you had bananas and milk, you've eaten what's in NutraSweet." The NAD contended that "because the three components of aspartame don't appear together naturally in any one food" the advertisement misled consumers (*FDA Consumer*, Jul–Aug 1987). The advertiser argued that statements included in the text such as "banana plants don't make NutraSweet" explained the facts accurately. However, the advertiser said that it would take into consideration NAD's concerns in future advertisements.

In 1991, once again, the Council of Better Business Bureaus took action against the NutraSweet Company, in response to a complaint filed by the Cumberland Packing Corporation, the manufacturer of Sweet'n Low, the saccharin-containing sweetener. Cumberland objected to an advertisement claiming that use of a NutraSweet product, Sugar Delight (a blend of aspartame and sugar) would "avoid [after] taste of sweeteners" (*Food Chemical News*, Dec 16, 1991). The ad showed a comparison with an unidentified pink-colored packet of a sweetener, readily identifiable as Sweet'n Low but lacking any printed identification on the packet. The NAD concluded that the ad claim "would be interpreted to mean that Sugar Delight contains no artificial sweeteners . . . some consumers might not understand the visual of the pink packet as a reference to sweeteners." The NutraSweet Company agreed to modify advertising claims for its product blend to indicate clearly that the product did contain a synthesized sweetener.

MONSANTO'S ANTI-COMPETITIVE PRACTICES

In 1991, the Canadian government's antitrust department asked its Competition Tribunal to order the Monsanto Company's NutraSweet unit to drop various anti-competitive marketing practices that restricted competition in Canada's aspartame market. The offensive practices included offering big discounts—about 40 percent—to soft drink producers and others if they would use NutraSweet's red-and-white-swirl logo on their products.

The ruling was hailed by a main competitor, the Holland Sweetener Company (owned jointly by Tosoh Corporation of Japan and DSM N.V. in Maastricht, the Netherlands). Holland claimed that NutraSweet's game plan was to drive Holland out of business, and then retain the monopoly. At the time, Holland was excluded from the U.S. aspartame market by NutraSweet's patent that ran until 1992.

The Competition Tribunal's hearings became a major test of the provisions in Canada's 1986 antitrust law dealing with abuse of dominant market position and with exclusive deals and tied sales. The tribunal found that NutraSweet was using its market strength to keep other suppliers out of the Canadian market, where NutraSweet accounted for about 95 percent of Canadian aspartame sales in 1989. The tribunal alleged that NutraSweet made use of its logo and U.S. patent protection to pressure its customers to rely exclusively on NutraSweet for aspartame supplies.

Similarly, Monsanto's anticompetitive practices were experienced in Europe. Also acting on a Holland Sweetener complaint, the European Commission investigated antidumping allegations against NutraSweet, with its aspartame selling at unfairly low prices in the European community.

ASPARTAME: A TRIUMPH OF "ENTREPRENEURIAL SCIENCE"

Many people use diet soft drinks and other aspartame-sweetened foods in hopes that these sugar-free products will help them lose weight, or maintain weight loss. Unfortunately, as with cyclamates and saccharin, aspartame does not help in weight loss. On the contrary, it stimulates appetite.

The brain chemical, serotonin, which is stimulated by sucrose, carries a

message that enough sugar has been consumed. Aspartame, and other synthesized sweeteners carry no such message. Aspartame actually may carry
the opposite message, causing the brain to believe that more sugar (or carbohydrate) is needed. Thus, more food is eaten and weight is increased.

Some nutrition and weight-control experts are concerned about the effects
of synthesized sweeteners on the insatiable 'sweet tooth.' Substituting a low-
calorie sweetener for sugar does nothing to curb the passion for sweets. It
merely perpetuates the likelihood that individuals will succumb to very sweet
high-calorie foods rather than to select nutrient-dense ones.

Early studies combined all the synthesized sweeteners in use for weight
loss studies. In a mortality study in 1982, the American Cancer Society found
that among 79,000 women, those who were long-term users of synthesized
sweeteners, were more likely than nonusers to gain weight over a year.

Similarly, S. D. Stellman and L. Garfinkel found that women who used
synthesized sweeteners were more apt to gain weight than women who did
not. The sweetener users gained weight faster, regardless of their weight at
the start of the study (*Journal of Preventive Medicine*, Mar 1986).

Some studies were conducted solely with aspartame. Dr. J. E. Blundell
(mentioned earlier in the chapter on saccharin) and A. J. Hill at the Biopsychology Laboratories at Leeds University in England conducted experiments
with ninety-five young adults, aged eighteen years to twenty-two years.
Compared to an intake of glucose or water, aspartame increased their desire
to eat and decreased their sense of satiety. The researchers concluded that
aspartame may produce "a residual hunger" that leads to increased food consumption. The sweetener may send ambiguous signals to the brain resulting
in "a loss of control over appetite" (*The New England Journal of Medicine*, May
10, 1986).

Oral stimulation with aspartame-containing chewing gum increases
hunger, according to the findings of Michael G. Tordoff and Annette M. Alleva, both at the Monell Chemical Senses Center in Philadelphia, Pennsylvania.
They conducted clinical tests with human volunteers: sixty healthy men and
sixty healthy women. The overall effect of using aspartame-containing chewing gum was that the desire to eat was increased by sweet stimulation in the
oral cavity (*Physiology and Behavior*, 1990).

Dr. Richard Wurtman, too, found that aspartame was useless as a diet aid.
In a letter to Dr. Sanford A. Miller, director of the FDA's Bureau of Foods,
Wurtman told Miller that "we and others will observe, when we examine
aspartame's appetitive effects, that, by blocking the serotonin rise, it causes
rats and people to increase their desire for, and elective consumption of, carbohydrates, a paradoxical action for a diet aid" (*Food Engineering*, Sept 1983).

Like saccharin, if aspartame had been classified as a drug rather than as a food additive, it might never have been approved. The required safety tests for a drug has a far higher standard. Also, a drug must be shown effective for its intended purpose. If aspartame had been presented as an effective aid for weight reduction, it would have failed. Aspartame would also have failed the safety test as a drug.

By 2008, forty-eight British Parliament members expressed "deep concern" about aspartame's toxicity, and urged its removal as a permissible additive. As a result, leading British supermarket chains pulled it from their shelves. Also, in 2008, the Hawaiian State Sentate urged the FDA to rescind aspartame approval.

After diligently reading widely from the medical literature, any open-minded reader will reach certain conclusions. The ADI level set for aspartame is unrealistic. Many people, especially young children, exceed it. Some people are affected adversely even at levels well below the ADI. Although PKU warnings may appear on labels, not every PKU carrier is aware of the condition. Aspartame is used with food and drink products that are nutrient-poor, and usually have other objectionable ingredients as well.

FDA Commissioner Arthur Hull Hayes defended aspartame approval. He assured the public with the same mantra that has been repeated ad nauseum. "Few compounds have withstood such detailed testing and repeated close scrutiny, and the process through which aspartame has gone should protect the public with additional confidence in its safety." Yet, as one FDA scientist frankly admitted, "It doesn't matter how many tests are done on a food additive. The proper question is, how many are valid? And do they prove the additive is safe?" This is the crux of the controversy.

According to law, if tests are inconclusive, the FDA is not supposed to approve an additive. Yet the FDA approved aspartame.

SHREWD OBSERVATIONS BY SENATOR METZENBAUM

". . . We don't need the company or the nonprofit institutes fronting for the company, telling us that this product is safe. I hope that message comes across loud and clear here today . . . I am frank to say that the NutraSweet Company, the food and beverage industry, and their various institutes, exert tremendous influence over scientific research and investigation. I want to make sure such work is genuinely independent.

"I do not believe that scientists who have raised concerns about safety should be excluded from the process . . ."

—U.S. Senator Howard M. Metzenbaum, from his opening statement at the Senate Hearings: NutraSweet: Health and Safety Concerns, November 3, 1987

The open-minded reader will be puzzled by the evidence. Why are there so many contradictory findings? Some studies seem to demonstrate harm from aspartame use, while others exonerate it. Dr. Walton, mentioned earlier, was puzzled by the contradictory findings. He conducted a survey of aspartame studies and the correlation of outcome depending on whether the studies were conducted independently, or funded by Searle, Ajinomoto, NutraSweet, and other groups with vested interests. Of the 166 studies related to aspartame safety for human use, published in peer-reviewed medical periodicals, Walton found that 74 were industry-funded, and all of these studies supported the safety of aspartame. Ninety-two of the studies were independently funded, and all of them showed adverse effects except for seven (of which four were from studies conducted by FDA staff members). Walton reported that all the studies exonerating aspartame "have severe design deficiencies which help to guarantee the 'desired' outcomes" (*Analysis Shows Nearly 100 Percent of Independent Research Finds Problems with Aspartame*, www.holisticmed.com/aspartame/100.html). Walton reported that the industry-supported studies are the ones cited in public relations and news reports from vested interest groups.

Walton's findings were strengthened by others who also investigated the relationship between funding sources and conclusions drawn in nutritional studies. In an article published in *PLoS Medicine* (Jan 2007) U. Lesser and associates reported on their worldwide literature search of three food subjects (soft drinks, juices, and milk) published between 1999 and 2003. The researchers evaluated funding sources and conclusions drawn from the studies. Unfavorable conclusions were 0 percent for all industry-funded studies, and 37 percent for non-industry-funded ones. The researchers concluded that industry-funded, nutrition-related scientific articles may bias conclusions that favor the sponsors' products. In another article related to the subject, published in the same issue, Martijn B. Katan, professor of nutrition at Vrije Universiteit, Amsterdam, the Netherlands, noted that "when an industry is the major sponsor of research on its own product, unfavorable effects of that product are less likely to be investigated."

H. J. Roberts, M.D., a physician who has been an independent crusader against aspartame since its inception, has written about the subsidized "entrepreneurial science" aimed at promoting specific products such as aspartame in his book *Aspartame (NutraSweet): Is it Safe?* (Charles Press Publishers, 1990). Roberts wrote that "Many are shocked to learn that payment for research services and testing may be made by contract . . . rather than by grants to scholars."

Roberts, personally, has experienced the effects of "entrepreneurial science," by having his letters-to-the-editor or his articles on aspartame rejected by the editors of some medical journals on the flimsy grounds that the subject is of no interest to the readership. These editors also reject his case studies as mere anecdotal evidence. What distinguishes the two? Roberts has been attacked verbally by industry-funded henchmen. Yet, because of his dedicated sense of mission, Roberts has been able to enlighten scores of people about the true nature of aspartame through his prodigious amounts of writing on the subject. As Roberts wrote in his book cited above, "I have made a desperate attempt to maintain my professional objectivity and integrity, without intent of malice, in pursuing this clinical and scientific probe." Later, he added, "I think it would be a tragedy if this issue is ignored . . . we could be inviting disastrous medical, psychological, and neurological problems . . . let's look at the problem NOW, instead of in five or ten years when we might be having a medical plague on our hands."

Chapter 14

NEOTAME: "SUPERASPARTAME"

The timing and self-serving corporate interests of this petition are suggested by the fact that the patent on aspartame expired several years ago. The fundamental issue is that Neotame, a synthetic variation of aspartame, requires extensive evaluation before the FDA should accept a superficial opinion about its purported safety, based largely on limited short-term date involving potentially flawed protocols that were almost totally funded by corporate contracts.

—H. J. ROBERTS, M.D., LETTER OF MARCH 3, 1998 TO DOCKETS MANAGEMENT BRANCH, FDA, PUBLIC COMMENTS ON PETITION FOR FDA APPROVAL OF NEOTAME

After the success of aspartame, researchers at the French Université Claude Bernard reported at a meeting of the American Chemical Society in 1995 about a derivative compound of L-aspartic acid that was up to 70,000 times sweeter than sucrose. According to Jean-Marie Tinti, as reported in *Food Chemical News* (Sept 4, 1995), the compound was "the most potent sweetener based on L-aspartic acid known."

Also, at the same meeting, another series of high-potency sweeteners, L-aspartyl-D-alpha-aminoalkanoyl-(S)-N-alpha-alkylbenzylamide were described by Dr. James Sweeney, a representative of the Coca-Cola Company. Sweeney noted that a number of compounds in the series of high-intensity sweeteners were more potent than aspartame. However, he added that "regulatory approval is a very long and expensive procedure. We're still trying to decide what to do with the sweeteners."

Neotame is a derivative of a dipeptide composed of two amino acids: aspartic acid and phenylalanine. If this composition sounds familiar, it should; it is somewhat similar to that of aspartame.

With neotame, both amino acids are in the natural L-configuration (left rotating under polarized light). There are three other possible isomers (substances composed of the same element and in the same proportion, but different in properties due to different arrangements of atoms), LD- (left and right); DD- (right and right); and DL- (right and left). These three isomers lack the sweet taste of neotame, with its configuration of LL- (left and left).

Neotame is produced by hydrogenating aspartame with 3,3-dimethylbutyl aldehyde. This action produces a chemical change that increases the sweetness level.

NEOTAME'S WINNING FEATURES

Tinti and colleague, Claude Nofre, prepared a series of compounds by substituting the terminal nitrogen of aspartame with a number of hydrophobic (not dissolving readily in water) groups, and determined their sweetness compared to a 2 percent sucrose solution. The findings were astonishing. One of the compounds, neotame, was 30 to 40 times sweeter than aspartame, and dubbed "superaspartame." Neotame was found to be 7,000 to 13,000 times sweeter than sucrose, depending on its application. It is far sweeter than any other noncaloric high-intensity sweetener in common use.

Of all the very high-intensity sweeteners that Tinti and Nofre examined and were screened by Monsanto, neotame was the one selected for further research and development. After more than sixteen years, development was completed and Monsanto petitioned the Food and Drug Administration (FDA) for its approval. The company had long-term plans and was eager to introduce neotame. For years, Monsanto's NutraSweet Company unit had held exclusive marketing rights to aspartame (NutraSweet). But ultimately competitors, including private-label manufacturers, had produced their own versions in a crowded and lucrative market of sweeteners.

Monsanto, in its annual report in 1998, described neotame as a compound "designed to deliver a naturally sweet taste like sugar, with no added calories, and to be used at significantly lower levels than other sweetening alternatives, providing potential cost savings."

In *Chemical & Engineering News*, a publication of the American Chemical Society (Jan 1999), Monsanto's development of neotame was regarded as "an effort to extend its hold on the 1 billion-dollar-per-year global market for aspartame sweeteners." The magazine noted that Monsanto "has exclusive rights to patents covering neotame, some of which will extend patent protection late into the second decade of the 21st century."

The patent rights on aspartame had expired in the late 1990s. It was thought that neotame, once approved, could replace up to 50 percent of the aspartame market share. As with aspartame, Monsanto would retain exclusive rights to the neotame patent that would cover the product; its manufacturing processes; and its various uses in foods, pharmaceuticals, and nutritional supplements. Monsanto termed this total control as "an extensive patent estate." Monsanto planned to petition for approval of neotame in other areas of the world.

PETITION TO FDA FOR APPROVAL OF NEOTAME

In 1997, Monsanto's sweetening business unit filed a food additive petition with the FDA for neotame's use as a tabletop sweetener. The FDA reviewed more than a hundred animal and human studies submitted to establish neotame's safety. Some of the studies were designed to detect any cancer-causing effects; others, for any adverse reproductive or neurological effects.

George Pauli, director of the FDA's Office of Premarket Approval (OPA) apportioned Monsanto's safety data among chemistry and toxicology reviewers. The experts judged that the submitted safety data in the petition lacked major elements. Complete pathological data, and data on neotame's functional effects on food were missing. The FDA requested that Monsanto supply the lacking information.

The studies showed that neotame is not metabolized the same as aspartame. Neotame results in far less phenylalanine release during the digestive process. Also, because neotame is so much sweeter than aspartame, products made with neotame would contain less of the added sweetener. However, neotame's role in phenylketonuria remains equivocal.

According to Harriett H. Butchko, M.D., vice president of Medical and Scientific Affairs at NutraSweet, neotame is metabolized quickly and is eliminated totally by the body via normal biological processes. Butchko emphasized that, unlike aspartame, no phenylalanine is formed in neotame's metabolism. Therefore, producers of the sweetener should not be required to print any cautionary warning about phenylketonuria (PKU) on the label. However, Butchko's statement does not match the FDA's assessment.

According to the FDA, neotame *does* form some phenylalaline during metabolism, albeit far less than aspartame. The agency estimated that the amount would be no more than 0.3 to 0.4 percent of the daily intake that is allowable for a child with PKU. Because the level is so low, the agency concluded that neotame would not pose a threat to children or adults with this disorder. According to Monsanto, neotame could be used safely by everyone, including children, pregnant and breastfeeding women, and diabetics.

Vigorous Opposition to Neotame Approval

In public comments received by the FDA's Dockets Management Branch, criticisms were raised about the safety of neotame, and protests about the FDA's consideration for its approval. Some of the concerns pertained to the inadequacy of the safety data that had been submitted. It was argued that additional data were needed to resolve the issue about the body weight gain of test animals consuming neotame. There was insufficient information concerning the toxic effect on growth, an issue that impacts on the establishment of a no-effect or no-adverse-effect level that must be evaluated. The critics contended that the issues could be resolved only through additional data.

H. J. Roberts, M.D., a long-time aspartame critic, had written letters of protest on March 3, 1998 (quoted at the beginning of this chapter), and February 25, 1999. In further protest, on April 7, 1999, Roberts wrote once again to the FDA's Dockets Management Branch, warning that the health hazards of neotame would not necessarily be observed in the rat and dog studies submitted by the petitioner, nor would they be discovered in the extremely short period of tests (only thirteen weeks) with healthy humans.

Roberts asserted that neotame (as well as aspartame) does affect glycemic control, contrary to the statement of the petitioner. In Roberts's clinical experience, he found that such products upset diabetes control and its complications. Roberts continued:

Corporate-sponsored researchers have no justification for their published 'negative' conclusions on this issue . . . [Also] it is erroneous to assume that a dietary concentration of less than 10 parts per billion (ppb) of each minor degradent . . . is innocuous. From my work on pesticides, there are several molecules in each cell [of the pesticide] even in parts per *trillion*, (emphasis supplied).

In Roberts's concluding statement to the FDA's Dockets Management Branch, he wrote:

I am a totally corporate-neutral physician who is concerned about the ongoing exposure of the population to aspartame and numerous other chemicals that were approved without adequate long-term pertinent studies by corporate-neutral investigators and politically neutral regulators. Let me repeat: *it will be a public health tragedy if the aspartame problem is allowed to be repeated in the absence of these safeguards*, (emphasis supplied).

Roberts's criticism of neotame was supported by the Aspartame Toxicity Information Center (www.holisticmed.com/aspertame). This group also urged the FDA not to approve the new sweetener, a potential repeat of the "aspartame fiasco" and an "upsetting development." The group challenged Monsanto's daily use estimate for neotame, calling the figures "clearly inaccurate." Accurate daily use estimates are crucial in order to make a realistic environmental or safety assessment of a food additive. The group suggested that if the FDA is interested in accurate estimates, the agency must require:

1. the Monsanto Company to make revisions to the estimate based on sales of tabletop sweeteners;

2. forward these revised estimates to concerned parties; and

3. allow a reasonable period of time for public analysis and comments on these new estimates. Any other action can be reasonably construed as a continued strong bias against the general public and [favoring] Monsanto.

The Aspartame Toxicity Information Center's statement was quoted by *Food Chemical News* (Apr 13, 1998). The same issue also quoted another group, the Aspartame Consumer Safety Network (ACSN) in Frisco, Texas, which expressed vigorous opposition to neotame approval, because the sweetener "is based on the aspartame formula." The ACSN reminded the public that the FDA's own toxicologists who had testified in 1987 at a Senate hearing, had charged that the safety tests submitted for aspartame approval had been falsified. The deaths of laboratory animals had been covered up, and unreported. The ACSN continued, "Based on over a decade of epidemiological research and work with consumer and health-care professionals, we urgently implore the FDA to unequivocally deny any form of approval of neotame."

Despite these various criticisms, in July 2002, the FDA approved neotame as a direct food additive for use as a general sweetener and flavor enhancer in a variety of products. In June 2003, the Food and Agricultural Organization (FAO)/World Health Organization (WHO) of the United Nations' Joint Expert Committee on Food Additives (JECFA) reviewed neotame favorably.

Monsanto submitted another petition to the FDA to extend neotame's use as a general purpose sweetener in any food or beverage product sold in the United States. According to Etienne Veber, vice president of Monsanto's sweetener business unit, the new petition "keeps us right on target for making submissions to other world areas . . ." (quoted in *Food Product Design*, Mar 1999).

After submitting the second petition, Monsanto sold rights to the petitions to the NutraSweet Company, the manufacturers of aspartame.

APPROVED NEOTAME SATURATES GLOBAL MARKET

The introduction of neotame was well received by food and beverage processors. Neotame, sweeter than other available noncaloric sweeteners, could cut manufacturing costs. Also, it added another bow to the quiver, by increasing the number of choices for sweeteners and sweetening blends in formulations.

Neotame has some characteristics that are more favorable than aspartame for food and beverage processors. It is less expensive then sucrose, fructose, corn syrup, or other commonly used sweeteners, as well as several other high-intensity sweeteners. Neotame can be used by itself, or blended with other nutritive or nonnutritive sweeteners.

In dry form, neotame is stable, even after five years of storage. It is more stable than aspartame in pH-neutral foods such as baked goods, and dairy products such as yogurt. Neotame is heat stable and can be used in cooking as well as its use as a tabletop sweetener.

Neotame is a water-soluble white crystalline powder, and reported to taste like sucrose. It has a clean taste with no bitter or metallic afternotes.

One of neotame's unusual features, according to Glenn A. Corliss, senior food scientist at NutraSweet, is its use in chewing gums. Neotame can extend the perception of sweetness in those products for a longer period than other sweeteners.

Neotame is used, too, as a flavor enhancer, to increase a product's overall sweetness. According to Bob Warren, director of marketing of Univar Food Ingredients, the exclusive distributor of neotame-based blends, neotame enhances flavors such as mint, vanilla, berry, and citrus. The neotame blends are reported to benefit the overall flavor profile of food formulations and, at the same time, offer opportunities to cut costs.

John Curry, vice president of Business Development at Sweetener Solutions in Savannah, Georgia, a strategic partner of the NutraSweet Company, noted that blending multiple high-intensity sweeteners is a relatively new practice in the United States. Curry observed that some manufacturers may not feel comfortable using neotame alone in the production process. Blends may help ease that apprehension by allowing for easy measurement and use; consistent sweetener ingredient dispersal; and cost savings that only neotame and Sweetener Solutions' blends bring to the bottom line.

By 2005, proprietary blends with neotame were made with other sweeteners, such as sucrose, polyols, and fiber-based maltodextrins. According to Curry, SucraSweet HIS 600, a popular blend containing neotame, acesulfame-K, and crystalline maltitol, is 600 times sweeter than sucrose.

After neotame's approval in the United States, its uses expanded globally. The sweetener became available in Latin American countries including Costa Rica, Ecuador, Guatemala, Mexico, Peru, Trinidad, and Tobago; in the Middle East including Iran; in Europe including Bulgaria, the Czech Republic, Poland, Romania, Slovakia, Russia; and in the Asia-Pacific area, Australia, New Zealand, the Philippines, and China.

Neotame has a share in the global sweetener market, which by 2005 reached an annual sale of some 50 billion dollars from sugar, HFCS, and other sweeteners. According to a Monsanto annual report, "neotame has a dynamic sales potential."

Chapter 15

ACESULFAME-K: AN UPSTART SWEETENER

During the '80s, Sweet'n Low in the pink packets and Equal in the blue packets have faced off for a place on the nation's table tops. Now the artificial-sweetener market is about to get more complicated. An upstart sweetener called Sweet One—the first new product since aspartame was introduced eight years ago—is beginning to hit sugar bowls . . . Sweet One . . . its biggest selling point: it is the only sugar substitute now on the market that doesn't require any kind of warning label. Aspartame cautions people with the rare genetic disease phenylketonuria against using it, while saccharin carries a cancer warning . . .

—THE WALL STREET JOURNAL, FEBRUARY 6, 1989

Acesulfame-K is a high-intensity synthesized sweetener, also known by its acronyms Ace-K and ACK. It is the potassium salt, in a white crystalline form, derived from acetoacetic acid. The abbreviation for potassium is K; hence Ace-K.

Ace-K was discovered by chance in 1967 by a chemist, Karl Clauss, employed at Hoechst, a pharmaceutical company in Frankfurt, West Germany. Working with a derivative of acetoacetic acid—as with chance discovery of sweeteners earlier—Clauss licked his finger in order to pick up a piece of paper. He noted an intensely sweet taste on his finger. As follow-up, the substance was investigated for a decade in Hoechst's research laboratories before it was ready for testing, approval, and marketing.

Hoechst conducted a range of toxicity and mutagenicity screening trials. Acute oral toxicity was very low, and the substance was considered to be virtually nontoxic. Feeding trials with rats showed no subchronic toxic effects. Long-term feeding trials with rats and mice, as well as a two-year study with dogs, revealed no toxic effects. Neither were there any adverse findings noted on rat reproduction, fertility, number of pups per litter, nor on the rates of birth, growth, or mortality.

Tests with human volunteers showed that Ace-K was excreted unaltered from its original form. Food and beverage studies showed that Ace-K was eliminated rapidly after consumption, mostly in the urine. There was no evidence that Ace-K accumulated in tissues or serum, even at different intake levels. Because Ace-K was not metabolized, it would not contribute calories to the diet. This feature might make it suitable for those on calorie-restricted diets as well as for diabetics.

In 1983, the United Kingdom's Food Additives and Contaminants Commission approved Ace-K use. The following year, FAO/WHO's Joint Expert Committee on Food Additives (JECFA) reviewed the safety data for Ace-K and added the sweetener to its list of safe food additives. Based on rat studies, JECFA gave Ace-K an acceptable daily intake (ADI) level of 15 milligrams per kilogram of body weight (mg/kg/bw). This amount would be equivalent to a person weighing 132 pounds and drinking about two gallons of Ace-K-sweetened beverages daily, or eating an equivalent amount of a half pound of sugar daily.

In 1985, the European Commission's Scientific Committee on Foods (SCF) published a comprehensive assessment of Ace-K. A committee of toxicology experts from European Economic Community member countries approved Ace-K use for foods and beverages. Based on dog studies, the experts assigned a level of 9 mg/kg/bw as a safe daily level. Note that this level was lower than JECFAs.

After these official actions, Ace-K was approved for food and beverage uses in many European countries. Petitions were filed elsewhere, including the United States.

The safety reviews in the United States did not go as smoothly as in Europe or elsewhere. Approval was delayed for several years. There was a range of objections raised by some critics.

SAFETY TESTING UNCONVINCING

In September 1987, the Center for Science in the Public Interest (CSPI) requested that the Food and Drug Administration (FDA) deny Ace-K approval. CSPI cited studies that raised safety concerns. In one study, the animals fed Ace-K developed lung and breast tumors. In another study, a group of diabetic rats experienced a rise in blood cholesterol level after consuming Ace-K. The FDA dismissed CSPI's objections and reported that the tumors were not due to Ace-K consumption. The tumors were in a normal range for tumors common in the strain of old-age rats used in the study.

Dr. Richard Wurtman, director of a clinical research center at the Massachusetts Institute of Technology (MIT) in Cambridge, earlier involved with aspartame, was critical of Ace-K. He charged that the new sweetener had not been tested adequately. He complained that the FDA did not require studies on the effects of such sweeteners on humans.

The following year, 1988, CSPI repeated its request that the FDA deny Ace-K approval. The FDA rejected CSPI's request, and granted approval for what would turn out to be only the initial approval by the FDA for Ace-K. Over time, the agency would grant a total of eight approvals, with incremental expansions for Ace-K uses.

In 1989, the FDA established an ADI for Ace-K, similar to the one established five years earlier by JECFA: 15 mg/kg/bw. The agency had chosen the more liberal ADI, over the more conservative 9 mg/kg/bw set by the EU.

Elsewhere, by 1989, more than fifty international safety studies with Ace-K had been conducted over a span of fifteen years.

In the United States additional petitions for Ace-K's expanded uses continued. In 1989, the FDA granted approval for its use in confections, including hard and soft candies. This approval was followed in 1990 for Ace-K's use in nonalcoholic soft drinks. Then, approvals were granted, in quick succession, for Ace-K's use as a general purpose sweetener and flavor enhancer, applicable to many new categories. Ultimately, Ace-K's expanded uses in the United States and elsewhere would lead to use of this sweetener in more than 4,000 different types of food and beverage products in about a hundred countries worldwide.

Meanwhile, in 1989, when Ace-K had barely begun to reach market shelves in the United States, CSPI maintained a steady assault on the FDA, by faulting the agency, and continuing to question the validity of the safety tests. CSPI charged that Hoechst's long-term mice studies were only eighty weeks in duration, but the U.S. National Toxicology Program (NTP) required 104 weeks for long-range studies. CSPI charged that Hoechst's tests with rats and mice were "seriously flawed." CSPI alleged an absence of complete histopathological data.

OTHER ISSUES OF CONCERN

CSPI raised other issues, too. There was possible contamination of Ace-K with methylene chloride (MC), an acknowledged carcinogenic solvent used in the initial stage of processing this sweetener. In the FDA's final rule report, the agency said that MC was present in the finished product of Ace-K at 20 parts per billion (ppb). This is only half the level at which the testing method was able to detect MC; detection was only as low as 40 parts per million (ppm). However, the FDA reported that MC is a compound that will volatilize out of

Ace-K before further purification of the product. The agency did not expect MC to remain as an impurity in the sweetener, even at a low level.

In earlier rulemaking, the FDA had addressed the issue of MC in Ace-K. The agency had estimated that the upper limit for a lifetime risk from MC exposure for an individual would be less than three parts in one hundred million. The FDA had concluded a "reasonable certainty" of no harm from Ace-K use in nonalcoholic beverages (reported in *Food Chemical News*, May 8, 1995).

Another issue concerned Ace-K's breakdown products, acetoacetic acid (AAA) and acetoacetamide-N-sulfonic acid (AAS). There was some possibility that these breakdown products might form in Ace-K-sweetened nonalcoholic beverages under certain storage conditions. Based on conservative assumptions, the FDA concluded that AAA formation was "highly unlikely to pose more than a neglible risk to consumers."

CSPI disagreed. Acidic products, such as carbonated beverages, could become toxic with AAA formation. CSPI cited studies showing that levels of 1 and 5 percent of AAA in the diet of rats causes cancerous growths (thyroid follicular cell adenomas) over a time period as brief as three months. The levels of AAA used in the animal studies were high. Humans would be exposed to much lower levels with Ace-K. Nevertheless, the findings suggested a need for adequate long-term studies.

Dr. Charles Capen (mentioned in Chapter 5), a consultant to Hoechst responded to CSPI's concerns and appeared to support them. After reviewing the animal pathology data in the studies, Capen said that AAA "has been shown to result in histologic changes in thyroid glands of three different animal species (rat, rabbit, and dog). The lesions developed quickly with extensive depletion of follicular colloid and collapse of follicles occurring in high-dose animals after only fourteen days of acetoacetic acid administration." He noted further, "In my experience, it is unusual for a xenobiotic [a substance foreign to the body] to result in the formation of adenomas in rats after only 90 days of treatment" (*Food Chemical News*, Mar 4, 1996).

FDA URGED TO REVOKE PAST APPROVALS OF ACE-K

CSPI continued to urge the FDA to withdrew its 1995 approval for certain applications of Ace-K with alcoholic beverages, and to evaluate properly the additive's potential carcinogenicity in long-term animal feeding tests. CSPI contended that "technical flaws render several key safety studies inadequate." CSPI charged that doses in a rat study were too low to demonstrate whether or not the sweetener would cause cancer. The earlier studies in which Ace-K appeared to induce tumors in rats fell short of FDA's own testing guidelines. CSPI repeated what it had told FDA in 1991: the agency should not consider increasing public exposure to Ace-K until the FDA could "fully resolve the outstanding safety concerns regarding the original approval." The FDA had rejected the argument in 1991. Once more, CSPI asked the FDA to "withdraw this approval and, instead, require that acesulfame potassium, including its breakdown products, be evaluated for carcinogenicity in properly conducted long-term animal feeding tests." CSPI contended that the petition should be reconsidered only after the tests were completed and evaluated.

CSPI's repeated requests were rejected, time after time. The body of evidence submitted by CSPI to the FDA was dismissed summarily each time by the FDA. Thwarted, CSPI stepped up its pressure to deny the latest Ace-K petition, by arranging for a well-publicized press conference. On July 31, 1986, CSPI spokespersons discussed its latest campaign against Ace-K. CSPI urged the NTP to conduct chronic toxicity tests so that FDA's decisions could be based on sound science. CSPI asked that the FDA reject Ace-K use in soft drinks, and to revoke its past approvals. Then, CSPI launched an impressive assault by reading the results of ten experts who independently had reviewed and evaluated data on Ace-K, and who criticized the tests conducted by Hoechst (by then, renamed Hoechst Celanese Corporation). All ten experts had concluded that Ace-K should never have been approved. The ten were prestigious in their own fields of expertize:

- David Rall, former director of the U.S. National Institute of Environmental Health Sciences and the National Toxicology Program

- Arthur Upton, former director of the National Cancer Institute

- Umberto Saffiotti, chief of the Laboratory of Experimental Pathology at the National Institutes of Health

- Marvin Schneiderman, former associate director of Field Studies and Statistics at the National Institutes of Health

- Lorenzo Tomatis, former director of the International Agency for Research on Cancer

- Ellen Silbergold, professor of toxicology at the University of Maryland

- Emmanuel Farber, professor of pathology at Jefferson Medical College, in Philadelphia, Pennsylvania

- J. D. Milbourn, World Health Organization

- Sidney Wolfe, director of Public Citizen's Health Research Group in Washington, D.C.

- Franklin Mirer, director of the Health and Safety Department of the United Auto Workers

There was unanimous agreement among these ten experts that safety testing for Ace-K was unconvincing. Dr. Rall termed the chronic toxicity data "clearly inadequate" and said that they "do not permit an assessment that use of this compound would provide a reasonable certainty of no harm. In fact, there are indications that it might be carcinogenic."

Dr. Upton agreed that Hoechst submitted data that failed to measure up to current standards and that large-scale consumption of the sweetener in soft drinks emphasizes that "appropriate steps to determine its safety should clearly be taken in advance."

Dr. Saffiotti stated that "such poor-quality tests should not be considered as acceptable evidence for an important public health evaluation" and that "rigorous bioassays should be performed."

Dr. Schneiderman found not only that the data were "seriously flawed" but they pointed to evidence of carcinogenicity of the sweetener.

Dr. Tomatis noted that a large proportion of children would be drinking soft drinks sweetened with Ace-K, which made it important to initiate as soon as possible "properly conducted long-term tests."

The other scientists enlisted by CSPI to review the toxicity tests expressed similar concerns, and urged that further tests be conducted (*Food Chemical News*, Aug 5, 1996).

The Hoechst Celanese Corporation responded promptly to the charges reported at the press conference. A company spokesman stated that Ace-K had been the focus of more than ninety safety studies. The sweetener had been approved as safe by various official organizations. Also, the sweetener had a track record of safe use for thirteen years.

Apparently, CSPI had been selective in the safety tests it had submitted to the ten experts to evaluate. Later, Drs. Upton and Farber were requested to review earlier safety data from the 1970s, submitted to them by Dr. Jon Simplicio, director of Scientific and Regulatory Affairs at Nutrinova, a manufacturer of Ace-K. Both Drs. Upton and Farber evaluated the earlier studies and retracted their previous evaluations presented at the press conference. Both reported that their prior concerns about Ace-K's safety were dispelled. In separate letters, Upton and Farber stated that the 1970s data from one rat study and from one mouse study had shown no genotoxicity, carcinogenicity, chronic pulmonary diseases or other serious adverse effects from the consumption of large doses of Ace-K. Upton reported that the rat and mouse tests "appear to have been well designed and carefully conducted." He wrote that he had been "unaware of these toxicological data" when earlier he had recommended further premarket testing. He was "now satisfied that further testing of the substance is no longer needed." Farber's response was similar to Upton's. According to Dr. Simplicio, CSPI had shown the ten experts only a small part of the studies, and showing only parts of the research misrepresented the whole body of work (*Food Chemical News*, Mar 23, 1998).

However, Dr. Saffiotti pointed out that the original safety tests for Ace-K, conducted in the 1970s, was a time when "the standard criteria for the design of animal carcinogenesis bioassays were still under development."

ACE-K BREAKS LOCK ON SWEETENER MARKET

When the FDA approved Ace-K in 1998 as a sweetener for use in dry foods, the sweetener was the new kid on the block. It competed with two other well-established concentrated sweeteners, aspartame and saccharin. The three were the main competitors in a billion-dollar-a-year market of synthetic sweeteners in the United States.

In order to achieve a toehold in this lucrative market, in August 1989, manufacturers of the newest entry, Ace-K launched a $5 million television advertising blitz, describing the sweetener as "the one you've been waiting for." The campaign predated the national availability of the new sweetener. In addition to the advertising campaign, potential consumers were given coupons and in-store samplings in attempts to wean them away from aspartame (priced competitively) and saccharin (only one-third the price of Ace-K).

Once Ace-K was available, competition stiffened. By October 1989, the trade magazine, *Prepared Foods* described the scene in the sporting terms of boxing. It was a "battle of the sweeteners," with aspartame and Ace-K duking it out, as they "maneuvre for heavyweight title." Aspartame "has captured the attention of consumers" but new high-intensity sweeteners such as Ace-K "will enter the ring and challenge this popularity." The article posed the question, "Will aspartame hold the crown or meet its match? Or will the showdown to determine America's leading sweetener end in a split decision?"

Ace-K was in one of the corners as "the first rival to challenge the aspartame dynasty" and "in the opposite corner" was aspartame. To reinforce the boxing theme, the graphics accompanying the article showed a pair of boxing gloves.

Ace-K promotion emphasized that it was sweeter than aspartame, and 200 times sweeter than sucrose. With greater sweetness, less Ace-K needed to be used and it could cut costs. Ace-K had no calories, aspartame had some. Ace-K was stable after long storage; aspartame deteriorated. Ace-K was stable after being heated; aspartame lost its potency. Ace-K required no warning label; aspartame required one.

Saccharin was less of a competitive threat than aspartame. Ace-K promotion downgraded saccharin, too. Ace-K had no aftertaste; saccharin had a bitter aftertaste. Ace-K required no warning label; saccharin required one. (Later, the warning label would be dropped.)

Sweetener Blends as Partial Sucrose Replacements

Although dieters accept the typical taste of diet products, they would appreciate a more regularlike taste, according to Bill Riha, Ph.D., head of technical and regulatory affairs at Nutrinova, Inc., in Frankfurt, Germany. In Riha's article "Blending Better Sweetener Systems" (*Functional Foods & Nutraceuticals,* Nov 2005), he noted that many weight-conscious consumers are unwilling to compromise on taste. Sugar or high-fructose corn syrup (HFCS) are the gold standards. Sweetening blends can result in the desired sugarlike taste by means of synergistic interactions of different sweeteners.

Among the sweetener blends as partial sucrose replacers are:

- sucrose, Ace-K, and aspartame
- HFCS (55 percent), Ace-K, and aspartame
- HFCS (42 percent), Ace-K, and aspartame
- sucrose, Ace-K, and sucralose
- HFCS (55 percent), Ace-K, and sucralose
- HFCS (42 percent), Ace-K, and sucralose
- sucrose and sucralose
- HFCS (42 percent) and sucralose
- sucrose and aspartame
- HFCS (42 percent) and aspartame
- HFCS (42 percent) and Ace-K

Processors benefit in blending various sweeteners together. As sucrose replacers, no one sweetener achieves all of its characteristics. Blended together, they can match it more closely. Also, due to the intensity of the sweetness, processors can use less, and achieve the same level of sweetness at a reduced cost. Also, there is a claim for greater "safety in numbers," because the amount of any one sweetener being consumed is smaller in a blend. According to Stanley Segall at Drexel University in Philadelphia, Pennsylvania, "When you have more sweeteners, they're often mixed together, so the amount you ingest of any one chemical becomes even smaller."

The possibility of chemical interactions of the various sweeteners, when combined, or when other ingredients are added to the sweeteners, has never been addressed. It deserves investigation. It is known, for example, that benzoate of soda and ascorbic acid—both added to some soft drinks—can produce benzene, a carcinogen.

Monsanto's patent on aspartame was due to expire in 1992. Meanwhile, the company vowed to protect its hefty 70 percent share of the synthetic sweetener market. Processors had complained that they had been gouged, and hailed the arrival of Ace-K as a new competitor that might break the lock on the market.

In subsequent years, that dream would become a reality, with the introduction of more sweeteners developed and introduced into the marketplace.

After many years of intense competition between Ace-K and aspartame, the two rivals discovered that by combining their sweeteners, there were mutual benefits. Twinsweet made by the Holland Sweetener Company in Marietta, Georgia, is a product that molecularly links 36 percent Ace-K with 64 percent aspartame on an equal-weight basis. Chemically, aspartame replaces Ace-K's potassium ion, and both sweeteners are linked together strongly by the ionic bond. Twinsweet is an odorless white crystalline powder that is reported to have a clean sugarlike taste. Depending on the concentration, it is about 200 to 400 times sweeter than sucrose. When Twinsweet is dissolved, it acts similar to a solution of aspartame or Ace-K. In solid form, it is completely different from a physical mixture of these two sweeteners, and may offer advantages over traditionally blended sweetening systems. Ironically, the two former competitors have been united in a beneficial arrangement.

Enrique Guardia, senior vice president for Technology at General Foods predicted, "With time, you will see no one sweetener with a monopoly on the market." Food technologists, especially, regarded the change as beneficial. Guardia continued (quoted in the *Wall Street Journal*, Feb 6, 1989):

> It's hellish to formulate a variety of low-calorie products with only one sweetener, and that's what food technologists have today with aspartame. The food technologist's dream is a kitchenful of sweeteners."

PROMOTING ACE-K

Promotion of Ace-K with consumers has emphasized the health aspects of this sweetener:

- Although Ace-K tastes like sugar, it is a low-calorie sweetener.

- Ace-K is suitable for reduced-calorie diets.

- The American Diabetes Association has had a policy of acknowledging that any nonnutritive sweetener, if approved by the FDA as safe, is safe for diabetic use.

- The American Dietetic Association reported that Ace-K is safe for use by pregnant women in amounts within acceptable daily intakes. The International Food Information Council Foundation added a caveat: "Pregnant women, however, should follow the advice of their physician[s] regarding their nutrition, including the use of low-calorie sweeteners."

- Bacteria in the mouth do not metabolize Ace-K. Therefore, the bacteria are unable to convert to plaque or harmful acids that lead to tooth decay.

- The potassium in Ace-K is present in an extremely small amount. A tabletop sweetener packet of Ace-K contains only 10 mg of potassium. In contrast, the average person ingests about 2,000 to 3,000 mg of potassium daily from a variety of foods. For example, one banana contains 400 mg of potassium; a sweet potato, 390 mg; and an orange, 252 mg.

- Ace-K contains sulfur. Some forms of sulfur, especially in sulfa drugs as well as in six sulfiting agents allowed as food additives, are acknowledged causes of allergic reactions, sometimes extremely severe, in individuals who are sensitive to them. However, there is no evidence that the sulfur contained in Ace-K induces allergic reactions.

ACE-K WINS APPROVAL

Over the years, in a series of petitions, Ace-K has been approved for use in the United States and elsewhere virtually for all applications with processed foods and beverages. It is used as a tabletop sweetener and in sugar substitute products in which nonnutritive sweeteners are used, in granulated, powdered, or liquid forms. Ace-K is used in dry bases for beverages, instant coffees and teas, dessert gelatins and puddings, nondairy creamers, chewing gums, and powdered mouthwashes. It is used in baked goods and baking mixes, including frostings, icings, toppings, and fillings for baked goods. In 1992, when the FDA approved Ace-K's use in soft and hard candies, the agency's actions conflicted with an earlier Compliance Policy Guide, instituted by the U.S. Congress in 1980. The guide barred the use of nonnutritive sweeteners in confections unless they were used for a practical function. Congress had adopted the clause to prevent "economic adulteration" of food by use of cheap fillers or stretchers to replace more costly ingredients. Later, the FDA decided that the purpose of using a nonnutritive sweetener such as Ace-K in confections was to reduce calories, and should not be regarded as economic adulteration.

Additional approved uses for Ace-K were in table syrups, including sweet sauces and toppings; yogurt and yogurt-type products; frozen and refrigerated desserts; nonalcoholic beverages, and beverage bases; diet soft drinks; and all alcoholic beverages, including beverage bases, wine coolers, cordials, and premixed cocktails. In 2002, Ace-K was approved as a general purpose sweetener and flavor enhancer.

ACE-K PRODUCTS

At first, Ace-K was produced by Hoechst, in Frankfurt, West Germany, as mentioned earlier, and sold throughout Europe and elsewhere by its trade name Sunett. Later, Ace-K was produced in the United States by American Hoechst Corporation (later renamed Hoechst Celanese Corporation) in Somerville, New Jersey. When Ace-K was launched in the United States its trade name was altered to Sunette. In 1994, the final "e" was dropped from the trade name, to become Sunett, and to conform with the European spelling.

Sweet One is an Ace-K tabletop sweetener, available in retail stores, in powder and tablet forms.

Twinsweet, a blend of Ace-K and aspartame, has already been discussed (see page 291).

DiabetiSweet, manufactured by Health Care Products in Amityville, New York, is a blend of Ace-K and the polyol, isomalt. According to the manufacturer, the product is granulated for consistency in baked goods. It has similar qualities to sucrose in baking and cooking, and leaves no aftertaste.

SugarLike, available from Bateman's Products in Rigby, Idaho, is a blend of Ace-K, polyols, inulin, and polydextrose. The product is intended for baking, cooking, and for tabletop use.

The use of Ace-K has continued to expand. It became the sweetener of choice for diet cola line extensions and for 7UP Plus in 2005. Nutrinova, the major Ace-K supplier, reported a greater than 20 percent increase in annual sales volume for the sweetener. Ultimately, Ace-K use became all-inclusive.

Chapter 16

SUCRALOSE: A SUCROSE DERIVATIVE, BUT NOT SUCROSE

*Artificial sweeteners will lead the growth in the food additive market,
concludes a new report by market analysts Freedonia. The market is
expected to grow 8.3 percent per year in the United States until 2008.
Sales will rise from $81 million in 1998 to $189 million in 2008,
Freedonia reports. New high-intensity sweeteners, such as sugar
derivative sucralose, are driving this growth.*

—"SWEET NEWS FOR SWEETENERS," *FUNCTIONAL FOODS & NUTRACEUTICALS,*
FEBRUARY 2005

In 1976, Tate & Lyle, in London, England, the world's largest independent sugar refiner, entered a collaborative arrangement with Queen Elizabeth College at the University of London, to search for ways to use sucrose as a chemical intermediary. One of the researchers, a foreign graduate student, Shashikant Phadnis, misunderstood a request to "test" a chlorinated sugar, as a request to "taste" a chlorinated sugar. This misunderstanding led to the chance discovery that many chlorinated sugars are intensely sweet—hundreds or even thousands of times sweeter than sucrose.

Following this discovery Tate & Lyle, Ltd., arranged with Johnson & Johnson, in New Brunswick, New Jersey, at the time the world's largest healthcare company, to develop and test one of the sweeterers from chlorinated sucrose. Johnson & Johnson acquired exclusive licensing rights, and formed a subsidiary company in 1980, named McNeil Nutritionals in Fort Washington, Pennsylvania, to work with the new sweetener. The chlorinated sucrose product would be termed sucralose, and after approval, would be marketed with the trade name, Splenda.

Sucralose is trichlorogalactosucrose (TGS), made from a complex patented process, with multiple steps involving the selective chlorination of sucrose. The process begins with blocking primary hydroxyls, followed by protecting the secondary hydroxyl groups as acetates. Then, in the final steps, the groups blocking the primary hydroxyls are removed, and an acetate group is moved from the fourth to the sixth position of the glucose portion of the sucrose. The chlorination at the fourth position causes an inversion to the galactose configuration found in sucralose. Chlorination also takes place at the first and sixth position of the fructose portion. These changed configurations result in the greatly increased sweetness intensity of sucralose.

According to McNeil's application to the Food and Drug Administration (FDA), sucralose is from 320 to 1,000 times sweeter than its parent compound, depending on its application. The average sweetness of sucralose is about 600 times greater than sucrose.

THE LURE OF SUCRALOSE

The new sweetener was found to have many attributes. It is a white, crystalline nonhygroscopic solid, and is highly soluble in water or alcohol. It is more resistant to acid or enzymatic hydrolysis than its parent compound, sucrose. It has a pleasant sweet taste, similar to sucrose, albeit much more intense. Compared to other synthesized sweeteners, sucralose appears to have more favorable characteristics. It is free of the bitter aftertaste of saccharin. It has a slight lingering aftertaste, but less than that of aspartame. Sucralose is very stable at low and at high temperatures. Unlike aspartame, sucralose can be used in cooking and baking.

Most consumed sucralose, about 85 percent, is not absorbed, and passes unchanged through the intestinal tract. According to McNeil's estimates, about 15 percent is absorbed. The FDA's estimates range from about 11 to 27 percent absorption. The low percentage of absorption makes it suitable for low-calorie foods and beverages, because it is considered as noncaloric. Also, unlike its parent compound, it is deemed noncariogenic.

When newly introduced, sucralose was attractive economically. At the time, it was believed that the new sweetener could help to offer relief from the problem of sugar quotas and price support for cane and beet sugar farmers. In 1985, the problem was plaguing the proposed farm bill. The manufacturers of sucralose would make use of sugar as its basic raw material. Foreign sugar, was selling for less than three cents a pound; domestic sugar, more than twenty cents a pound. To circumvent the sugar quotas and high support prices from 1982 to 1985, large U.S. companies had been importing considerably large amounts of a product from Canada that consisted of 94 percent sucrose and 6 percent fructose. This blend was sold as a food product, not as sugar.

Meanwhile, Tate & Lyle bought into Western Sugar and Beatrice Foods, and invested 5 million pounds (sterling) to research its patented sweetener, sucralose.

APPROVALS FOR SUCRALOSE USE

In March 1987, the FDA accepted for filing McNeil's petition (under its exclusive license from Tate & Lyle) for approval of sucralose as a nonnutritive sweetener, first for use in chewing gums and marshmallows; and later, for a broad range of products. Lyle & Tate also filed petitions in Canada and the United Kingdom.

The FDA began its procedure to evaluate the safety data in the sucralose petition. While the FDA was engaged in this work, Canada approved sucralose, in 1991 as a sweetener and flavor enhancer in fifteen food categories, for a wide range of foods and beverages. Tate & Lyle agreed to conduct postmarket surveillance of sucralose in Canada, after the company achieved a full market penetration.

In 1992, the Australian National Food Authority endorsed sucralose while the sweetener was undergoing additional regulatory review. The sweetener was under review, as well, in the United Kingdom and European Union (EU).

The WHO/FAO's Joint Expert Committee on Food Additives (JECFA) reviewed sucralose and established an acceptable daily intake (ADI) of up to 15 milligrams per kilogram of body weight daily (0–15 mg/kg/bw/day).

By this time, the synthetic sweetener market in the United States had reached an annual sales figure of $1.5 billion. The sucralose sponsors were eager to compete. Also, processors of diet soft drinks expressed keen anticipation. While waiting for its share in this lucrative market as the FDA reviewed data, Tate & Lyle announced an intial advertising budget of $25 million.

SUCRALOSE SAFETY IS CHALLENGED

The regulatory process would be thwarted, repeatedly. On May 10, 1991, Dr. Michael Jacobson, executive director of the Center for Science in the Public Interest (CSPI) and Lisa Y. Lefferts, a staff scientist at the Center, along with a consulting toxicologist, Dr. Judith Bellin, wrote a joint letter to the FDA, urging the agency not to approve sucralose for all its petitioned uses, due to some unresolved toxicological concerns. Jacobson and his cohorts had reviewed some of the submitted data and were concerned about the sweetener's effect on the thymus gland, which in turn could adversely affect the immune system from functioning properly. Also, Jacobson and his cohorts felt that based on sucralose's possible effects on the thymus and kidney, JECFA's ADI was set too high. They urged the FDA to set a lower limit. "If sucralose is approved at all," they wrote, "it should be approved for only very limited uses, so that a consumer would not exceed 0.2 mg/kg/[bw]/day." Also, the group called for studies of sucralose's possible effects on diabetic animals and people. "The lack of an effect of sucralose on glucose metabolism in normal subjects does not satisfactorily establish that sucralose is safe for diabetics."

Another concern was a breakdown product of sucralose, 1,6-dichlorofructose. In the Ames test (for mutagenicity), this compound is mutagenic. It produces lymphoma in mice, and is cytogenic in human lymphocyte tests.

Bellin recommended that the FDA obtain an expert review of all thymus histology slides in oral feeding studies, including those from a two-generational rat study. Further, Bellin urged that "adequate studies of immune system function" be conducted, and that possible immune function effects of sucralose be evaluated in a clinical study. She suggested an additional study to clear up contradictory findings in different types of tests, in order to arrive at a more accurate ADI estimate. Also, she recommended more studies with type 1 and type 2 diabetes. The group expressed concern about kidney effects, cecal enlargements, and secondary renal changes, and challenged the adequacy of the submitted study of rat reproductive and developmental toxicity (*Food Chemical News*, May 20, 1991).

In response, the FDA rejected CSPI's challenge on the thymus and cecal/renal changes. The agency did not consider them to be toxicologically significant effects of sucralose.

Then, CSPI charged that sucralose caused much greater reduction in thymus weight in rats than did caloric restriction.

This time, McNeil responded, and told CSPI that the amount of thymus weight decrease seen in stressed rats is not greater than would be expected, based on decreased food intake and on animal age.

Jacobson remained unconvinced. He wrote another letter to the FDA on September 26, 1991. Jacobson granted that the thymus gland does atrophy with age, but "there is no adequate data available on the effect of sucralose on thymus weight in rats younger than twelve weeks. In rats older than twelve weeks of age, sucralose consistently causes more change in relative thymus weight than does underfeeding."

Bellin added that the "FDA should be urged to obtain an impartial blinded expert review of all thymus histology slides in the oral feeding studies, including those from the two generation rat study." This was a repetition of Bellin's earlier plea. Also, she recommended that the FDA require adequate immune system function studies in the control group and in the sucralose-fed rats, and in humans, too; require a study to clarify the different effects on the thymus and body weight, depending on the mode of administering sucralose; and require studies on insulin secretion and action, and glucose metabolism in types 1 and 2 diabetes.

Additional Safety Concerns Delay Approval

CSPI raised additional issues. McNeil had stated that the half-life for sucralose in humans is twelve hours; CSPI contended it was actually twenty-four hours. Furthermore, sucralose may never be excreted entirely from the body, even of periodic users. CSPI charged that the potential human exposure levels to sucralose breakdown products appeared to be grossly underestimated. One of the breakdown products (1,6-dichloro-1,6-dideoxyfructose) is a germ cell mutagen. Another breakdown product, not yet identified, has antifertility activity. Early involution of the thymus in laboratory animals fed sucralose may indicate that the sweetener is immunotoxic. To resolve this concern, it would be necessary to determine the differential lymphocyte count with the natural killer cell activity.

CSPI suggested that if sucralose were to be approved, doubtless many diabetics would be using it. Many diabetics have a predisposition to autoimmune diseases. Therefore, they might be at special risk.

Jacobson also raised the question as to whether the breakdown product that shows mutagenic activity might also be a carcinogen. In another letter to the FDA, on December 11, 1992, Jacobson noted that McNeil's tests found DNA-binding in several tissues. Could the mutagenicity and immunotoxicity have a synergistic effect with the body unable to kill the mutagen-transformed cells? Jacobson asked the FDA if McNeil had conducted any test to assess these risks. Jacobson wrote that "such chemicals could generate an impossible-to-detect trait of 'genetic time bombs' whose effects may not be manifested for several generations. The FDA should not approve additives that pose any significant risk of genetic damage."

Then, CSPI—a group that appeared to be the sole voice in the wilderness—was given bizarre support. An anonymous individual, referred to merely as R. Smith (the equivalent of John Doe) was represented by a law firm, Malkins Jenner, in London. England. The client, through his lawyers, focused on studies with sucralose, conducted by Life Science Research, Ltd., in Suffolk, England. In addition to correspondence with the FDA, Malkins Jenner sent the same questions to the agency's counterparts in the United Kingdom, Canada, Australia, and other countries—wherever sucralose was approved or under review.

The lawyers noted that in the study conducted by Life Science Research only two dose levels of sucralose had been used. The lower dose level was a 3 percent dose of sucralose. Therefore, the result was that a no-effect level was established. Also, the animals were significantly older than rats used in earlier research. The study relied heavily on only one or two previous papers to explain the results as being a consequence of reduced palatability of the test diets.

The lawyers expressed safety concerns about immunotoxicology, developmental toxicity, antifertility effects, physiological effects attributed by the sweetener's sponsor to reduced palatability, and effects on galactosemic individuals, on the enzyme galactosyltransferase, and the long half-life of the product in humans. The lawyers noted that the European Commission's Scientific Committee on Foods had raised similar questions regarding the safety of the sweetener and had requested additional studies prior to approval.

The lawyers claimed that the use of the name "sucralose" is deceptive and may mislead consumers. The sweetener is a chlorinated version of a novel disaccharide, fructogalactose. The common name should not misrepresent the disaccharide makeup of the material. It should accurately reflect the presence of chlorine, and should avoid confusion with sucrose.

McNeil charged that the actions of Malkins Jenner were "competitively motivated," according to *Food Chemical News* (Mar 2, 1992).

FDA PRESSURED TO APPROVE SUCRALOSE

The FDA had to take time from its review process to answer questions and refute charges raised by Jacobson and Malkins Jenner. Meanwhile, the agency was being pressured by food and beverage processors, the petitioner, and even the American Diabetes Association, to take prompt action. By 1993, Russia had approved sucralose. Then Australia followed. The National Food Authority in Australia granted sucralose the broadest initial approval that had ever been granted to a low-calorie sweetener in Australia. Then, the sweetener was approved in Mexico.

By 1994, the FDA's delay in sucrose approval caused Senator Harlan Mathews (D-TN) to suggest to his fellow senators that a new award, the Golden Grinch (after Dr. Seuss' character) should be created for "federal agencies whose stubborn regulations and uncompromising behavior steal jobs, economic growth and progress from the American people." His first suggested recipient was the FDA, which Mathews said "has indulged in an extensive and unreasonable series of delays in approving sucralose noncalorie sweetener for U.S. consumption" (*Food Chemical News*, Aug 29, 1994).

One sucralose processing plant in Tennessee was operating at a reduced capacity. Another plant, built specifically to process sucralose in Newport, Tennessee, remained idle. Because of what many critics viewed as the FDA's "cumbersome process" for food additive petition review, any third party could delay approval of an additive indefinitely merely by repeatedly submitting its interpretation of data. Each time this occurs, the agency needs to stop the review process for response. Critics charged that sham petitioning was being used to create unwarranted delays. Anonymous submissions, made late in the food additive review process sabotaged the procedure. The FDA was urged to place a strict limit on the time for filing comments.

The Institute of Medicine (IOM) of the National Academy of Sciences (NAS) considered sham petitioning an "improper use of administrative procedures by firms seeking to delay or prevent entry into the market of a would-be competitor." Sucralose was considered to be a case in point.

Since the first petition filed in 1987, the FDA had reviewed data on more than 110 studies with animals and with humans. McNeil had continued to comply with FDA's requests for additional studies. McNeil had completed a six-month clinical study in diabetic patients. Between 1995 and 1997, McNeil had conducted a better controlled study in a larger pool of people, reanalyzed the original study, and had conducted additional studies. The newer studies alleviated the concerns arising from the original study.

The FDA concluded that sucralose is poorly absorbed after it is taken into the body. Thirty-six percent or less is absorbed in rats, mice, rabbits, dogs, and humans. The studies revealed a longer half-life of sucrose in the rabbit, but the FDA determined that the pharmacokinetics of sucralose in the rabbit differs significantly from that of humans and other tested species. (The pharmacokinetics of a substance usually concerns drugs, but it can be applied to food additives, too. It is the process by which a substance is absorbed, distributed, metabolized, and eliminated by the body.) In reviewing the metabolic studies of sucralose in rats, mice, dogs, and rabbits, the FDA found that the metabolic profile of the sweetener in rats was most similar to the profile in humans. The FDA concluded that the rat is the most appropriate experimental model to establish a safe level of sucralose use by humans.

Based on the results of two-generational reproductive toxicity studies, the FDA concluded that sucralose does not cause any reproductive effects in rats in doses up to 3 percent of the diet. Based on a teratology study in rats, the FDA determined that sucralose did not cause maternal toxicity, embryo toxicity, or fetal toxicity. Nor did sucralose induce terata (birth defects) in rats at dose levels up to 2,000 mg/kg/bw/day. Another teratology study, in rabbits, failed to show any teratogenicity.

The FDA's evaluations also confirmed the safety of sucralose's breakdown products. Based on results of a two-generational reproductive toxicity study in rats, the FDA concluded that these substances, given in the rat diet at levels up to 2,000 parts per million (ppm), caused no alteration in the reproductive performance of the animals over two generations. They did not produce terata in rats when administered at doses up to 270 mg/kg/bw/day.

The FDA also reviewed male fertility studies of sucralose and its breakdown products in rats. No effect on fertility or other reproductive parameters were observed in either male or female rats.

McNeil also conducted a combined toxicity/carcinogenicity study in rats, and a carcinogenicity study in mice, to evaluate the chronic toxicity and carcinogenic potential of sucralose when given to rodents over most of their lifetime. The rat study included an in utero phase as well. A one-year study on sucralose was conducted with dogs to assess the effects of the sweetener in a nonrodent species. In addition, a two-year carcinogenicity study in rats was conducted to study the chronic toxicity and carcinogenic potential of sucralose breakdown products. The results were negative.

McNeil had complied with all FDA requests for further studies. Many of the studies were in response to issues raised by Jacobson and Malkins Jenner. Ultimately, the FDA was satisfied. The agency established an ADI for sucralose, using the rat as the model for establishing a safe level for human ingestion. Using the no-observed-effect level of 500 mg/kg/bw/day, and applying a hundredfold safety factor, the FDA established an ADI of 5 mg/kg/bw/day for sucralose—far lower than the ADI established by JECFA (up to 15 mg/kg/bw/day), but higher than requested by Bellin (0.2 mg/kg/bw/day).

FDA FINALLY APPROVES SUCRALOSE

Finally, on August 12, 1997, the FDA approved use of sucralose as a general purpose sweetener. Sixteen months after the initial regulatory approval, sucralose was approved for use in fifteen food and beverage categories. Sucralose received the broadest initial FDA approval ever given to a low-calorie sweetener. It included baked goods, baking mixes, beverages including soft drinks, dairy products, chewing gums, and processed fruits and fruit juices.

By the time that the FDA approved sucralose, twenty-six countries worldwide already were using the sweetener.

SALES OF SUCRALOSE SOAR

After sucralose was approved in the United States many food and beverage processors switched from aspartame to sucralose in their formulations. The Royal Crown Cola Company was the first to use sucralose in its diet soft drinks. Allen Flavors in Edison, New Jersey, was instrumental in developing sucralose-sweetened, award-winning coffee drinks made by Ferolito, Vultaggio & Sons (FV&S). John Balboni, executive vice president of Marketing and Business Development for FV&S, told *Prepared Foods* (Apr 1999) that "sucralose blended well with coffee and offered a stability at high temperatures that additives like aspartame do not, and allows the product to sustain a consistency in quality. If we had used aspartame in Blue Luna [the coffee drink product] we'd be looking at a shelf life of about six months, while with sucralose, it's more in the nine to twelve month range."

McNeil won the 1999 Institute of Food Technology Industrial Achievement Award for sucralose. The award is given to recognize and honor developers of an outstanding food process or product that represents a significant advance in application of food production. However, McNeil won the 2005 Rotten Apple Award from the Order of Professional Dietitians of Quebec, Canada. This award is bestowed on companies that cause the most confusion about food products. The group cited McNeil's print advertisement "Dance of the Splenda Plum Fairy" that featured a young child eating cookies. The advertisement boasted that Splenda is "an excellent reason to spoil your loved ones." The award was given "for marketing that evokes the idea that their product can . . . be given to children without limitation . . ."

"CAN'T GET ENOUGH SUCRALOSE?"

"In this day of excess factory capacity, London-based ingredients supplier Tate & Lyle has an enviable problem on its hands. It can't make enough sucralose fast enough. Running out of capacity at its sole sucralose plant in McIntosh, Alabama, Tate & Lyle, which has sole worldwide manufacturing rights, in November started rationing the artificial sweetener, allegedly accepting no new customers and keeping existing customers to within a few percentages of what they were getting earlier in the year.

"Driven by both low-carb dieting and the consumer acceptance of the sweetener, which is sold for consumer use as Splenda, sales of sucralose have grown 126 percent in the past two years while rival sugar substitutes have declined by 8 percent, according to research from Mintel International Group. The shortage apparently has caused some problems for food processors . . . Tate & Lyle announced plans for a $75 million expansion of the McIntosh plant plus a $175 million new plant in Singapore, but neither will be online until 2006."

—Food Processing, February 2005

By 1999, the FDA approved additional uses of sucralose as a general purpose sweetener. Sales of sucralose soared, creating shortages (see inset above). The advertising campaign to woo food and beverage processors as well as the general public to sucralose use was affecting sellers of competitive synthetic noncaloric sweeteners as well as caloric ones. By 2004, segments of both groups challenged McNeil.

Merisant, the manufacturer of an aspartame product, Equal, filed a false advertising complaint against McNeil, the makers of Splenda, in late 2004 in the Philadelphia federal court. Merisant charged that McNeil was misleading consumers by claiming that their product, sucralose, was "made from sugar, so it tastes like sugar." Instead, Merisant reported, the claim should read, "made from dextrose, maltodextrin, and 4-chloro-d-deoxy-(-D-galactopyra-nosyl-1,6, di-deoxyl)-D-fructofuranoside." A McNeil spokeswoman retorted that consumers are not misled. Merisant sought unspecified damages and advertising to clarify that Splenda is a synthetic product.

During the same period of time, the Sugar Association sued Johnson & Johnson, the parent company of McNeil, and declared that Splenda is not a sugar, but rather is a highly-processed artificial sweetener. Claiming that in order to help American consumers make informed decisions about the food they eat, the Sugar Association filed a lawsuit seeking a nationwide injunction preventing Johnson & Johnson from misleading the public about the chemical product, Splenda. The head of marketing for Johnson & Johnson had stated that it is a declarative fact that this product is made from sugar, so it tastes like sugar. The Sugar Association disagreed, claiming that the product does not taste like sugar. In fact, the base ingredient of Splenda is about 600 times sweeter than sugar, and does not taste like sugar. Furthermore, the Sugar Association argued, Splenda is not natural, as consumers have been led to believe. Rather, the product:

> . . . is a highly-processed chemical sweetener, created with chlorine and other chemicals, being marketed through a shrewd advertising campaign designed to misinform consumers. Johnson & Johnson has reportedly spent in excess of $100 million to establish Splenda in the minds of Americans as being a natural, zero-calorie sugar. Once consumers learn the facts/truth about Splenda, there is significant concern expressed about the product and its misleading advertising. The Sugar Association aims to correct this falsehood and welcomes other organizations that seek to protect the public's trust for accurate food labeling and advertising to join us (Press release, Sugar Association, Dec 10, 2004).

The Sugar Association's contentions were taken a step further. In 2007, Merisant, manufacturer of Equal (aspartame) sued its competitor, McNeil Nutritionals, marketer of Splenda (sucralose). By then, Splenda had toppled Equal and NutraSweet, which previously had dominated the synthetic sweetener market. In the legal suit, Merisant contended that Splenda's advertising statements that its product is "made from sugar, so it tastes like sugar" misleads millions of people, and also gives Splenda an unfair competitive advantage by making people wrongly believe that Splenda is more natural than other synthetic sweeteners.

Merisant noted that when McNeil launched Splenda in 2001, it used that phrase. The following year, for a while another phrase was added, "but it's not sugar." However, that phrase caused sales to fall, and the phrase was dropped. The advertisements returned to the original phrase, and the sales rose again.

After sucralose was introduced into the food supply, a long list of adverse reactions to the sweetener were reported. The symptoms bear close resemblance to those induced by aspartame. According to Dr. Joseph Mercola (an osteopathic physician and surgeon who is a popular lecturer on health topics), individuals who have consumed sucralose have reported: flushing, redness and/or a burning feeling of the skin; rash and/or itching; swelling; blisters or welts; nausea; stomach cramps; dry heaves; feelings of food poisoning; bloated abdomen; diarrhea; vomiting; body or chest pain; headache; seeing spots; dulled senses; becoming withdrawn and/or losing interest in usual activities; feeling forgetful; moodiness; unexplained crying; feeling depressed; altered emotional state such as feeling irate, impatient, hypersensitive; trouble concentrating/stayng in focus; seizures; shaking; feeling faint; anxiety; shaky feeling; panic attacks; and mental or emotional breakdown (www.mercola.com, access date: Mar 1, 2007).

Despite all the setbacks and challenges, by 2006 Splenda brand sucralose became the world's fastest growing seller of high-intensity sweeteners. It had captured 26 percent of the global market, second only to aspartame's (declining) 44 percent. Splenda is used not only in packets and bulk but also in nearly 4,500 other consumer products. In less than a decade, Splenda dominated the American market for synthetic sweeteners, with sales in 2006 of $212 million. It overshadowed Equal's sales of only $40 million.

Chapter 17

ALITAME: A HIGH-INTENSITY SWEETENER IN LIMBO

Learn to labor and to wait.

—LONGFELLOW, "A PSALM OF LIFE"

In 1979, an intensely sweet, odorless white crystalline powder was discovered and developed at Pfizer Central Research in Groton, Connecticut. The powder, named alitame, is a member of an amide series, L-α-aspartyl-D-alanine. The alanine carboxyl group ends as an amide in a novel amine, thietane. The structure of this amide is responsible for alitame's intense sweetness. Although the composition of food can change the perceived sweetness of a food product, generally alitame is perceived to be about 2,000 sweeter than sucrose; 12 times sweeter than aspartame; and 6 times sweeter then saccharin.

RESULTS OF SAFETY STUDIES

In 1986, Pfizer petitioned the Food and Drug Administration (FDA) for approval of alitame, in sixteen broad categories. Two decades later, the agency has not given any conclusive ruling, and the sweetener remains under review.

To determine alitame's safety, the compound has undergone extensive animal studies and some human studies. In long-term studies with three animal species (mice, rats, and dogs), consumption of alitame at levels greater than 300 times the mean daily human dietary intake showed no adverse effects. The calculations were made with an extremely unlikely scenario in which alitame would be the sole sweetener used in the food supply. Additional two-year studies with two animal species (rats and mice) given high daily doses did not demonstrate any cancer-inducing effects of the sweetener. Nor did mutagenic studies or reproductive studies reveal any adverse effects. Teratogenic studies, at dosages more than 1,000 times the amount that might be consumed daily over a long period, did not show any harmful embryonic effects, or any adverse effects that might lead to the development of defective offspring.

In studies with human volunteers, at daily doses up to 44 times the estimated average human intake over a set period of time, no changes were noted in blood chemistry or other measurements.

By 1989, Pfizer's safety studies were completed. Based on various studies, Pfizer concluded that alitame was safe for its intended uses in the human food supply.

The FDA requested Pfizer to repeat an animal study. Completion of the requested study was lengthy, and would require years to complete. Thus, approval was pushed further along into the future.

According to Ray Glowasky, a Pfizer associate, the delays in approval were due to test protocols rather than safety issues. Some observers have been less sanguine. They regarded the footdragging by the federal agency as a response to pressures exerted by producers of aspartame to keep its lion's share of the high-intensity sweetener market.

ALITAME'S ATTRIBUTES

Alitame resembles aspartame somewhat, but with some distinct differences. Like aspartame, alitame is based on amino acids (building blocks of protein), in contrast to carbohydrate-based caloric sugars from cane, beet, corn, or other plant foods. Unlike the carbohydrate-based sugars, amino-acid based sweeteners do not ferment in the mouth, and are regarded as noncariogenic.

Alitame, like aspartame, has L-aspartic acid (an amino acid) as one component. The body metabolizes L-aspartic acid. However, alitame, unlike aspartame, does not contain L-phenylalanine (another amino acid) that poses a problem for phenylketonurics (PKU carriers) who cannot metabolize it. Instead, alitame's other amino acid is D-alanine, which being in the D-form, passes through the body largely unmetabolized.

Alitame is reported to be more stable than aspartame in food products over a broad pH range. The sweetness of alitame does not degrade or dissipate when food products are heated. Little potency is lost, even after long storage of alitame-sweetened foods and beverages. Because of its chemical structure, alitame may react with food components such as reducing sugars and certain flavorings.

Unlike some other synthesized sweeteners—for example, saccharin—alitame does not leave an unpleasant aftertaste, but has what is described as "clean sweetness" with no "off notes." But off-flavors can develop during the storage of alitame-sweetened liquid foods in the presence, even at low levels, of preservatives such as sodium bisulfite, ascorbic acid, or erythorbic acid.

Use of a high-intensity sweetener such as alitame makes it necessary to use a bulking agent to replace the 'body' normally supplied by sugar in foods and beverages. Pfizer manufactures polydextrose, a bulking agent approved for this purpose in 1981. If alitame ever wins FDA approval, Pfizer will be able to use its own bulking agent to provide body to its sweetener. Other substances, such as cellulose and sorbitol, also are used as bulking agents in low-calorie food products in which sucrose has been reduced or eliminated. However, food products with high-intensity sweeteners such as alitame will not necessarily be calorie-reduced, if the caloric sugar is replaced by bulking and texturizing agents of similar caloric value.

A PRODUCT IN LIMBO

If alitame ever wins approval for use in the United States, Pfizer will sell it under the trade name Novasweet. At present, the sweetener remains in limbo in the United States. Meanwhile, alitame has won official approval for use in Australia, New Zealand, China, Indonesia, Mexico, Colombia, and Chile. It is marketed in those countries by Cultor Food Science, and its trade name is Aclame. It has a wide range of applications with foods and beverages. It is suitable, too, for toiletries and pharmaceuticals.

Part Four

A New Generation of Sweeteners

Chapter 18

TREHALOSE, TAGATOSE, AND AGAVE NECTAR

There are three things which the public will always clamour for,
sooner or later; namely, novelty, novelty, novelty.
—THOMAS HOOD, *ANNOUNCEMENT OF COMIC ANNUAL*, 1836

A new generation of sweeteners has been stimulated by the never-ending search for "natural" alternatives. Food components such as cornstarch, dairy byproducts, and plant saps are among the substances being utlized to develop novelty niche products that add to the ever-expanding sweetener market.

TREHALOSE

Trehalose is found naturally in many foods, such as honey, shellfish, and mushrooms. However, commercial trehalose is produced by treating cornstarch with enzymes.

Trehalose is a disaccharide, consisting of two glucose molecules linked together in such a way that they do not expose reducing ends. This structure is novel. The lack of reducing ends makes trehalose a non-reducing sugar, so it can be used to stabilize amino acids without triggering a Maillard reaction (browning) even in acidic foods.

For decades, trehalose had been used in pharmaceuticals and specialty applications. However, it was costly to produce. A Japanese biotechnology group, Hayashibara Company, Ltd., patented a more efficient method of producing commercial trehalose from liquified cornstarch, in a multi-stage enzymatic process. Since 1994, trehalose has been produced and consumed in increasing amounts. Much of its consumption is in Japan, but it is used as well in more than forty other countries.

On behalf of Hayashibara, Bioresco sought approval for trehalose from the European Union (EU). Bioresco is a Swiss consulting company that advises companies on scientific and regulatory issues concerning food and food products. Some member states raised objections. In an early evaluation, the United Kingdom had noted that trehalose was not authorized for infant formulas and follow-on formulas. Italy also raised concerns about this issue. France requested more information on the enzymes used to produce trehalose. The EU responded by assuring that no residual enzymes were detected in the finished product. The United Kingdom conducted its own assessment, and concluded that the sweetener was safe for human consumption.

By 2001, the EU had evaluated trehalose as a "novel ingredient" and concluded that it could be authorized "without prejudice to specific requirements of EU law concerning the composition of foods for particular nutritional uses," (quoted in *Food Chemical News*, Jul 2, 2001). The draft commission decision was referred to its Standing Committee on Foodstuffs for final approval, and the EU authorized trehalose use in 2001.

In 2002, a letter from the Food and Drug Administration (FDA) to Hayashibara gave notification of "no objection" to the petition for Generally Recognized as Safe (GRAS) status of trehalose, and with no restriction on its use in foods. Cargill Health & Food Technologies in Wayzata, Minnesota, obtained exclusive rights from Hayashibara to manufacture and sell trehalose under the brand name, Ascend, throughout the Americas and Europe. By 2004, trehalose was approved for use worldwide.

Metabolism of Trehalose

Trehalose is metabolized completely to glucose molecules and absorbed in the small intestine. However, unlike glucose, it induces only a low insulin response. It is metabolized slowly. It provides energy over a sustained period of time and also stabilizes blood sugar. Although the insulin response is low, the glucose response is normal. This feature suggests that the sweetener might be useful for weight control.

A small percentage of people are genetically prone to have a deficiency of trehalase, the enzyme needed to metabolize trehalose. In these rare instances, such individuals may experience gastrointestinal distress after consuming trehalose-containing food, whether the sweetener is naturally occurring or added as a manufactured sweetener.

Attractiveness of Trehalose

Trehalose is reported to be about 45 percent as sweet as sucrose. It has a clean taste with no aftertaste. It is an attractive sweetener for food and beverage processors. In addition to its attributes as a sweetener, it can function as a flavor enhancer, color stabilizer, humectant, and texturizer. It is clear in solution and will not distort the natural color of a product. Trehalose is promoted as an ideal ingredient in beverages (especially sports beverages), nutritional bars, bakery products, ice creams, and confections. It stabilizes proteins during freeze-thaw cycles, a characteristic that makes it useful with processed meats and poultry; frozen fish; surimi (restructured fish products); and dried foods.

On April 6, 1999, Hayashibara was granted a U.S. patent for a high-trehalose-containing syrup. The product is supersaturated in trehalose, and contains another dissolved saccharide in an amount at least equal to that of trehalose. The saccharide, which may be a reducing or non-reducing monosaccharide or oligosaccharide, acts to prevent crystallization of the syrup. Now, with trehalose available to processors in both clear liquid form and in syrup form, this sweetener will have even wider applications.

TAGATOSE

Tagatose is made from a dairy byproduct, whey, by a patented process. The lactose (milk sugar) in the whey is hydrolyzed to galactose (another milk sugar). Then, under alkaline conditions, the galactose is converted to tagatose, and is concentrated and crystallized in a process similar to the one that converts fructose to sucrose.

Because tagatose is dairy-derived, it is being promoted as a "natural sweetener," although the end product actually is a synthesized substance.

Tagatose is a monosaccharide in structure. It has the same chemical structure as fructose, but its molecular arrangement differs slightly. Tagatose is a sterioisomer (a mirror image) of fructose.

Characteristics of Tagatose

Tagatose has several characteristics that appear to have health effects. Only about 20 percent of the ingested tagatose is absorbed. Consumed at high levels, tagatose has been reported to cause gastrointestinal distress, including flatulence, diarrhea, and nausea. The major portion of ingested tagatose passes into the colon where it is fermented. It is considered to be a prebiotic by stimulating the beneficial bacteria in the digestive tract. Physiologically, it acts as a fiber and is suited to low-carbohydrate foods. Tagatose has a low glycemic index rating (see Chapter 20). The insulin response to tagatose is only 3 percent as much as the insulin response to glucose. Thus, tagatose is promoted as being suitable for diabetics.

Tagatose is a carbohydrate that is fermented slowly by oral microorganisms that lead to dental decay. The FDA concluded that there was significant scientific agreement on the relationship between slowly fermented carbohydrate sugar substitutes and the nonpromotion of dental caries. The agency approved a dental health claim for tagatose. The food and beverage processors who use tagatose in their products are permitted to use a health claim that the sweetener "does not promote tooth decay," or "may reduce the risk of tooth decay."

Development of Tagatose

Tagatose research and development spanned more than a decade, before it became available commercially in 2003. Its history has taken numerous twists and turns.

Tagatose was discovered in 1988 by scientists working for Biospherics in Beltsville, Maryland. Later, the company was renamed Spherix.

In 1992, Pfizer announced a joint venture with Biospherics to commercialize D-tagatose as a noncaloric bulking agent, Sugaree.

In 1996, MD Foods, which later merged with Swedish Arla amba, formed Arla Foods and bought the rights to tagatose from Spherix. Arla Foods located in Viby, Denmark was among the largest dairy suppliers in Europe. Spherix announced that it would produce its own tagatose and market it with the trade name Naturlose, intended for nonfood uses.

In September 1999, Spherix was awarded a patent for the use of tagatose to treat anemia and hemophilia. The company reported that the low-calorie sweetener improved blood factors in these two diseases. They based this claim on analysis of a ninety-day rat study using relatively high doses of the sweetener. The FDA approval for tagatose use with drugs was expected to follow its approval with foods.

The first commercial production of tagatose was in May 2003, resulting from a joint effort of Arla Foods and Nordzucker, a German company that is one of the largest sugar suppliers in Europe. In turn, this led to a joint venture company, SweetGredients, which became the sole commercial supply source of the sweetener using the combined capabilities of Arla and Nordzucker.

After this development, Spherix had a legal dispute with Arla Foods concerning the new sweetener. The wrangle delayed tagatose entry into the U.S. market.

Tagatose Gains Acceptance

In May 2001, Arla Foods submitted a self-affirming GRAS petition, which the FDA accepted. Such a petition, if accepted, exempts a manufacturer from any FDA requirements of premarket or food additive approval. In October 2001, the FDA approved tagatose use as a bulk sweetener, humectant, texturizer, or stabilizer in a range of food products, including "light," "low-calorie," "sugar-free," "sugarless," "low-fat," and "reduced-fat" products. The FDA's approval was based on the sweetener's clearance after an evaluation by the agency's own expert panel.

The FAO/WHO's Joint Expert Committee on Food Additives (JECFA) also conducted a safety evaluation of tagatose, and deemed it safe. This action opened up markets for the sweetener globally.

Applications of Tagatose

In anticipation of official approval, the William Wrigley Jr. Company had already filed in 1997 for U.S. and international patents to use tagatose in chewing gums. After approval, in 2003, 7-Eleven, Inc., become the first American soft drink manufacturer to use tagatose. The company used Naturlose, the trade name given to tagatose and available from Biospherics. The Kellogg Company in Battle Creek, Michigan, received a U.S. patent for the use of tagatose in its ready-to-eat cereals, other convenience foods, and also functional foods. The patent award does not necessarily signify that the company actually will incorporate the substance into its products. Arla Food Ingredients, Inc., in New Jersey, became the U.S. subsidiary of the European Arla to make Gaio available in the United States to food processors.

After tagatose approval in the United States and Europe, marketing efforts for regulatory approval developed in Asian-Pacific countries, notably Korea, Japan, Australia, and New Zealand. Some South American countries also became interested in tagatose.

A Tagatose Spinoff

A tagatose spinoff entered the marketplace. Swiss Diet Shugr is the trade name for a proprietary blend of liquid tagatose and erythritol, plus maltodextrin, and a trace amount of sucralose (less than .005 grams per teaspoonful of Shugr). The tagatose adds some prebiotic fiber that benefits digestion. It is reported that the patented formulation tastes somewhat like sucrose, and lacks the common aftertaste of other "zero-calorie" sweeteners. The product is reported to be noncariogenic and safe for diabetics. Swiss Research in Los Angeles, California makes the product available and is the distributor. The product is pricey. In 2005, one 3.4-ounce bottle retailed from $10 to 13.

AGAVE NECTAR

The sap from agave and maguey plants, both indigenous to Mesoamerica, have long provided sweetening agents to the people of the area. Both are currently in commercial production, on a modest scale, as concentrated sweeteners from plants.

The agave plant has been used for thousands of years as food and fiber.

Agave tequilana weber—traditionally gathered to make tequila—also provides a nectar that can sweeten many foods and beverages. The juice is pressed from the agave, then filtered and heated to produce a sweet juice that is comprised mainly of fructose, with a small amount of glucose. The clarified juice is concentrated to a thin syrup that is shelf stable. The light-colored agave nectar is demineralized and has a bland flavor; the amber-colored nectar, which retains its mineral content, has a molasseslike flavor.

Due to the predominance of fructose in agave nectar, this sweetener is 42 percent sweeter than sucrose, but has the same caloric value. Thus, a smaller amount of agave nectar can produce a degree of sweetness in foods and beverages comparable to sucrose, but contributes fewer calories to the product.

Agave nectar has a relatively low glycemic index rating (see Chapter 20.) Jennie Brand-Miller, Ph.D., professor of nutrition and biochemistry at the University of Sydney in Australia, an authority on the glycemic index, tested samples of light-colored agave nectars. She found that their glycemic index was relatively low. Therefore, the nectars would be absorbed slowly by the body, and not spike highs and lows in insulin production.

According to Roland von Dorp, president of Western Commerce Corporation in City of Industry, California, distributor of agave nectar, "Agave's glycemic index of 11 is one of the lowest ever seen" for sweeteners. He added, "it would be suitable for diabetics as long as they monitor their carbohydrate intake."

Agave ingredients are certified organic by Quality Assurance International in San Diego, California. Organic agave syrup is supplied by Industrial-izadora Integral Del Agave, S.A. de C.V., Mexico.

The concentrated juice from another plant, *Agave atrovirens*, is processed from the giant maguey, the largest of all century plants. The sap from the plant has been used for over 2,000 years in Mexico, and was considered to be a food for the gods. Its importance in religious and cultural ceremonies was reflected in rituals and legends. In modern times, the sap is gathered from the central highlands of Mexico's interior.

The maguey plant is hearty. It thrives in high altitudes in dry, cold climates inhospitable to many other plants. Fully mature, agave plants can weigh up to two tons, and individual leaves can weigh about 110 pounds.

The maguey life cycle begins with sprouts ("mecuates") that appear in large numbers at the base of the plants. The sprouts can be transplanted and cultivated, thus assuring survival of the species.

The plant matures within eight to twelve years and reaches a productive state. The first sign of maturity begins with the center section becoming more slender and elongated. This change signals that the plant is ready to send up a flower stalk that can reach up to twenty feet in height. To prevent its emergence, the large part of the compact central section is cut off, allowed to heal for several months, and then reopened, The fibrous pulp is removed, and the sap gathered twice daily for several months, until the flow of sap ends.

It is reported that only one-fourth of a teaspoonful of the concentrated juice (containing five calories) is required to replace one teaspoonful of sucrose (containing sixteen calories). The concentrated juice, a thick dark-amber-colored liquid, is stable at room temperature and does not crystallize. Agave fructose syrups are available from Good Food, Honey Brook, Pennsylvania.

Chapter 19

DESIGNING NEW SWEETENERS: A NEW ERA MAY BE AT HAND

In time, I am confident that an artificial sweetener meeting all the criteria of safety, stability, solubility, and taste will be found. Ideally, it will have the taste of sucrose and the pharmacology of pure mountain water.

—MARVIN K. COOK, CONSULTING CHEMIST, "NATURAL AND SYNTHETIC SWEETENERS," *DRUG & COSMETIC INDUSTRY,* SEPTEMBER 1975

In the early 1990s, the NutraSweet Company engaged in a systematic search to create new synthetic sweeteners by using methods of computer design. The pharmaceutical industry already was using this technique, but using it to create synthetic sweeteners was a new application. It was a logical extension, because synthetic sweeteners had been developed and manufactured by some leading pharmaceutical companies, including Searle, Johnson & Johnson, and McNeil.

By using information already gained about developed sweeteners, analogs might be created. The first step in developing a new sweetener by means of computer design is to increase the potencies of a known sweetener by a factor of 10 to 100.

FROM COMPUTER MODEL TO MOLECULE

The NutraSweet scientists used computer design methods to develop a sweet-taste receptor model. They reviewed previous sweeteners. As early as 1948, suosan, derived from beta-alanine, was found to be 400 times sweeter than sucrose. In 1973, α-L-aspartyl-p-cyanoanilide derivatives had been described as being 3,000 times sweeter than sucrose. In 1986, guanidines were found to be 170,000 times sweeter than sucrose. Building on information gained about these earlier undeveloped synthetic sweeteners, as well as knowledge about aspartame, the NutraSweet scientists were able to develop a computerized sweet-taste receptor model. Reexamining suosan in the receptor model showed that the sweetener lacked the large hydrophobic recognition unit common to a large number of high-intensity sweeteners. Using that finding and methods that had been developed for drug design, the researchers found a new series of suosan-related sweeteners that were up to 20,000 sweeter than sucrose.

The next step was to design a totally new sweet-tasting molecule. Enhanced computer capabilities and a better understanding of biological message transduction applied to the taste of sweetness looked promising. It caused the researchers to report that "a new era may be at hand" (*Chemical & Engineering News*, Apr 30, 1990).

In 1991, the NutraSweet Company described its work with a new high-intensity sweetener 10,000 times sweeter than sucrose, and far sweeter than its existing product, NutraSweet (aspartame). A company representative would not speculate on any timetable for petitioning the Food and Drug Administration (FDA) for approval of this sweetener, which was given a code name, SC-45647.

By the mid-1990s, members of the research and development division of the Coca-Cola Company in Atlanta, Georgia, also were using computer models to design improved sweeteners for their drinks. Using comparative molecular field analysis, they studied a group of structurally diverse sweeteners in an attempt to design a new series of aspartame analogs. The result was the creation of L-aspartyl-D-amino acid amide sweeteners that were five times more stable than aspartame, in a typical beverage with a low pH (ph 3.0 to ph 4.0). The amide portion of the sweetener was derived from *a*-alkyl-substituted benzylamine. The most potent member of the series of analogs was L-aspartyl-D-*a*-aminobutyric acid (S-*a*-ethylbenzylamide), about 2,000 times sweeter than sucrose. Several compounds in this series were found to be more potent than aspartame. However, there were no plans at the time to commercialize them.

According to Robert M. Mazur, a senior research fellow at NutraSweet, future sweetener research must move in two directions, perhaps simultaneously. The research must develop new methods to assess potential long-term toxicity of new sweeteners and their breakdown products. Also, research should depend on natural substances as starting materials. Mazur predicted that "a huge upsurge in the quality and quantity of research very much like that now found in the pharmaceutical industry" will occur (*Chemical & Engineering News*, Apr 30, 1990).

RTI-001

In 1985, at the annual meeting of the American Chemical Society, Herbert H. Saltzman, a senior research chemist and his colleagues at Research Triangle

Institute in Triangle Park, North Carolina, reported that they had synthesized a new peptide sweetener. It was an aspartame spinoff.

The researchers had worked from 1980 to 1983, funded by the National Institute for Dental Research (NIDR) of the National Institutes of Health (NIH). The NIDR hoped to find noncariogenic sucrose substitutes. Saltzman and his colleagues had synthesized and tested five classes of compounds in hopes of finding a compound that would be nontoxic, noncariogenic, and sucroselike in taste and stability for food preparation and storage. They had synthesized and tested fourteen different dipeptides and amides. In safety tests, all of the compounds were examined for mutagenicity in bacteria (using the Ames test), and for acute oral toxicity in mice. In addition to observing the animals, they had tested for signs of liver and kidney damage. All tests were negative.

Among the compounds examined, DL-amino malonyl-D-alaine isopropyl ester was the most promising candidate. It was given a code name of RTI-001. Although it was only half as sweet as aspartame, it was still 58 times sweeter than sucrose. It did not deteriorate as did aspartame, at room temperature after thirty-six days.

Because RTI-001 is a mixture of two sterioisomers (mirror images), only one of the isomers is likely to be sweet. Saltzman suggested that once the sweet isomer is isolated and developed, it would match aspartame in its level of sweetness, but have greater stability, safety, and leave no undesirable aftertaste or sidetaste.

To date, RTI-001 has not been developed for commercial use. Federal funding for the project ran out. The Research Triangle Institute was unable to find additional funding for further development of the sweetener. A commercial manufacturing process would need to be developed, and then, a lengthy process for FDA approval. Meanwhile, sugar alternatives promoted by large corporations, with deep pockets and clout, were flooding the marketplace with their products. The future looked unpromising that RTI-001 or other new synthesized sweeteners would enter an already highly competititive market.

A-SILFAM-K

Other synthetic sweeteners in various stages of development remain in limbo. One is acetosulfam, also known as A-Silfam-K, a cyclic sulfoamide, related to saccharin. In the 1970s, Hoechst, a pharmaceutical company in West Germany, had been researching it. As discussed earlier, Hoeschst developed acesulfame-K (Ace-K). The taste of the sweetener was similar to saccharin, but it had only half the sweetening power of saccharin. It was stable, and was about 130 times sweeter than sucrose.

A SWEETNESS MODIFIER

Chemical compounds that do not have any flavor of their own can activate or block taste receptors in the mouth. Such chemical compounds can replicate or enhance the taste of sugar (as well as other tastes in food). By adding one of these chemical compounds to a sweet product—for example, cake—the amount of sugar in the formulation can be reduced by one-third to one-half, yet the cake will still retain the same perceived sweetness level.

Senomyx, a biotechnology company in San Diego, California, has been researching these chemical compounds. Many of the techniques used by Senomyx are the same as those used in biotechnology to develop new drugs. Using the human genome sequence, Senomyx has identified hundreds of taste receptors on the tongue or in the mouth that are responsible for taste recognition. The chemical compounds can activate the receptors in a way that intensifies the taste of sugar or other tastes. The ongoing research and development is supported by $30 million from major food and beverage processors such as Kraft Foods, Nestlé, the Coca-Cola Company, Campbell Soup, and Cadbury Schweppes. In return, these companies will have exclusive rights to use the chemical compounds in their products. Senomyx will collect 1 to 4 percent royalties from product sales. It was projected that a sugar modulator might be available from Senomyx in the marketplace in the near future. Royalties from food product sales are expected to reach $50 million annually, beginning with its inception.

These large food and beverage companies are interested in Senomyx because it could be very cost effective. For example, its addition in a minuscule amount to a soft drink would allow a manufacturer to reduce the sugar content of the product by as much as 40 percent, without altering the sweetness perception in the drink.

Because the chemical compound will be used in less than one part per million (ppm) Senomyx expects that it will be able to bypass the FDA's lengthy approval process required for food additives. The company submitted a three-month study with rats, and was able to receive a self-affirmed Generally Recognized as Safe (GRAS) status approval by the Flavor and Extract Manufacturers Association (FEMA) in less than eighteen months.

Senomyx claims that the compound, used at a low level would pose no safety risk. However, Dr. Michael Jacobson, executive director of the Center for Science in the Public Interest (CSPI), challenged this assertion. As quoted in the New York Times (Apr 6, 2005), Jacobson said, "A three-month study is completely inadequate. What you want is at least a two-year study on several species of animals." Nor is it necessarily true that the sweetness modifier would be safe at a low level. Numerous substances below ppm, and even some at parts per billion or parts per trillion have been shown to be unsafe and to induce harm.

By using the sweetness modifier at what Senomyx considers a "low use" level, the chemical compound will be listed on labels as an artificial flavor. Clearly, this is a misnomer.

SRI OXIME V

Stanford Research Institute (SRI) was researching a synthetic aldoxime sweetener derived from petrochemicals. Using the acronym of the institute, the product was called SRI oxime V. It was a modified version of perillartin, an intensely sweet derivative of perillaldehyde, an aldoxime nonnutritive sweetener used since 1920 in Japan, where it is known as perillo sugar. The sweetener is synthesized from perilla, a perennial herb, as well as from other plants.

At SRI, the research and development team attempted to produce a clean-tasting compound that would pass safety tests. SRI oxime V appeared to be applicable for all uses, including sweet concentrates, baked goods, and acidic soft drinks. The sweetener was reported to be 450 times sweeter than sucrose, and without the offtaste of saccharin. Presently, the project is in limbo.

NONABSORBABLE LEACHED POLYMERS

One approach in developing new sweeteners was to develop nonabsorbable leashed polymers. The approach was based on the knowledge that protein sweeteners, such as thaumatin and monellin (see Chapters 8 and 10) have such large molecules that they do not penetrate the taste cell, yet they are intensely sweet. This indicates that the sweet taste response can be extracellular as well.

This information led to an innovative approach for nonabsorbed sweeteners, begun in 1972 by a group of researchers at Dynapol, a high technology company in California. The promise was that once sweetness has been savored, the role of the sweetener is completed. The sweetener is no longer needed during the digestive process. Yet, the physiological damage may come after sweeteners are absorbed through the gastrointestinal tract lining and move into the bloodstream and internal organs. To prevent this absorption, small molecules of the sweetener were leashed to much larger molecules, called polymer carriers, which are not absorbed. The sweetener, attached to the polymer carrier, passes intact through the gastrointestinal tract, unabsorbed, and is excreted.

Dynapol had been funded partly by NIDH in its search for noncariogenic sweeteners, with additional funding by a major soft-drink manufacturer. Dynapol also had been investigating analogs of DHC (see Chapter 9), and had been attempting to develop a system to leash synthetic food colors and synthetic food antioxidants to nonabsorbable polymers. The intention was to prevent such compounds of questionable safety from being absorbed in the gastrointestinal tract.

Finding a taste quality in the nonabsorbed sweeteners proved to be a major obstacle, and kept Dynapol's sweetener research years behind their progress with food colors and food antioxidants. It proved difficult to bind sweeteners to larger molecules that could reach the taste buds, have an acceptable flavor, and yet remain unabsorbed by the body. Additional problems arose, including the clearance of safety tests to FDA's satisfaction, and the cost competitiveness with other sweeteners.

SUGAR-BASED DRUGS?

Some drugs are protein-based. There is interest in developing sugar-based drugs, too. Sugars form a class of molecules that may be the raw materials for drugs to treat a range of health problems, including infections, inflammations, and cancers.

Usually, proteins made by the body are coated with sugars. In order for protein-based bioengineered drugs to work properly, the sugar coating must be correct.

Protein-based drugs are simpler to design, compared with sugars that are more complex. Amino acids, the building blocks of proteins, link together, end to and. However, with sugars, all of them are composed of carbon, hydrogen, and oxygen, arranged in particular types of ring patterns. For example, glucose is a single ring (monosaccharide); sucrose, a double ring (disaccharide); and more complex sugars can have dozens of rings linked in a long chain (polysaccharides). The sugar rings can link together at several different locations on the ring. With proteins, there are only twenty-four possible combinations of four amino acids on a ring. But, with sugars, four sugar rings can be linked in about 35,000 different combinations. Although each one would have the same chemical formula, it would have a different shape and function. With sugars, it is challenging to get the rings to link together in a precise way that is desired.

With genetic engineering, it is possible to implant a specific gene into an organism to produce a specific protein. But sugars are not produced by genes but by enzymes—proteins that act as organic catalysts and are, themselves, produced by genes. In order to engineer organisms to produce a specific sugar, it is necessary to know which specific enzymes are needed, and then implant the gene for these enzymes.

In future, the old ditty about "a spoonful of sugar helps the medicine go down" may need modification. A spoonful of the medicine itself may be sugar-based.

LEFT-ROTATING SUGAR

Exploiting left-rotating sugar has been another approach in seeking to develop a nonabsorbable sweetener. The normal geometric arrangement of sugar is right-rotating. Under polarized light, the molecules can be seen rotating to the right. During our human evolution we developed enzymes capable of metabolizing right-rotating sugar molecules, but not left-rotating ones. Right-rotating substances are designated by D- (dextrarotatory), and left-rotating substances by L- (levorotatory). Thus, while both right- and left-rotating sugars may have identical chemical components, the former is caloric and digestible; the latter, noncaloric and nondigestible.

In the 1970s, this difference was explored by a company that acquired a patent for a sweetening process involving left-rotating sugars that would not be absorbed. However, a wide chasm can exist between patent acquisition and marketing approval. Extensive studies are required for toxicological tests, and for the physiological effects of extra bulk from nonabsorbed molecules traveling through the digestive tract. The left-rotating sugar, limited to laboratory study, failed to guarantee its economic feasibility in commercial production.

D-FORM AMINO ACIDS

Two unnatural forms of amino acids, D-tryptophan and D-phenylalanine, have been suggested as potential sweeteners. L- is the natural form for both these amino acids. Pharmaceutical chemists, searching for an antifungal enzyme, by chance discovered an intensely sweet compound. It was a chlorinated derivative of tryptophan in the D- form: D-6-chlorotryptophan. This substance, about 1,300 times sweeter than sucrose, was found to leave no perceptible aftertaste. Very few toxicological tests were performed, possibly because it held less promise for commercial applications than other substances under investigation at the time. No work in progress has been reported on this substance.

PS 99 AND PS 100

In 1988, General Foods was awarded a patent for two amino acid-based sweeteners. The compounds were dipeptide esters that are high-intensity sweeteners, from 2,000 times to 2,500 times sweeter then sucrose. According to the company, the sweeteners had a clean sugarlike taste, with no aftertaste. They were stable at high temperatures, and over a wide pH range. The sweeteners were code named PS 99 and PS 100. The company announced that it was conducting further research to establish both the safety and performance of these sweeteners before petitioning the FDA for approval. These sweeteners never reached the marketplace.

GLYCINE AND KYNURENINE

Glycine, another amino acid, was used to mask the bitterness of saccharin until the FDA prohibited this use, and retracted glycine's GRAS status. Its safety as a food additive appeared questionable. In experiments, glycine fed at high levels, suppressed rat growth, reduced body weight, increased liver weight, and induced some cases of paralysis of the cervix. The agency gave manufacturers six months to prove that glycine, used in combination with saccharin, was safe. Despite glycine's dubious safety, the FDA cleared glycine's use as a masking agent for saccharin, when used in beverages and beverage bases, up to a level of two-tenths of a percent in the finished beverage. Glycine was allowed, too, as a stabilizer in edible fats, up to a level of two-hundredths of a percent of the fats.

Glycine has the ability to mask bitterness and saltiness in flavor systems. Technical texts describe glycine as a flavor enhancer, improver, and potentiator, and as a substance that acts synergistically with other flavors. In some foods, glycine acts as a preservative and antimicrobial agent. It can act as an antioxidant and stabilizer for emulsifiers and for vitamin C.

The Meat Inspection Division of the U.S. Department of Agriculture (USDA) allows glycine to be used to retard rancidity in rendered animal fats, or a combination of animal and vegetable fats, up to a level of one-hundredth of a percent; and a combination of glycine and synthetic antioxidants, up to two-hundredths of a percent.

The U.S. Department of the Treasury's Bureau of Alcohol, Tobacco and Firearms (BATF) cleared the use of glycine as a yeast food to aid in wine fermentation, up to 10 pounds of glycine per 1,000 gallons of wine. Glycine also enhances the fruity flavor in wine by shortening the aging process and by reducing any undesirable yeasty flavor. Glycine acts as a clarifying agent, and eliminates harsh, undesirable flavors in beer.

The masking effect of glycine could improve the taste of products containing potassium chloride (a salt substitute) as well as products containing some of the more bitter hydrolyzed vegetable proteins (HVPs), and improve the flavor of foods such as tofu.

Many of the research projects on glycine's properties and its utilization were conducted in Japan, where glycine's use is permitted for practically any application. In the United States, glycine as a sweetening agent is made available to food and beverage processors by the Organic Chemicals Division of W. R. Grace and Company.

Another amino acid, produced in the body by tryptophan, is kynurenine. This amino acid was found to be 30 to 50 times sweeter than sucrose. Its metabolites, N-acetyl and N-formyl derivatives, were studied, but not developed as sweeteners.

EFFORTS TO DEVELOP ADDITIONAL FUTURE SWEETENERS

The need to design an ever-expanding array of sweeteners for food and beverage products is questionable. The idea of rendering undesirable substances nonabsorbable is not in the best interest of consumers. Even if the leashed polymers pass safety tests, this approach should be rejected. It encourages poor dietary patterns. Our alimentary tracts should not serve as delivery systems for highly processed concoctions of low or no nutritive value.

There is ample evidence concerning synthetic sweeteners that should make us wary. From the earlier cyclamate and saccharin fiascos and experience with dulcin, synthetic sweeteners have had a poor safety record. The NIDR would make better use of taxpayers' money if it invested in educating the public about the importance of wise food choices for dental health rather than funding to develop noncariogenic sweeteners for undesirable foods and drinks.

Efforts to develop additional future sweeteners are wasted. Naturally derived sweeteners are not necessarily a solution, as demonstrated with the problems developing from high levels of licorice consumption, or even the natural sugars in foods for some individuals. (See Apendix D.) Taste-altering perception of sweetness is not the answer. We lack information about possible long-range health effects resulting from chronically distorted taste perception. Irreversible damage might be inflicted.

We do not need more alternative sweeteners. We do need a lower consumption of all sugars and sweeteners, and of all types of foods and beverages that require the addition of sugars and sweeteners, especially at high levels.

Part Five

MORE REASONS TO MINIMIZE SWEETENER USE

Chapter 20

SUGARS AND THE GLYCEMIC INDEX: NOT A HAPPY STORY

*"The slow energy-releasing properties of oats give them
an ideal low score on the glycemic index—the GI diet
being the fashionable health plan of the moment."*
—"TIME TO DO PORRIDGE" BY SANDRA SMITH, *THE GUARDIAN WEEKLY* (ENGLAND),
APRIL 10, 2005

Until the release of the U.S. Department of Agriculture's (USDA) 2005 version of its Dietary Guidelines and nutritional pyramid, the agency had emphasized carbohydrates—up to twelve servings a day from the bread/cereal group. The agency made no distinction between whole grains and refined flours, nor any mention about the sweetness levels in many baked goods. Americans gorged on pastas and breads, and felt virtuous. Sports people practiced carbohydrate loading. Ultimately, the high-carb craze was recognized as an important factor in the alarming rise in obesity. The pendulum swung to the low-carb craze. It harmonized with a growing interest in the glycemic index. Food processors are offered "low-glycemic ingredients to fill the low-carb market demands," as advertised in a full-page back cover of *Food Technology* (Mar 2005). Food trade journals offer many ingredients described as low carb or low glycemic. Sweetening ingredients such as lactitol and xylitol are being offered because of their very low-glycemic indices, compared to a traditional sweetener such as glucose.

CONCEPT OF THE GLYCEMIC INDEX

The glycemic index (GI) was devised to help consumers know how specific foods affect blood sugar levels. Foods with high numbers—70 to 100 in the index—raise blood sugar and should be eaten sparingly; those from 56 to 69 are intermediate, and should be eaten moderately; and those at 55 or lower, can be eaten freely. As one could expect, the GI is not a happy story for sugars; all are high in GI values. However, they do differ, one from another on the index.

The GI values were developed by Jennie Brand-Miller, Ph.D., professor of human nutrition, School of Molecular and Microbial Biosciences, at the University of Sydney, Australia. She felt that GI values would be useful to learn about the health significance of the glycemic response to specific foods.

As practical examples, Brand-Miller reported that various types of rice show a wide difference in GI values, based on the availability of the starch. The soft rice in many Chinese dishes has a high GI value; the GI of basmati rice is low. In general, Brand-Miller recommended the avoidance of corn syrups, glucose, and maltodextrins as sweeteners due to their high GI values. She suggested substituting acidic fruits, whenever possible, as sweeteners. Also, she advised consumers to choose breads and other baked goods made with whole grains. Such products have lower GI values than their counterparts made with refined grains and lacking in dietary fibers.

Professor David Jenkins, Department of Nutritional Sciences at the University of Toronto, Canada, is credited with popularizing the GI in 1981. Jenkins defined GI in lofty academic terms quoted in *Food Product Design* (Apr 2005) as:

> . . . the incremental area under the blood-glucose response curve elicited by a 50 gram available carbohydrate portion of a test food expressed as a percentage of the response elicited by the same amount of carbohydrate from a reference food taken by the same subject.

Jenkins added that the reference food should be taken on three occasions to reduce variability. Carbohydrates that are digested and absorbed quickly have high GI values; those that are digested and absorbed more slowly have lower GI values. Thus, GI serves as a scale to rank an available carboydrate according to its effect on blood glucose (blood sugar).

TOOL FOR MANAGING DIABETES, WEIGHT, AND GENERAL HEALTH

Knowing the GI values of sugars is especially important for diabetics, prediabetics, and insulin-resistant individuals. Prediabetics are persons with elevated blood sugar levels, but who are not yet considered to be active diabetics. The insulin resistance syndrome (also known as Metabolic Syndrome or Syndrome X) is a health condition in which there is a clustering of conditions: abdominal fat, high blood pressure, and elevated cholesterol. All three signal significantly increased risks for diabetes development and coronary artery diseases. Epidemiological data suggest that a high dietary glycemic load from refined carbohydrates increases the risk of coronary heart disease *independent* of known coronary disease risk factors.

By 2005, the Centers for Disease Control and Prevention (CDC) considered diabetes to be of epidemic proportions in the United States afflicting 18.2 million people. The CDC projected that over their lifetime, one out of three Americans born in 2000 will develop diabetes. An additional 41 million people, by 2005, were prediabetic, and another 49 to 69 million people were insulin resistant, according to CDC's estimates. The agency regards obesity as a factor in diabetic development, and found that all ages were affected. The CDC reported that two-thirds of American adults were overweight; plus 5.3 million teenagers; 3.9 million young children; and even 10 percent of infants.

Controlling blood sugar in diabetes involves monitoring the types and amounts of foods eaten. The GI is a tool that can help diabetics manage their blood glucose levels. Different carbohydrates raise blood glucose differently. Sugars, which are simple carbohydrates, raise blood glucose rapidly to a level that is too high, and then drops it rapidly to a level that is too low. Whole grains, which are complex carbohydrates, raise blood glucose more slowly to a favorable level, and sustain the level for some time.

Interest in the GI is not limited to diabetics. It appeals to a broader audience. The role of carbohydrates became a hot issue in the late 1990s and into the 2000s when the popular Atkins Diet, South Beach Diet, Zone Diet, and others, led to the "low-carb" diet craze. Food and beverage processors responded by using some sweeteners with lower GI values, and replaced some sucrose in their formulations so that products could be promoted as "low-carb" and "low glycemic." The popular diets had drawbacks, but they succeeded in making many people aware of the health problems that can develop from high intake of simple carbohydrates such as sugars. Many people began to avoid products containing refined sugars and refined flours, recognizing the role of these constituents in raising blood sugar levels, promoting weight gain, and increasing the risks of diabetes and cardiovascular diseases.

Food and beverage processors flooded the marketplace with low-carb products, and more low-sugar, no-sugar, and sugar-free products. These were accompanied by nutritional supplements and functional foods purportedly developed to balance blood sugar levels, lead to weight loss, and an increase in energy. The National Marketing Institute (NMI) reported in *Functional Foods & Nutraceuticals* (Jun 2005) that the year 2004 heralded "breakthrough" awareness of the GI, and predicted that interest in it would continue to grow. The interest and awareness in the GI was reflected in market trends. Sales of low-carb food and beverage products rose 144 percent in 2004, as tracked by Information Resources, Inc. (IRI). Also, NMI reported that by 2004, about 10 percent of consumers followed a low-carb diet, of which 12.8 percent were on a low-sugar diet. Not surprisingly, interest was growing rapidly for reduced-sugar and sugar-free products. A 2004 survey by the Calorie Control Council (CCC) showed that 84 percent of the respondents regularly used foods and beverages considered to be low calorie, reduced sugar, and sugar free.

AWARENESS OF GI VALUES INCREASING

Sugar closely followed fat and calories as label information that consumers seek most commonly. Recent market trends show that, typically, more than half of all consumers monitor the sugar content of their diets. Some 44 percent usually check labels for types of sugars, and 38 percent prefer foods with no added sugars. One in five parents seek no-sugar-added products for their children. The IRI reported that in the period from 2003 to 2004, increased sales of diet candies soared 62 percent; increased sugar-substitute sales rose 16 percent; and increased low-calorie soft drink sales gained 9 percent.

Consumer awareness of GI values, which led to a negative perception of sugars, caused some manufacturers to change their formulations. For example, Slim-Fast cut sugar by 40 percent in its Optima Shake Mix. Food manufacturers also reformulated. By 2005, General Mills reduced added sugar by a hefty 75 percent in its Trix cereals. The new version of Kellogg's Frosted Flakes contained one-third less sugar than the former product. Tasty Baking introduced sugar-free, lower net-carb snack cake products in its line of Sensables. Stonyfield Farm launched MOOye Over Sugar Yogurt, which contains 50 percent less sugar and net carbs than its regular low-fat yogurt. Stonyfield Farm claimed to use no artificial sweeteners in its products. Instead, their flavored yogurts contain naturally milled organic sugar and fruits. Nana's Cookie Bars were among a new group of products promoted as containing "no refined sugar."

The NMI noted that one-third of adults surveyed had heard of the term GI. However, their depth of understanding was limited. Some 22 percent of the respondents viewed favorably labels indicating that the products had a low GI, but they did not understand what GI signified. Only 2 percent of respondents reported that they actually sought GI information on labels. This low percentage may reflect the lack of meaningfulness and relevance of GI information on labels. Nevertheless, due to promotion, interest in GI appears to be increasing. HealthFocus's 2005 Trends Report noted that six out of ten consumers wanted more information on blood sugar controls and 50 percent of them wanted to learn more about the GI.

In response, sweetener producers have made available to food and beverage processors several types of products that are regarded to be low-glycemic. They include products mentioned earlier such as Swiss Research's Shugr; Cargill's Eridex; and Danisco's Litesse made of polydextrose, lactitol, xylitol, and tagatose. Roxler International's BeFlora Plus powders are sweet blends of prebiotic oligofructose fiber and fructose, with sprouted mung bean extract, grown in an acesulfame-K enriched medium.

SHORTCOMINGS OF THE GI CONCEPT

Different factors can affect the GI value of a food:

- The type of sugar in a food can lower its GI value. At 100, glucose and corn syrups have the highest GI values of any food; sucrose—consisting of half glucose and half fructose—has a GI value of 65 (considered moderate); fructose and polyols have lower GI values (below 50).

- The type of starch in the food affects GI values. For example, amylose is harder to digest than amylopectin. Therefore, starchy foods with high amounts of amylose have a lower GI value.

- The method of cooking affects GI values. For example white-flour spaghetti, boiled five minutes, has a GI value of 341; the same spaghetti, boiled ten to fifteen minutes, has a GI value of 40.

- The temperature at which a cooked starchy food is consumed influences GI values. In a study, two meals containing cooked potato were fed to nine human subjects with varied degrees of insulin sensitivity. In one meal the potatoes were served hot at 83.6°C (about 180°F), and in the other meal, the potatoes were served cold at 26°C (about 78.8°F). The cooling of the potatoes resulted in a significantly lower mean blood glucose level and serum triglyceride concentration in the subjects, compared with the hot potatoes. Cooling a cooked food may change the chemical structure of the starch, thereby slowing down the rate at which it is digested. Diabetics who have difficulty controlling their glucose levels might benefit by chilling starchy foods such as potato salad and tabouli before eating them.

- The method of processing food affects GI values. The more extensively the food has been processed, the higher is its GI value. For example, finely milled flour is higher in GI value than coarse stone-ground flour. White bread has a high GI value of 73; pumpernickel bread, a lower GI value of 46.

- The fat content affects GI value. Fat in food slows gastric emptying, and slows the rate at which carbohydrates are absorbed. The GI value of French fried potatoes is high at 75. If they are fried in fat, their carbohydrate absorption might be slowed down, but they would not necessarily be healthier, even though their GI value would be lower. Baked potatoes have a higher GI value than French fried potatoes (85 and 75 respectively). Yet, the nutritional superiority of the former is undeniably greater than of the latter.

- Acidity affects GI values. Acid, like fat, slows gastric emptying, and slows the rate at which carbohydrates are absorbed. Lemon juice or vinegar with salad, or sourdough in breads, are beneficial.

- Protein affects GI values. Like fat and acid, protein delays gastric emptying.

- Fiber affects GI values. The viscous property of soluble fiber thickens gastric content, slows digestion, and decreases absorption.

- Mixed meals affect GI values. Consumption of foods with low GI values along with other foods with higher GI values, will change total GI values. This feature demonstrates the difficulties in trying to determine the GI values in food consumption.

The GI concept has its critics. The American Diabetes Association (ADA) opposes the use of GI as a consumer tool.

The American Institute for Cancer Research (AICR) has been reluctant to endorse the GI concept. As reported in *Food Product Design* (Apr 2005), AICR stated that:

> . . . due to insufficient evidence of clinical efficiency and persistent concerns regarding how glycemic index values are determined, AIRC cautions the public not to make dietary changes based solely on this interesting, but still unproven concept.

The AICR had concerns about methology and standardization, and questioned how the GI values are tested and measured. The organization was critical of "using one reference food—not two reference foods—as the standard for calculating GI values to avoid inconsistencies in GI tables." Another AICR concern was about variability of the GI:

> . . . whether it's due to the physical structure of the carbohydrates, the inclusion of carbohydrates in the mixed meal, or the variation of an individual's blood sugar response to a carbohydrate, needs to be clarified so that the appropriate dietary guidance on GI can be provided.

The GI is based on available carbohydrate. Critics question the accuracy of calculating available carbohydrate. For example, variations exist within subject sources. Jenkins, cited earlier, reported that there is a variation of about 25 percent among healthy individuals. There is variation, too, between subjects. At least ten people need to be tested and pooled in order to establish a reasonably accurate GI value. Also, there are source variations. For example, differences exist between venous and capillary blood samples. It is necessary to recognize these differences when blood glucose levels are measured.

AN ALTERNATIVE TO THE GI

Because of the shortcomings of the GI concept, in 1997, researchers at Harvard University in Cambridge, Massachusetts, developed a concept of the glycemic load (GL) to express the amount of available carbohydrate per serving of food. The GL is still related to GI values. GL equals GI, multiplied by the number of carbohydrate grams per serving. Using this method of measurement, available carbohydrate still needs to be determined. Because there is no global uniformity in the calculation of available carbohydrates, and no accurate tables or methods to determine them, there remains the same potential for inaccuracies, both in GI and GL values.

The U.S. Food and Nutrition Board did not make any recommendation for use of the GI in its most recent report updating the daily intake of nutrients. However, the board reported that:

> The principle of slowing carbohydrate absorption, which may underpin the positive findings made in relation to GI, is a potentially important principle with respect to the beneficial health effects of carbohydrates. Further research in this area is needed, (quoted in *Functional Foods & Nutraceuticals*, Jun 2005).

IDENTIFYING LOW GI FOODS

The GI is only one of several recent attempts to educate consumers about foods and their effects on blood sugar levels. "Glycemic load," "zero carbs," "net carbs," and "slow carbs" (the amount of absorbed carbohydrates) are some of the terms used. They create confusion, and the confusion is compounded by a wide range of definitions for carbohydrates used by different governments. For example, for labeling purposes, the United States has decided not to include polyols as sugars, even though they are caloric sugars, albeit low-caloric ones. (For more information about sugar polyols, see Chapter 5.) In Europe, polyols are included among the metabolizable carbohydrates. In the United States carbohydrates are not yet defined officially, but the subject of carbohydrate labeling is considered to be a top priority for the FDA. Over the years, terms such as "digestibility and undigestibility," "available, bioavailable, and unavailable," "nonstarch polysaccharides," "complex and simple carbohydrates" have been used. The variety of terms has added to the confusion.

To clarify and unify definitions, in late 2004, the AACC International (formerly the American Association of Cereal Chemists) convened a committee, assigned to formulate a carbohydrate definition that could be used for labeling purposes. The committee included the GI in its discussion. It reached a concensus on definitions:

- Available (net) carbohydrates can be absorbed as monosaccharide and metabolized by the body.

- Glycemic carbohydrate is the portion of available carbohydrate that can elicit a blood-glucose response expressed as equivalent grams of glucose per serving, or per 100 grams of food.

- Glycemic response is the change in blood-glucose concentration induced by ingested food.

Gareth Hughes, business manager of Glycemic Index, Ltd., Australia, discussed the GI symbol program at a February 2005 AACC International Symposium. The symbol is sponsored by Glycemic Index, Ltd., a nonprofit organization formed jointly by the University of Sydney, Diabetes Australia, and the Juvenile Diabetes Research Foundation, also in Australia.

Central to the program is the GI-tested certification mark. A certified clinical laboratory tests a food product according to strict nutritional criteria before granting the certification mark. Australia's program, launched in 2000, is recognized by 67 percent of all shoppers in mainstream Australian food stores. To date, the program has nineteen licensees, seven of which are large multinational companies. The major products in Australia that bear the GI-tested certification mark are breads and yogurts. The movement of using the GI as an educational tool has spread to Sweden, South Africa, and Japan. In 2004, currently, Tesco, based in the United Kingdom and the largest grocery homeshopping service in the world, adopted the program. Tesco hopes to educate consumers about the GI by distributing brochures and recipes to shoppers. Glycemic Index, Ltd., hopes to establish partnerships in New Zealand, North America, and with the European Union. If the program succeeds, it may persuade consumers to select foods with low GI values, and limit intake of products with high levels of sugars and refined flours.

According to Kantha Shelke, ingredients editor of *Food Processing,* in an article titled "Must-Have Healthful Ingredients" (September 2005):

Increased use of testing for the glycemic index (GI) of foods is a development that could signal the next big trend in healthful foods. GI is a tool not just for managing diabetes but also weight and general health . . . While food processors revamp their product portfolio and carefully pace their efforts to make mainstream foods healthier, one thing is clear: Health is the future of food, and healthful ingredients are going to be powerful market drivers for a long time.

Chapter 21

SUGAR CONSUMPTION STATISTICS: DECEPTIVE AND CONFUSING

The seeming truth which cunning time puts on to trap the wisest.
—SHAKESPEARE, *THE MERCHANT OF VENICE*, ACT 3, SCENE 2, LINE 100

How much sugar does the average American consume? It would appear that this simple question could be answered straightforwardly. But the official responses misrepresent facts, mislead the public, and they have significant health implications as the basis for public policy.

According to a joint statement issued by L. Jackson Brown, D.D.S., chief epidemiologist at the National Institute of Dental Research (NIDR) at the National Institute of Dental Health (NIDH), and two economists from the University of Connecticut, Americans have been able to reduce their dental bills due to a decline in the per capita consumption of refined sugar—a drop of 33 percent during the 1980s. This was good news, because it is acknowledged generally that the amount of refined sugar eaten is related to the development of tooth decay—the greater the consumption, the more the likelihood of decay.

Unfortunately, the news was deceptive. There had *not* been a drop in sugar consumption; on the contrary, consumption had been rising steadily, year by year. This trend was of great concern to researchers and health professionals, who regard high sugar consumption as a serious health risk. Any improvement in dental health should be attributed to factors other than lowered sugar consumption.

SWEET TALK

What accounted for the discrepancy? Semantics. By formulating an inexplicable and arbitrary definition, the U.S. Department of Agriculture (USDA) had decreed that the term "refined sugar" solely denotes sucrose (table sugar derived from cane or beet), but excludes other caloric sugars—also refined—such as high-fructose corn syrup (HFCS), glucose, and dextrose, as well as some minor caloric sugars such as honey and edible syrups—all designated by the USDA as "sweeteners." The agency chose to ignore completely the low-caloric sweeteners, polyols, in its statistics.

This limited definition of "refined sugar" is unscientific because all caloric sugars are detrimental to teeth. With apologies to writer Gertrude Stein: sugar is sugar is sugar. Although economists may not be expected to recognize this fact, surely NIDR researchers should acknowledge the potentially damaging effects of all caloric sugars. Additionally, evidence from researchers at the USDA, and elsewhere, demonstrate the potentially harmful effects of high sugar consumption—the importance of which may be overlooked given the rosy but deceptive reporting.

What are the facts? It is true that refined sugar (sucrose) consumption, as defined by the USDA, has been declining steadily, from 83.6 pounds per person annually in 1980; to 64.6 pounds in 1994; to 61.9 pounds, in 2005. However, this decline should not be trumpeted, because it is only part of the story.

The figures for sucrose consumption are inextricably intertwined with those of corn sweeteners, mainly HFCS. The decline in sucrose consumption occurred at the same time as the rise in corn sweetener consumption. Ultimately, corn sweetener use *surpassed* sucrose use, as corn sweeteners became partial, and finally, total replacers of sucrose in many applications.

For an accurate set of figures, it is necessary to examine the figures for sucrose *and* corn sweeteners for the same years. In 1980, the corn sweetener consumption was 48.6 pounds per person; by 1998, it had risen to 83.5 pounds—nearly double. The total of sucrose and corn sweeteners, the two major sweeteners, increased from 123.2 pounds per person in 1980 to 179.8 pounds (an all-time high) in 1999; and by 2004, to 140.3 pounds. When *all* caloric sweeteners are added—including sucrose, HFCS, glucose, dextrose, honey, and edible syrups—the total for 1980 was 124.4 pounds per person, for 2005, 141.5 pounds. These figures are supplied by the USDA's Sugar and Sweeteners Outlook report compiled by its Economic Research Service (ERS).

The figures go higher when low-caloric sweeteners such as polyols and others are included. The ERS, in a separate 1991 tabulation, cited total annual sugar and sweetener consumption at 164.9 pounds per person. This is truly a staggering amount. Because segments of the population, either because of health reasons or choice, consume but little sugar or sweeteners, other segments may eat far more than the 164.9 pound average. The information may have been a source of embarrassment. Or economic and/or political pressure may have been applied. After the 1991 tabulation, such total consumption figures, if gathered, were not made available to the public.

In addition to the contradictory figures of the NIDR and the USDA regarding total sugar consumption, other groups also have misrepresented and grossly underestimated actual caloric sugar consumption. In a leaflet, "Sweet Talk: Facts About Sweeteners," the American Dietetic Association (ADA) reported that "the average American consumes almost 43 pounds of caloric sweeteners each year, mostly from corn syrup and table sugar." How did the ADA arrive at this low number? Apparently, it was based on information supplied by a trade group, the Sugar Association in a consumer fact sheet, stating that:

> . . . the U.S. Department of Agriculture reports disappearances not con-sumption, figures for sweeteners. [The] USDA estimates that in 1993, about 65 pounds of sugar (cane or beet), 79 pounds of corn sweeteners, and 1 pound of other sweeteners (honey, maple syrup) per capita were delivered into the food supply. That adds up to a total nutritive sweeten-er usage of about 145 pounds per capita.

So far, so good. But then, by a deft disappearing act, the total consumption was reduced drastically by over 100 pounds:

> As disappearance data, these numbers do not account for waste, sugars used up in fermentation as in bread baking, or use in pet foods . . . the Food and Drug Administration estimated that the amount of added sweeteners (sugar + corn sweeteners + other) Americans actually con-sume is considerably less than disappearance—about 43 pounds per person, or about 11 percent of total calories.

Despite the conflicting data, dietitians, physicians, and healthcare profes-sionals repeat the ADA's deceptive sugar consumption numbers. In turn, these numbers are repeated by food writers and read widely by the public.

ACTUAL CONSUMPTION NUMBERS
PROVOKE FIERCE INDUSTRY LOBBYING

When a joint report of the World Health Organization (WHO) and the Food and Agriculture Organization (FAO) linked obesity and excessive sugar con-sumption, especially in soft drinks, the sugar lobby reacted promptly. The lob-byists were especially incensed by the participation of U.S. government scientists in the preparation of the report, which reflected long-standing scien-tific and medical concerns. It appeared likely that U.S. regulatory actions might follow as a growing movement called for antiobesity measures. According to Chris Mooney, in *The Republican War on Science*, the sugar lobby-ists took their case to the U.S. Department of Health & Human Services (HHS) and received a sympathetic hearing. Mooney wrote that William Steiger, a godson of George Bush, Sr., used the Data Quality Act as his "bludgeon of choice" to attack the WHO/FAO report, even though researchers in his own department had participated in its preparation, and had endorsed the report as a reliable basis for policy recommendations.

With the cooperation of friendly George W. Bush officials, the sugar lobbyists as well as food and beverage processors deployed many administrative and bureaucratic maneuvers to discredit the unwelcome conclusions made by qualified scientists, and to block any regulatory action. As Mooney wrote:

> . . . by calling for unnecessary levels of scientific review, nit-picking over well-founded conclusions, attacking individual scientists, and even employing political threats, food interests did whatever they could to discredit the WHO/FAO report. They had political help in this process from the Bush administration, and in a sense, the strategy paid off.

The World Health Assembly omitted any reference to the disputed document in the global strategy for diet and health that it issued in 2004.

DECONSTRUCTING DIETARY ADVICE FOR SUGAR CONSUMPTION

According to Dr. Marion Nestle, professor and chair of the Department of Nutrition and Food Studies at New York University, and a contributor to the 2000 Dietary Guidelines, sugar was one of the more contentious issues. In her book *Food Politics: How the Food Industry Influences Nutrition and Health* (University of California Press, 2002), Nestle traces the progression of the dietary recommendation regarding sugar, as a mild recommendation that progressively is weakened. The committee's September 1999 draft report was: "*Go easy* on beverages and foods high in *added* sugars." The committee's February 2000 draft report was softened to: "Choose beverages and foods that *limit* your intake of sugars." Finally, the watered-down version of May 2000: "Choose beverages and foods to *moderate* your intake of sugars" (emphases supplied).

As Nestle explained, "go easy" means "eat less"—an anathema to the food and beverage interests; "added" separates less desirable processed foods with added sugars from more desirable foods such as fruits and vegetables that contain sugars naturally. The ultimate wording of "choose" is positive; "go easy" is restrictive.

Nestle claimed that investigative reporting revealed "fierce industry lobbying to retain the 1995 Dietary Goals' wording 'Choose a diet moderate in sugars.' Nestle commented that "sugar trade associations viewed *limit* as a potential disaster for their $26 billion annual industry, and their lobbyists induced thirty senators, half from sugar-growing states, to question whether the USDA had the right to change the sugar guidelines based on existing science.'"

STRICTER SUGAR LABEL REQUIREMENTS NEEDED

The information about sugar and sweeteners on the food label is another aspect of confusion and deception for the unsuspecting consumer. There is no differentiation made between sugars and sweeteners added to food from those sugars that are naturally present in foods.

On August 15, 2005, the Sugar Association submitted a petition to the FDA regarding the nutrition labeling for sugar and sweeteners. The petition requested that the FDA eliminate the current uninformative label and introduce a more informative one, similar to the mandatory labeling law for *trans* fats, effective January 1, 2006. A more informative label would differentiate between caloric sugar such as sucrose, and the high-intensity sweeteners, on the nutrition facts panel of labels.

Since 1994, food and beverage processors are required to include the term "sugar" on the nutrient facts panel for products containing added sugar. The Sugar Association petitioned the FDA to reconsider this regulation, and pointed out:

> FDA's current food labeling regulations have led to consumer confusion about the identities of the sweeteners in their foods and beverages and the calories contributed by these ingredients . . . For this reason, the Sugar Association is requesting FDA to eliminate mandatory labeling of added sugar on the nutrition facts panel and to prohibit reduced-sugar claims. If FDA decides not to accede to this request, then the Sugar Association strongly encourages FDA to change the 'sugar' category on the panel to 'sugars/syrups' and to mandate that high-intensity sweeteners and sugar alcohols [polyols] be mandatory on the nutrition facts panel so consumers know what type of sweetener products include.

Currently, the nutrition facts panel merely lists the vague term "sugars" without revealing that this term may include syrups derived from cornstarch, or other nonsucrose sugars, and high-intensity synthetic sweeteners. The term allows food companies to use the term "sugar" for any monosaccharide or disaccharide used in the product for nutrient-content claims. Such labels are misleading, says Cheryl Digges, director of Public Policy and Education at the Sugar Association. "Consumers don't know that 56 percent of their products contain other sweeteners than sucrose," Digges reported to *Food Product Design* (Oct 2005).

According to the Sugar Association, most consumers are unaware of the different sweeteners other than that sugars are present in many food and beverage products they consume. *Of the twenty-three sweeteners available to processors, consumers recognize only five* (emphasis added).

Digges continued:

Consumer education has not kept up with the industry. We want consumers to understand what is in their products and disclose exactly what sugars they are consuming. Especially with the FDA's "Calories Count" initiative. It is important for consumers to recognize this. Just because labels are claiming 50 percent less sugar does not mean less calories. Many times, sugarless products actually have as many, if not more, calories than full-sugar products.

Currently, FDA regulations permit reduced-sugar claims without giving information about the ingredients that replace sugar, which can affect the total caloric content of a product. According to Digges, "This means that products can be labeled as containing 'less sugar' when, in fact, the products contain no sugar and are manufactured with other 'sugars' such as corn syrup."

A CAMPAIGN TO BOOST SUGAR'S IMAGE

In a sidebar accompanying an article on sweeteners in *Food Product Design* (Feb 2001), Malaika Geuka Wells wrote in "Sugar's Sweet Surprise":

Adding more sugar to your morning coffee may actually help you perform better throughout the day. A recent study of 20 men and women between the ages of 60 and 82 suggests that eating carbohydrates in the morning contributes to enhanced memory and task performance. The results of the study are published in the September 20 issue of the *American Journal of Clinical Nutrition*. According to the study, consumption of carbohydrates, including glucose, potatoes or barley, is directly linked to improved cognition, especially in those with poor glucose regulation and poor cognition. After a short fast on four separate mornings, test participants ate either a placebo or 50 grams of carbohydrates as glucose, potatoes, or barley. Cognitive tests were given three times, at 15, 60, and 105 minutes after the carbohydrate consumption, after which blood glucose and serum insulin were measured. Of the 10 men and 10 women tested, subjects who ate carbohydrates performed better at delayed paragraph and word-list recall compared to subjects who were given the placebo . . . While these studies do not give license to obsessively consume sweets, they do scientifically support a beneficial relationship between glucose consumption and cognitive retention.

Another reason prompting the Sugar Association's petition are the 2005 figures from the USDA showing that sucrose consumption has decreased by

40 percent over the past thirty years, from 95.7 pounds per person annually in 1974 to 61.9 pounds per person annually in 2005. The reason for this decline, according to the Sugar Association, is that consumers believe that sugar consumption leads to obesity, which has stimulated many low-sugar and no-sugar diet trends, and in turn, has led to the rise of high-intensity sweeteners in food products—noted by the Sugar Association as a billion-dollar-annual market in the United States.

With high-intensity sweeteners growing in popularity, due in part to trendy diets and health-conscious consumers, the sugar industry is placing more importance on which sweeteners are included in a product, and how much is being used. Digges noted, "It's not only important for the label terminology to change, but we also want the amount of artificial sweeteners or sugar alcohols to be claimed in the nutrition panel, as well." Having stricter label requirements make manufacturers accountable for reporting the amount of any or a combination of sweeteners added to food and beverage products.

In May 2005, the Sugar Association launched a $3 million advertising campaign in hopes of boosting its image. The campaign praises sugar as a natural sweetener, and clears up what it considers a common misconception. According to the Association, many people believe that a teaspoonful of sugar contains about 76 calories; it contains only 15 calories.

Despite this advertising blitz, the ADA continues to maintain that a diet high in sugar contributes to empty calories, which can lead to obesity and health issues, and displaces more nutritious foods that contain naturally occurring sugars. These statements are accurate, but then the ADA offers poor advice. The ADA suggests that the use of high-intensity synthetic sweeteners, as part of a calorie-controlled diet, is beneficial in maintaining health and losing weight. Not so. The recommendation represents one more deceptive and confusing piece of information about sugars and sweeteners given to consumers.

The public is unaware of the financial ties between the ADA and the sugar and sweetener interests. In each issue of the Journal of the American Dietetic Association are "Nutrition Fact Sheets" intended for duplication and distribution to patients. When the topics concern sugars and sweeteners, the materials are supplied by a "sponsor," the Sugar Association. Also, the ADA devotes a full inner back page in its journal issue near the end of the year to thank its sponsors. "These organizations have provided generous financial support for the mission and goals of the Association, the ongoing professional education to its members and the Food and Nutrition Conference & Expo." Among its sponsors in 2005 were the Sugar Association, Equal (produced by Merisant), the Coca-Cola Company, Wrigley, and the International Food Information Council (funded by numerous food and beverage manufacturers).

Chapter 22

AVOIDING THE SWEETENER TRAP: SIMPLE STRATEGIES

For people seeking optimum health . . . the (best) approach would be to avoid both sugar and artificial sweeteners. Doing so allows one's taste buds to be reawakened to the natural sweet taste of whole foods.

—ALAN R. GABY, M.D., (EDITORIAL) *TOWNSEND LETTER*
FOR DOCTOR & PATIENTS, MAY 2005

The public is tempted everywhere with sweetened food and beverage products. Advertising and easy accessibility to these products ensure their sales and consumption. They are affordable and tasty. A glazed doughnut is more sexy than an apple, and a soft drink, more than plain water. How can one avoid the sweetener trap?

CHOOSE NUTRITIOUS SOURCES OF SWEETS

A good diet of basic whole foods (quality protein foods, fruits and vegetables, whole grains, dairy products, and nuts/seeds) provide all the naturally occurring sugar that the body requires. Fruits are sweet. Even some vegetables, notably sweet potatoes, carrots, parsnips, beets, squash, and pumpkin, are sweet. Select fruits in season and use them for desserts and for between-meal snacks. Many common fruits, including oranges, apples, pears, and bananas, are available everywhere year-round. Even ones that used to be seasonal, such as cherries and grapes, are available out of season from countries such as Chile and Mexico. Several types of berries, notably blueberries, strawberries, blackberries, and raspberries, can be purchased out of season, frozen, without sugar or syrup.

The U.S. Department of Agriculture (USDA) launched a program of "Five A Day" servings of vegetables and fruits. Many health professionals feel that five servings daily is far too little, and they have recommended doubling the number. Yet, many Americans fail to eat even five servings daily, and if it is from the fruit category, some people eat none, or others only consume fruit in juice form.

Few fruits require any added sweetening. Some rare exceptions may be tart raspberries, acrid rhubarb, and acidic lemon. The season for raspberries and rhubarb is brief, lemons are used as flavoring rather than as fruit.

Dried fruits need to be eaten in limited quantities because of the concentration of their sugars. A tablespoon of raisins or currants, or two or three minced dried apricots, prunes, dried dates, or figs, soaked overnight along with soaking wholegrain cereal (such as steel-cut oats, brown rice, barley, buckwheat, bulghur, quinoa, amaranth, or others) will sweeten the cooked cereal sufficiently so that additional sweetening is not necessary.

If dried fruits are used as snacks, they also need to be eaten in limited amounts, and accompanied by fluid intake to restore the lost moisture. Also, due to their stickiness and adhesion to the teeth, prompt tooth brushing and flossing after eating a dried fruit snack is prudent.

Eating a variety of whole fruits is laudable; drinking fruit juices is undesirable. Products such as frozen concentrates of unsweetened frozen juices, as well as refrigerated cartons of pasteurized unsweetened fruit juices, and cans of unsweetened fruit juices fill grocery shelves. These products—though better than fruit drinks with as little as 10 percent fruit juice, or synthetic fruit drinks with no real fruit juice—are inferior to whole fruits. In producing the juice, nutrient losses occur, and dietary fiber is removed. Also, one can drink more juice than eat whole fruit, resulting in too great an intake of fruit sugars. Fruit juices are high-profit products for producers and sellers, and processed juices have long shelf life. For these reasons, shun fruit juices and fruit drinks, and choose whole fruits.

The practice of giving a nighttime bottle containing apple juice to an infant is discouraged by pediatricians and dentists. The natural sugar contained in the apple juice, held in the oral cavity of the sleeping infant, can lead to tooth decay. Also, pediatricians frown on the practice by some parents to substitute apple juice for milk with toddlers. The substitution lowers the nutrient intake, and also can induce gastrointestinal discomfort, including diarrhea in young children.

Some consumers select fruit juice-sweetened jellies, jams, and preserves with the mistaken notion that these products are superior to their common counterparts. Not so. The fruit juices used by processors as sweeteners have undergone extreme modification to make them bland and colorless, so that they will not change the color or flavor of the jellies, jams, and preserves. Consumers pay more for such products, yet the products fail to have added value.

For many Americans, dietary habits have developed with a pattern of consuming desserts three times daily: Danish pastry at breakfast; pie at lunch; cake at supper; and possibly a between-meal snack of cookies, candies, or doughnuts, washed down with a sweetened beverage at meals and with snacks. Many people consider this pattern "normal." Yet formerly, desserts were not daily occurrences, but rather occasional treats.

For those who feel that a meal is incomplete without dessert, or that between-meal snacks must be sweet food, fruit is the ideal choice. Fruits can be eaten by themselves, or combined with other high-nutrient foods. Fruits combine well with unflavored yogurt or with natural cheeses (if dairy foods are tolerated). Examples are a ripe pear and Cheddar cheese; an apple and Swiss cheese; or grapes and Gouda cheese.

Recent information about the values of nuts and seeds make these basic foods desirable as part of the diet. They combine well with fruits for desserts or snacks. Examples are walnuts with a banana; almonds with an orange; or sunflower seeds with a wedge of cantaloupe. (Tree nuts and ground nuts such as peanuts are not tolerated by all.)

All of these simple desserts and snack suggestions require a minimum of preparation. They satisfy the palate, and are readily available in food stores. They are less costly than sweetened food and beverage products, and they are nutrient-dense. As you wean yourself away from sweetened food and beverage products, your palate will come to appreciate the subtle flavors of sweetness in whole foods. The formerly relished seven-layer cake or fudge may become cloyingly sweet.

PROTECTING CHILDREN FROM THE SWEETNER TRAP

As an age group, children are the greatest sweetener consumers. Lifetime habits form early. Good eating habits contribute to lifetime health. Yet, marketing lures children to foods that contribute to poor eating habits.

Children, especially, have been targeted for the sale of highly processed, highly sweetened foods and beverages. Formerly, the federal government regarded young children in need of protection from the wiles of the marketplace. Young children were regarded as being vulnerable because they had not yet developed skills to make mature judgments. With the growth of the concept of "free market" accompanied by "laissez faire," controls vanished. Young children, whose third word uttered, after momma and poppa, was McDonald's, became subjects of marketing goods.

A landmark report, "Food Marketing to Children and Youth: Threat or Opportunity?" was issued in December 2005 by the Institute of Medicine (IOM). A committee comprised of health professionals reviewed 120 studies to explore the connection between TV advertising and overweight children. The report related the epidemic of childhood obesity to the food, beverage, and advertising industries. Key facts in the report noted:

- There is strong evidence that marketing foods and beverages to children influences their preferences.

- The dominant focus of marketing to children and youth is on foods and beverages high in calories and low in nutrients, and is sharply out of balance with healthful diets. Marketing (has) become multi-faceted and sophisticated.

- Given the media and marketing environment that envelope over children's lives, there is a surprising paucity of research on ways [that] may be used to promote health.

The report found that the youngest children are the most vulnerable. To reduce childhood obesity, the report recommended a long-term campaign to educate the public about making healthy food choices. The campaign would be financed by public and private funds (the latter from the very industries considered to be responsible for the increased number of overweight and obese children).

The report recommended that if food and beverage marketers did not *voluntarily* shift the emphasis of TV advertising aimed at children to health foods from high-calorie low-nutrient products, Congress should *mandate* changes.

Industry responses were limited. Although poor food and beverage choices (including those with high amounts or sugars and sweeteners) represent only one factor in the multifaceted problem of obesity, many of the affected industries chose to stress parental responsibility, and more physical exercise as the appropriate solutions. These actions only nibble around the edge of the problem: For example, McDonald's, beginning in 2006, started to list nutritional facts on its packaging and wrappers of Big Mac, french fries, salad, and Apple Dippers. However, the listing is limited to calories, proteins, fat, carbohydrates, and sodium in percentages of daily values (DV) and grams/milligrams. Sugar is hidden in the carbohydrate listing. Even if curious consumers read the labels, they will not be informed about the sugar content of the products.

As for "parental responsibility" even the most concerned of parents wage a losing battle in an unlevel playing field, against the powerful and monied forces marketing to their children, and the few good choices being offered.

Parental concerns have been increasing, and actions, both individual and group, have developed around the issue of the quality of foods served to their children in school lunchrooms. In many locations, there are attempts to upgrade the food and beverage offerings, but such efforts face many obstacles. In some instances, parents have targeted the undesirable offerings in school vending machines. Here, too, such efforts face many obstacles. However, as of 2007, there have been a few notable success stories. Early on, at the urgings, mainly of parents, public school systems in the counties of Mont-gomery, Fairfax, and Arlington, all in Virginia, were successful in imposing restrictions on what could be sold in school vending machines, and the hours of sales not to be in competition with the time for serving school lunches. These pioneering efforts cascaded into a widespread movement everywhere in the country. The American Bottlers Association (ABA) issued guidelines in August 2005 for a voluntary limitation of soft drink offerings in vending machines to no more than 50 percent of the options in high schools. The state of California went further by enacting legislation banning *all* soft drinks in vending machines in *all* state public schools.

In early 2006, the soft drink industry responded to the mounting criticism against the practice of supplying soft drinks in school vending machines. The industry announced that by 2008, it would stock school vending machines with bottled water, sports drinks, fruit juices, and diet soft drinks nationwide. This move preempted any federally mandated proposal that might be made. Yet the action would not incur any monetary loss. The manufacturers of soft drinks also process the other bottled drinks.

"The American concept of a normal diet has gotten out of wack," reported Samuel S. Gidding, M.D., professor of pediatric cardiology at Jefferson Medical College in Philadelphia, Pennsylvania, and chair of a committee responsible for writing guidelines issued by the American Heart Association (AHA) in Septem-ber 2005. Worried that children are not receiving a healthy diet and are learning lifestyle-related behavior that increases the risks of heart disease and stroke in adulthood, the AHA issued new recommendations for feeding and exercise *beginning at birth.* The guidelines were intended to encourage parents and clini-cians to take a "primordial preventive" approach, beginning in infancy (*Circula-tion,* 2005). Giddings reported that "what used to be considered child's food was nutritious, but now it tends to be treats or high-calorie, low-nutrition snacks."

The new guidelines pointed out that on any given day one-third of nine-teen-month to twenty-four-month-old children consume *no* fruit; two-thirds eat baked desserts; one-fifth munch on candy; and nearly half drink sweet-ened beverages. Giddings said, "Poor nutrition and bad eating habits are tied to the obesity epidemic."

Previous AHA recommendations were not intended for children younger than two years of age, but continuing research prompted the inclusion of infants under two years of age in the new guidelines. Among the high points of the recommendations are:

• Infants should be fed breastmilk exclusively in the first four to six months of life, and with some breastfeeding continued until the infant is a year old.

• The diets of older children should follow the general guidelines for adults:

daily consumption of fruits and vegetables; consumption of whole grains rather than refined ones; and reduction of sugar intake.

The recommendations for parents and other caregivers are:

- Control what food is available to children, when the food can be eaten, its nutrient quality, and portion size.

- Teach children about food and nutrition, while shopping or cooking.

- Counteract inaccurate information emanating from the media and other influences.

- Serve as role models for the children and lead by example.

Giddings said that "parents have lost control of their children's diets. We want parents to regain control of the kitchen and recognize the dietary needs of their children."

Another reflection of the impact of poor diets, of which highly sweetened foods and beverages play a role, is the alarming rate of diabetic development in young children as well as in the adult population. In a remarkable in-depth exploration of the diabetic epidemic in New York City, a lengthy four-part series presented an apocalyptic scenario, on the front pages of the *New York Times* (Jan 9–12, 2006). The problem was described as one emerging into a full-blown crisis. New York City is not unique. In part four of the series, the focus was on food choices. In New York City, the school breakfast program serves children fat-free chocolate milk, a reduced-fat doughnut, a packaged cereal, and fruit juice. The total sugar content of this meal is 47 grams, an issue that is ignored with a misplaced concern solely on fat. All four components of the meal are food and beverage products that are profitable for the suppliers but do little good for the children.

Because the taste buds of so many young children have been perverted by intensely sweetened items, their appetites run to sweeter, high-calorie foods. Although New York City mandates that schools serve fruit such as a banana or apple as part of the lunch program, often the fruits are not eaten. They become plate waste.

At the end of 2005, a legal case was being built to relate childhood obesity to the sale of soft drinks in school vending machines. A coalition of the same group of lawyers who successfully sued tobacco companies, led by Richard A. Daynard and Stephen A. Sheller, announced plans to file a class action lawsuit against soft-drink manufacturers for selling their sugar-containing products in schools. The lawyers were joined by the Center for Science in the Public Interest (CSPI). The lawyers had been preparing their case for more than two years, and planned to file the lawsuit in Massachusetts, where some of the nation's most plaintiff-friendly regulations exist. Massachusetts is one of the few states where plaintiffs in a consumer-protection case do not have to demonstrate actual damage—only that a violation has occurred.

In an interview with the *Washington Post* (Dec 2, 2005) Daynard said, "The idea is to get soda machines out of schools because they [the sodas] are clearly making a substantial contribution to the obesity epidemic." The legal basis of the suit will use the concept of "attractive nuisance," Daynard explained. "If someone has something on his land like a swimming pool that he knows is attractive to kids and dangerous, then he has some obligation to keep the kids away from it. You want to keep kids away from dangerous objects, and [soda in] a soda machine is demonstrated to be a dangerous object for kids."

PROTECTING ADULTS FROM THE SWEETENER TRAP

For adults, too, the high intake of sugars and sweeteners has become more recognized as a health risk. Dr. Wolfgang C. Winkelmayer and his colleagues at Brigham and Women's Hospital and Harvard Medical School, funded by a grant from the National Institues of Health (NIH) as well as other independent organizations, found that both sugar-containing and diet-cola beverages consistently were associated with hypertension in all groups of women studied. Caffeine was not a factor in the drinks, but the added sugars and sweeteners were. The greater number of diet drinks consumed, the greater the risk of high blood pressure.

Rat studies by S. B. Choi and colleagues, reported in 2002, found an increase in consumption of cola drinks increased insulin resistance in the animals. Human studies reported by M.B. Schulze and colleagues showed an increased risk of diabetes from the intake of cola drinks. These studies attributed the increased risks in insulin resistance and diabetes to the glycemic load from high-fructose corn syrup (HFCS) used in these drinks. Winkelmayer and his colleagues concluded that if the sugars and sweeteners used in the cola drinks are causally related to high blood pressure, "they may have considerable impact on public health" (*Journal of the American Medical Association*, Nov 9, 2005).

The lesson from this study, as well as from others, is to reduce—or better yet, eliminate—soft drink consumption. If coffee, tea, or other hot beverages are used, reduce or eliminate sugars and sweeteners added to these beverages.

Avoiding the sweetener trap is relatively simple, provided one has an incentive to maintain or restore good health. For some, changing eating habits is a difficult challenge. For such individuals, making small, incremental changes may be all that can be achieved: less sweetening in hot beverages, a reduction in the number of candy bars, cookies, or soft drinks consumed; eating more fruits, and so forth. For others, who are highly motivated, dietary changes may be more extensive: avoidance of all soft drinks and other pre-sweetened processed drinks; eating more fruits; and eliminating all sugar- or sweetener-added products, except on rare occasions.

For individuals on good diets, the sweetening problem is not even an issue. Whole basic foods (whatever is tolerated), such as quality protein foods from animal sources, fruits, vegetables, dairy products, whole grains, and nuts and seeds, do not require added sugars or sweeteners. For individuals making good food choices, the sweetener trap will not be sprung.

Appendix A

ACRONYMS USED IN TEXT

Parent organizations and renamed organizations are in parentheses following the acronyms.

AAA: acetoacetic acid

AACC: American Association of Cereal Chemists (renamed AACC International)

AAEM: American Academy of Environmental Medicine

AAS: acetocetamide-N-sulfonic acid

ABA: American Bottlers Association

ACS: American Chemical Society

ACSH: American Council on Science and Health

ACSN: Aspartame Consumer Safety Network

ADA: American Diabetes Association

ADA: American Dietetic Association

ADI: Acceptable daily intake

AMA: The American Medical Association

ARMS: Adverse Reaction Monitoring System (FDA)

ARS: Agricultural Research Service (USDA)

BATF: Bureau of Alcohol, Tobacco and Firearms (U.S. Department of Treasury; renamed Bureau of Alcohol, Tobacco, Firearms, and Explosives, AFT for short, and transferrred to the Department of Justice under the Homeland Security Act)

CCC: Calorie Control Council

CCG: California Canners and Growers

CDC: Centers for Disease Control and Prevention (USPHS, under the U.S. Department of Health and Human Services)

CFSAN: Center for Food Safety and Applied Nutrition (FDA)

CNI: Community Nutrition Institute

CSPI: Center for Science in the Public Interest

DSHEA: Dietary Supplement, Health and Education Act (FDA)

DV: Daily value

EEC: European Economic Community (now known as the European Union or EU)

ELISHAs: Enzyme-linked immunosorbent assays

EPA: Environmental Protection Agency

ERS: Economic Research Service (USDA)

EU: European Union (formerly known as the European Economic Community or EEC)

FAO: Food and Agriculture Organization (United Nations or UN)

FASEB: Federation of American Societies for Experimental Biology

FDA: Food and Drug Administration (HHS)

FEMA: Flavor and Extract Manufacturers Association

FTC: Federal Trade Commission

GALT: Galactose-1-phosphate uridyl transferase

GAO: General Accountability Office (formerly General Accounting Office)

GI: Glycemic Index

GRAS: Generally Recognized As Safe

HDLs: High-density lipoproteins

HEW: U.S. Department of Health, Education and Welfare (renamed U.S. Department of Health and Human Services

HFCS: High-fructose corn syrup

HHS: Department of Health and Human Services (formerly named Department of Health, Education and Welfare)

IARC: International Agency for Research on Cancer

IFIC: International Food Information Council Foundation

IFT: Institute of Food Technologists

ILSI: International Life Sciences Institute

IND: Investigational New Drug (FDA)

IRDC: International Research and Development Corporation

IRI: Information Resources, Inc.

IRS: Internal Revenue Service (U.S. Department of the Treasury)

ISRF: International Sugar Research Foundation

JECFA: Joint Expert Committee on Food Additives (UN)

kg: Kilogram(s)

LDLs: Low-density lipoproteins

MC: Methylene chloride

mcg: Microgram(s)

mg: Milligram(s)

MIT: Massachusetts Institute of Technology

MSG: monosodium glutamate

NAD: National Advertising Division (Better Business Bureaus)

NAS: National Academy of Sciences (renamed the National Academies)

Natl Inst Child Health: National Institute of Child Health (NIH)

NCI: National Cancer Institute (NIH)

NCTR: The National Center for Toxicological Research (FDA)

NIDR: National Institute of Dental Research (NIH)

NIEHS: National Institute of Environmental Health Sciences (NIH)

NIH: National Institutes of Health

NIHS: National Institutes of Health Sciences (NIH)

NIOSH: National Institute of Occupational Safety and Health (HHS)

NMI: National Marketing Institute

NSDA: National Soft Drinks Association

NSF: National Science Foundation

NTIS: National Technical Information Service (U.S. Department of Commerce)

NTP: National Toxicology Program (EPA)

OPA: Office of Premarket Approval (FDA)

OTA: Office of Technological Assessment

PBI: Public Board of Inquiry (FDA)

PHS: U.S. Public Health Service (HHS)

PKU: Phenylketonuria

RCT: Research Corporation Technologies

SGOT: Serum glutamic-oxaloacetic transaminase

SRI: Stanford Research Institute (Stanford University)

UAREP: Universities Associated for Research and Education in Pathology

USDA: U.S. Department of Agriculture

WARF: Wisconsin Alumni Research Foundation (University of Wisconsin)

WHO: World Health Organization

Appendix B

GLOSSARY OF SWEETENER TERMS

AAA: *See* acetoacetic acid.

Abrusides: Intensely sweet principles found in the leaves of two subtropical plants, *Abrus precatorius* and *Abrus fruticulosus.* The compounds are triterpene glycosides.

Ace-K: *See* acesulfame K.

Acesulfame K (Ace-K): A high-intensity sweetener derived from acetoacetic acid.

Acetoacetic acid (AAA): The base of the high-intensity sweetener, acesulfame-K.

ACK: *See* acesulfame-K.

Affination: The treatment of raw sugar crystals with a heavy syrup to remove the adhering molasses film.

Agave: Agave (*Agave tequilane weber*) and the great maguey (*Agave strovirens*) are plants that have sweet principles in their sap that can be processed into edible syrup. Dark agave syrup retains more minerals than light-colored syrup, which goes trhough a filtration process to remove some natural solids.

Alitame: A synthetic high-intensity sweetener comprised of an amide series.

Alternan: A carbohydrate polymer made by transforming sugar into a noncaloric sweetener by means of the enzyme, alpha-d-glucansucrase. Alternan is classified chemically as dextran.

Amasake: A starter, called koji, that breaks down the polysaccharides in sweet brown rice to disaccharides, and gives the resulting product a sweet taste.

Amylase: A saccharifying enzyme.

Arabinose: A crystalline sugar widely distributed in plants, usually polysaccharides. It is found especially in the gums of the cherry tree, mequite, western red cedar, and sapote. It is produced commercially from glucose. Arabinose is used as a culture medium for certain bacteria. It is known, too, as pectin sugar.

Artificial sweeteners: Synthesized compounds, such as cyclamates, saccharin, and aspartame that usually are noncaloric or low in calories, and highly intense in their sweetening power.

Aspartame: A high-intensity, low-calorie synthesized sweetener, composed of two amino acids: aspartic acid and phenylalanine. Chemically, the compound is the methyl ester of L- aspartyl-L-phenylalanine.

Barbados molasses: A popular flavorsome molasses that is usually unsulfured.

Barbados sugar: *See* muscovados.

Beet sugar: A refined carbohydrate processed from sugar beets. It is a disaccharide.

Bernadame: A synthesized high-intensity sweetener that is being researched but is not in commercial production.

Blackstrap molasses: The residue obtained from the manufacture of raw, or refined sugar, that contains some nutrients. It is bitter and needs to be combined with sweeter sugars. It consists of more than half sucrose. A typical composition is 54 percent sucrose, and lesser amounts of glucose and fructose.

Blend: A mixture, or solution, of two or more sugars or sweeteners combined in a prescribed ratio. By using two or more sugars, the same level of sweetness may be achieved with less quantity due to synergism.

Bottlers' sugar: Any liquid or granulated sugar that meets the quality standards of the American Bottlers of Carbonated Beverages.

Brazzein: A high-intensity sweetener derived from the plant, *Pentadiplandra brazzeana.*

Brix: A scale of measurement commonly used to designate the sugar concentration in a water solution. The solid's weight is expressed as a percentage of the total weight.

Brown sugar: A sugar with a soft grain and coated with a film of molasses syrup. It is a byproduct of the refining process, and consists of about 91 to 96 percent sucrose.

Buttered syrup: Buttered syrup is a type of pancake syrup containing a small amount of maple syrup, blended with other sugars.

Calcium salt of saccharin: One form of the synthesized sweetener, saccharin.

Cane sugar: Also known as sucrose, a refined sugar processed from sugarcane. It is a disaccharide. Commonly, it is called sugar, white sugar, or table sugar.

Cane syrup: A syrup made from concentrated untreated cane, that is produced without the use or lime, sulfur, or bleach. It is known, also, as pure ribbon cane syrup. It is in limited production and is available from specialty outlets.

Caramel: A food additive made from burnt sugar and used to color foods and beverages.

Caramelized sugar: A brittle, brown, and somewhat bitter substance produced commercially by heating dextrose with a small amount of ammonia or ammonium salts, and used as a coloring agent in carbonated beverages, bakery products, confections, and liquors. It is a suspected carcinogen, possibly due to the processing technique.

Carbohydrates: Molecular compounds that are comprised of carbon, hydrogen, and oxygen. Sugars are examples of simple carbohydrates; whole grains, of complex carbohydrates.

Carob: A pod from a tree in the locust family, grown mainly in the Mediterranean region. The pod, dried, toasted, and pulverized, is used as a chocolate substitute. Carob is known, too, as St. John's bread. The quality of the product varies considerably.

Carrelame: Carrelame is a synthesized high-intensity sweetener that is being researched, but is not in commercial production.

Cerebrose: *See* galactose.

Char: An adsorptive and decoloring agent used in sugar refining.

Coarse sugar: A sugar that has a crystal size larger than table sugar. Usually, it is processed from the purest sugar liquor. It is highly resistant to color change during its natural breakdown to fructose and glucose (*see* invert sugar) at high temperatures, making it useful in the manufacture of fondants, confections, and liquors.

Coconut sugar: A sugar made from the sap of coconut flowers. It is not as sweet as other plant-derived sweeteners. It is sold in Asian markets in paste form. It is known, too, as palm sugar.

Comogenization: A process for producing blends with corn syrup. Ingredients are combined in set ratios and subjected to heat, pasteurization, and fine-mesh filtration.

Complex carbohydrates: A type of carbohydrate found in whole grains and in legumes (beans) that releases its sugar relatively slowly into the body. Also called polysaccharides.

Confectioner's sugar: A granulated sugar pulverized to an extremely fine powder, and then sifted for rapid solution in cold liquids. It is called icing sugar, too.

Cornstarch: A finely textured flour made from pulverized corn by means of hydrolysis, and converted to corn sweeteners such as dextrose; conventional corn syrups; and to 42 percent, 55 percent, and 90 percent high-fructose corn syrups.

Corn sugar: *See* dextrose.

Corn syrup solids: Solids that are produced from corn syrup which is sprayed or vacuum-drum-dried to lower the moisture content in order to form granular, semi-crystalline products. The solids are moderately hygroscopic (absorbing moisture) and they are moderately sweet. The solids also are known as glucose solids.

Corn syrups: Corn syrups are produced commercially by the partial hydrolysis of cornstarch, and then converted by the action of enzymes and/or acids, and then clarified, decolored, and evaporated to form clear, concentrated, aqueous solutions. Light corn syrups may contain 19 percent glucose, 2 percent fructose, and the remainder, other carbohydrates. Unmixed corn syrups are only 30 percent as sweet as sucrose; enzymatically converted ones, 60 percent as sweet as sucrose. Corn syrups also are called glucose.

Crystalline fructose (CF): A monosaccharide (the simplest form of carbohydrate) that is usually produced commercially from sucrose.

Cyclamates: Synthesized sweeteners made from either the sodium or calcium salts of cyclohexylsulfamic acid. Cyclamates were banned from use in the United States in 1969.

Cyclohexanol: A metabolite (a breakdown product) of cyclamate.

Cyclohexanone: A metabolite of cyclamate.

Cyclohexyhydroxylamine: A metabolite of cyclamate.

Cyclohexylamine: A breakdown product of cyclamate.

Date sugar: A product made from dried, ground dates. It resembles brown sugar in appearance, and in its "caking" characteristic. The supply is limited and erratic from specialty outlets.

Dememara sugar: A light-brown sugar, popular in England, with large crystals that have a slightly sticky texture. Raw cane dememara is exported from Malawi.

Desugarization: An industrial process that extracts sugar from beet molasses. The process is more difficult than with cane molasses, and it has not achieved broad commercial application. A desugarization facility, commonly close to a refining facility, can recover much of the sugar from beet molasses. The process allows about 10 percent of the residual sugar to be extracted from sugar beets.

Dextran: A sugar that is produced commercially by bacterial growth on a sucrose substrate. It is used in soft-centered confections, and as a partial replacer for barley malt. Medically, dextran is used as the principal blood-plasma expander in hospitals.

Dextrinize: To dextrinize is to convert starch into dextrins.

Dextrins: Substances produced commercially by the hydrolysis of cornstarch, and converted by the action of heat and acids or enzymes, to maltose or glucose. The process is used in making syrups and beers.

Dextrose: A monosaccharide produced commercially by the complete hydrolysis of starch. Historically, dextrose has been produced mainly from cornstarch, which is then converted by the action of heat and acids or enzymes to produce a sweetener used in food and beverage products, and to make caramel coloring. Dextrose also is called glucose, corn sugar, or grape sugar. To a chemist, the term dextrose is synonymous with glucose. To the public, glucose usually means corn syrup, or a glucose-type syrup produced from sorghum, wheat, or potato starch.

DHC: *See* dihydrochalcones.

Diastase: A mixture of enzymes obtained from malt and used to convert starch to maltose. Diastase converts at least 50 times the weight of certain starches into sugars (dextrins and maltose). It is known, also, as maltin.

Diastatic malt: A processed malt that is dried at a lower temperature than conventional malt, in order to retain its enzymatic activity. It is used with baked goods, in which these enzymes transform starch, aid the fermentation, and produce soluble proteins utilized by the yeast. This malt also contributes nutrients, flavor, appearance, and helps to maintain freshness in baked goods.

Dihydrochalcones (DHC): A type of flavonoid found in citrus rinds, which are high-intensity sweeteners from plants. Examples include neohesperidin, prunin, hesperidin, and naringin dihydrochalcones.

Disaccharide: A double sugar, consisting of two simple sugars combined and broken down during the digestion to simple sugars, and then absorbed. Examples are sucrose (glucose and sucrose), lactose (glucose and galastose), and maltose (two units of glucose).

Dried corn syrup: Granulated glucose.

Dried glucose syrup: Granulated glucose in syrup form.

Dulcin: An early synthesized high-intensity sweetener, used for more than fifty years, until long overdue testing showed that it caused liver cancer in dogs. Dulcin was banned for use in the United States in 1950. Chemically, dulcin is ethoxyphenylurea, $C_9H_{12}N_2O_2$.

Erythritol: A processed polyol sweetener, based on wheat or cornstarch, that is hydrolyzed to glucose, and then is fermented to produce a crystalline powder.

Ethyl maltol: A form of the sweetener, maltol.

Floc: An insoluble material formed in a sugar solution that settles out slowly.

Fondant sugar: A creamy mass of cooked and uncooked sugar used as a base for candy and icing. Dried fondant sugar is produced by direct crystallization.

Formose: Synthesized sugars that are produced by converting formaldehyde to a complex mixture of high-molecular weight purified carbohydrates. The chemical structure of these sugars is branched, and not found in nature. Formose sugars are not approved for use.

Fructase: The enzyme that metabolizes fructose.

Fructose: A very sweet natural sugar found in many fruits, in honey, and is the sole sugar in blood and human semen. Fructose is a monosaccharide. Fructose also is called levulose, or fruit sugar. It is produced commercially by the hydrolysis of sucrose. Chemically, fructose is $C_6H_{12}O_6$. Commercial fructose is present in considerable quantities in combination with dextrose and sucrose in invert sugars.

Fructose syrup: A misleading term for high-fructose corn syrup (HFCS). It is processed from corn, not from fruit.

Fruit sugar: *See* fructose.

Galactase: The enzyme that metabolizes galactose.

Galactose: A naturally occurring sugar, but produced commercially in right-rotating form by the hydrolysis of lactose, melibiose, raffinose, or certain polysaccharides such as agar or pectin. It is produced in left-rotating form from flaxseed mucilage. It is less soluble and less sweet than glucose. Medically, galactose is used in a liver function test. Galactose is known, also, as brain sugar or cerebrose. Chemically, galactose is $C_6H_{17}O_6$.

Galactosemia: A health condition in which individuals are intolerant to galactose because they are deficient in galactase. (See Appendix D.)

GI: *See* glycemic index.

Glucose: A sugar that occurs naturally and in a free state in fruits and other plants, in polysaccharides, cellulose, and in starch. Glucose is produced commercially by the hydrolysis of cornstarch. Glucose is a monosaccharide, and is known, too, as dextrose, blood sugar, grape sugar, and corn sugar. Chemically, glucose is $C_6H_{12}O_6$. Commercially produced glucose should not be confused with glucose, found in glycogen and in human blood, which is a vital source of energy for humans as well as other living organisms.

Glucose solids: Nearly colorless substances made from starch, or a starch-containing substance. When made from corn, glucose solids are known as corn syrup solids.

Glucose syrup: A liquid solution of glucose, produced commercially by the hydrolysis of cornstarch.

Glycemic index (GI): A ranking system used to measure the relative ability of a carbohydrate to raise blood glucose levels.

Glycine: A naturally occurring amino acid that formerly was used to mask saccharin's bitterness. Glycine had been on the GRAS list (Generally Recognized as Safe) as a food additive, but was removed from the list after animal studies demonstrated its adverse effects. Further use of glycine with saccharin was forbidden. However, it is used as a sweetening agent by food and beverage manufacturers in numerous applications. Chemically, glycine is $C_2H_5NO_2$.

Glycogen: A polysaccharide made from a long chain of glucose molecules that serves as the cellular storehouse for glucose. Glycogen makes glucose readily available for energy turnover in cells. Athletes, for example, depend on glycogen stores for an energy supply during prolonged, vigorous activity.

Glycoproteins: Large complex compounds comprised of sugars attached to protein.

Golden syrup: A British equivalency of corn syrup that is used in cooking, baking, and for toppings and spreads.

Granulated sugar: Refined sucrose in crystalline form. There are many different types available to food and beverage processors and professional bakers. The types differ in crystal size, and they provide functional characteristics appropriate to the processing needs.

Grape sugar: *See* glucose.

Hernandulcin: A high-intensity sweetener from the leaves and blossoms of *Lippia dulcin Trev.* found in Central America.

Hexahydric alcohols: *See* polyols.

Hexahydroxy alcohols: *See* polyols.

Hexahydroxyl alcohols: *See* polyols.

Hexitols: *See* polyols.

HFCS: *See* high-fructose corn syrups.

High-fructose corn syrups (HFCSs): High-fructose corn syrups (HFCSs) are produced commercially by the hydrolysis of dextrose, and converted by the action of heat and enzymes to fructose, and then further processed to produce high-fructose corn syrups. HFCSs are sweeter than invert sugar, which they frequently replace.

Honey: A natural sweetener produced from the gathered nectars of blossoms and converted by the enzymes of the bees into invert sugar. The composition and flavor of honey varies, depending on the nectar sources. Among its main components are two sugars, fructose and glucose, with smaller amounts of sucrose and maltose.

HSH: *See* hydrogenated starch hydrolysate.

Hydrogenated glucose: Hydrogenated glucose is produced commercially by the hydrolysis of cornstarch.

Hydrogenated starch hydrolysate (HSH): A polyol sugar that is produced commercially by the hydrolysis of starch.

Hydrolysis: A chemical reaction in water, in which a bond in the reactant (other than the water) is split, and hydrogen and hydroxyl are added, with two or more new compounds formed.

Hydrometer: A calibrated floating instrument used to measure the density of a liquid sweetener.

Hygroscopic: Refers to a characteristic of a substance that absorbs moisture readily. If the substance resists moisture absorption, it is nonhygroscopic.

Icing sugar: *See* confectioner's sugar.

Imitation maple syrup: Imitation maple syrup is a blend of inexpensive syrups, which may or may not contain real maple syrup. If maple syrup is present in the blend, it comprises a miniscule amount of the total product. It is known, also, as pancake blend or pancake syrup, or waffle blend or waffle syrup.

Insulin Resistance Syndrome (IRS): A health condition marked by abdominal fat, high blood pressure, and elevated cholesterol. It is considered to be a health risk. It is known, also, as Syndrome X.

Inulin: A tasteless polysaccharide that occurs instead of starch in many plants, especially in the tubers and roots of the Jerusalem artichoke, dahlia, and chicory. Inulin is a fructooligosaccharide (FOS) which acts as a prebiotic. It stimulates the growth of bifidobacteria in the lower intestine, which in turn protects against food pathogens, and yields byproducts that stimulate the human immune system. Consumed at a high level, inulin has a laxative effect. Inulin is produced commercially by hydrolysis to yield fructose. Food processors use inulin to replace polyols, and to substitute for sugar in chocolates and other confections. Medically, inulin is used in a kidney function test.

Invertase: An enzyme capable of converting sucrose to invert sugar.

Invert sugar: A sugar that is a mixture of equal parts glucose and fructose, and is found naturally in fruits and honey. It is produced commercially by hydrolysis of sucrose with acid or enzymes. Invert sugar is used to retard the crystallization of sugar, and to retain moisture in food products. Invert sugar is used as a syrup in foods. Medically, it is used in intravenous feeding solutions.

Isomalt: A polyol derived from isomaltulose.

Isomaltose: A syrupy disaccharide made from dextran by acid hydrolysis.

Iso-sorbide: *See* sorbitol.

Lactase: An enzyme needed to metabolize the milk sugar, lactose. If an individual has a lactase deficiency, the condition is known as lactose intolerance, or lactose malabsorption. (See Appendix D.)

Lactate esters: Sugar-derived solvents that are highly miscible (easily mixed in any proportions). They are considered to be naturally occurring constituents of foods and beverages. Traces are identified in California sherry and in Spanish sherry. One form, ethyl lactate, is used as a flavoring agent.

Lactitol: A polyol made by hydrogenating lactose.

Lactose: Milk sugar present in the milk of all mammals. It is a disaccharide. Human milk consists of 7 percent lactose; cow's milk, 4.8 percent lactose.

Lactulose: An isomerized form of whey lactose, but more soluble and sweeter. (An isomerized form is a mirror image.) Lactulose is considered to be nonnutritive. In some cases, its humectant property makes it useful as a sucrose substitute. At high levels, lactulose is laxative.

L-altrose: A nonnutritive sweetener made by fermenting readily available substances. Some strains of the bacterium *Butyrivibrio fibrisolvens* are used with a carbohydrate-containing nutrient medium to produce this sweetener.

Levulose: One of two simple sugars formed in sucrose inversion. It is a monosaccharide. Levulose also is called fructose or fruit sugar.

Licorice (*Glycyrrhiza glabra*): A substance derived from the long, thick, sweet roots of a perennial leguminous plant grown in the Mediterranean region. The source of licorice extract used as a flavoring agent for foods, beverages, and tobacco, and also to mask unpleasant flavors in drugs, has been used increasingly as a sweetening agent. Ammoniated glycyrrhizin (an active principle) is about 50 times sweeter than sucrose. One pound of licorice added to 100 pounds of sucrose yields a sweetness level equivalent to 200 pounds of sucrose. Licorice, used at a high level, can induce high blood pressure and potassium depletion.

Liquid sugar: Sugar in a solution, such as sucrose in water. Liquid sugar was developed before current methods of sugar processing made it practical to transport and handle granulated sugar. Liquid sugar is a common form of sugar used by food and beverage processors because the liquid can be blended easily with other ingredients, and bulk handling of the liquid is economical. There are several types of liquid sugar.

Liquor: Liquor is a term applied generally to partially concentrated sugar solutions and syrups.

Lo Han: Lo A Chinese calabash plant, related to the cucumber or melon family, from which a sweetener can be extracted. The sweetener is available commercially, and is being used increasingly in food and beverage products. Other varieties or spellings include Luo Han Guo, Luo Han Kuo, Lu Han Gu, and Luo Han Go.

Lugdoname: A synthesized high-intensity sweetener, but it is not available in commercial production.

Maguey: *See* agave.

Malt: A sweetener produced commercially by steeping grain (usually barley) in water to soften and germinate it. Enzymes convert the grain's starch into sugar. The resulting form is kiln-dried, ground, and used as a nutrient, and by brewers and distillers in their products.

Malt extract: A powder, produced from barley, that contains diastase, dextrin, dextrose, protein, and salts. It is used in baked goods, processed cereals, and confections.

Malt sugar: *See* maltose.

Malt syrup: A nondiastatic syrup extracted from barley malt and concentrated into a liquid form.

Maltin: *See* diastase.

Maltitol: A polyol sugar.

Maltitol syrups: Syrups made from maltitol, a polyol.

Maltitritol: A highly hydrogenated form of saccharides.

Maltodextrins: A sweetener formed from carbohydrates hydrolyzed from wheat and barley. The process for producing them is similar to that for producing corn syrups, but the conversion is stopped at an earlier stage.

Maltol: A crystallized compound found especially in the bark of young larch trees, pine needles, chicory, wood tars and their oils, and in roasted malt. Maltol is used as a flavoring agent to give a "fresh-baked" odor and flavor to bakery products. Chemically, maltol is $C_6H_6O_3$.

Maltose: A sugar formed by two glucose units linked together. Maltose develops in sprouted grains, but commercially it is produced by the hydrolysis of starch. Maltose is a disaccharide, and is a fermentable reducing sugar that is useful in brewing, distilling, and in food processing. Maltose also is known as malt sugar. Chemically, maltose is $C_{12}H_{22}O_{11}H_2O$.

Maltose syrup: A liquid solution of maltose.

Manna sugar: *See* mannitol.

Mannite: *See* mannitol.

Mannitol: A polyol found as mannose in chicory and in roasted malt.

Mannose: A crystalline sweetener primarily from manna ash that is reduced to mannitol. Chemically, mannose is $C_6H_{12}0_6$.

Maple sugar: A granulated form of maple syrup made by boiling the syrup to the hard sugar stage and immediately stirring the syrup to promote crystallization.

Maple syrup: The concentrated sap from the maple tree, consisting mainly of sucrose, with water and a small amount of invert sugar and malic acid. It is produced by evaporating the surplus water. What sets maple syrup apart from other syrups is its distinctive flavor.

Milk sugar: Lactose, a disaccharide.

Miraculin: An intensely sweet glycoprotein in the miracle berry (*Synsepalum dulcificum*) with a large molecule and a molecular weight of 42,000. Miraculin is a high-intensity sweetener.

Molasses: The syrup obtained by evaporation and partial inversion of clarified or unclarified sugarcane juice. Molasses is the edible byproduct resulting from the manufacture of sucrose. Some, but not all, of the crystallizable sugar in the sugarcane juice is removed in the evaporation.

Monellin: A high-intensity sweetener from the serendipity berry (*Dioscoreophyllum cumminsii*).

Monosaccharide: A simple sugar in molecular structure. Examples include arabinose, dextrose, galactose, glucose, levulose (fructose), mannose, and xylose. Monosaccharides are the digestive end products of polysaccharides.

Muscovados: Unrefined raw sugar obtained from sugarcane juice, and exported mainly from Mauritius. This is a specialty brown sugar popular with the British. The sugar is very dark brown, with an especially strong molasses flavor. The crystals are slightly coarser and stickier in texture than ordinary brown sugar. It is known also as Barbados sugar.

Naringin: A bitter substance found in citrus rind that, when synthesized into neohesperidin, becomes intensely sweet.

Natural sugars: Sugars that are present naturally in foods, and also in breastmilk. Examples include fructose, lactose, and galactose.

Neohesperidin dihydrochalcones: *See* dihydrochalcones.

Neosugar: A nonnutritive, nondigestible sweetener manufactured from sucrose by a fungal enzyme. At present, it is used in Japan.

Neotame: A synthesized high-intensity sweetener composed of the amino acids, aspartic acid and phenylalanine—the same basic components of aspartame.

Nigerian berry (*Dioscoreophyllum cumminsii*): Also known as the serendipity berry. The plant contains a principle that is intensely sweet. It has a molecular weight of about 44,000.

Noncentrifuged sugars: Crude sugars made from sugarcane juice by evaporation and draining off the molasses. Some local names include muscovado, panocha, and papelon.

Nondiastatic malt: Extracted from barley malt and made into a concentrated syrup. It is known, too, as malt syrup.

Nonnutritive sweeteners: Synthesized noncaloric sweeteners such as cyclamates and saccharin.

Oligosaccharides: A chain consisting of fructose molecules found in many fruits and vegetables. Generally, they are mixtures of monosaccharides, disaccharides, or polysaccharides. Unlike starch or simple sugars, oligosaccharides do not ferment into acids, and thus they are not cariogenic. They act as prebiotics that selectively stimulate the growth and/or activity of certain beneficial bacterial species in the colon, and their physiological effects are somewhat similar to dietary fiber and are indigestible by humans.

Painted sugar: White sugar sprayed with brown-colored syrup.

Palm sugar: *See* coconut sugar.

Pancake blend: A mixture of syrups that may or may not contain a very small percentage of maple syrup. The blend also is termed imitation maple syrup, pancake syrup, waffle blend, or waffle syrup.

Pancake syrup: *See* pancake blend.

Pectin sugar: A product obtained as a powder or syrup that is extracted from citrus peel, dried apple powder, or dried sugar beet slices. It is used mainly in jellies, pharmaceuticals, and cosmetics. *Also see* arabinose.

Perillartine: A naturally occurring aldoxime present in the oil of *Perilla namkemonsis* Deone. (An aldoxime is an oxime of an aldehyde. An oxime is a group of compounds composed of carbon, nitrogen, oxygen, and hydrogen.) Perillartine is a high-intensity sweetener. Aldoxime analogs have been synthesized and reported to be superior to perillartine.

Pineapple syrup: A clarified, concentrated fruit sugar derived from byproducts of pineapple processing, namely the shells and outer portions of the pineapple. This product may be termed as pineapple syrup on the listing of ingredients on labels, although the description is somewhat misleading.

Policosanol: A mixture of long-chain primary alcohols isolated from sugar cane wax, and used to lower cholesterol and to treat atherosclerotic diseases.

Polyalcohols: *See* polyols.

Polyhedric alcohols: *See* polyols.

Polyols: Sugar alcohols such as sorbitol, mannitol, erythritol, xylitol, and others. They also are known as hexitols and hexahydroxyl alcohols.

Polysaccharides: Multiple sugars consisting of simple sugars that come together as a plant develops and grows. They are found in grains, dried peas, beans, rice, potatoes, unripe bananas and apples, old sweet corn, glycogen, cellulose, and hemicellulose.

Polysugars: *See* polyols.

Potato starch sugar: A sugar that is produced commercially by hydrolysis, using enzymes with the waste from potato processing. Potato starch slurry, called "white water" from potato cuttings is converted to a syrup for use on potatoes before they are fried.

Prebiotic: A nondigestlble food substance that stimulates the growth of beneficial bacteria that are present naturally in the colon.

Probiotic: A culture of beneficial bacteria that reside in a healthy colon and tend to suppress inflammatory responses.

PS 99: An amino-acid based high-intensity sweetener patented in 1988 by General Foods, USA, but to date, is not available.

PS 100: PS 100 is an amino-acid based high-intensity sweetener patented in 1988 by General Foods, USA, but to date, is not available.

Raffinose: An inulin-type oligosaccharide from chicory root that is reported to improve the functional wellbeing of infants.

Rapadura sugar: Dehydrated canesugar juice.

Rare sugars: *See* polyols.

Raw sugar: Newly formed crystals, coated with molasses, resulting from the boiling of sugarcane juice. See muscovados.

Reducing sugars: A general term for certain sugars such as dextrose, levulose, and others, that are oxidized readily by alkaline copper sulfate.

Refined sugar: Sugar with most of the undesirable impurities removed. Along with the removal, nutrients present at low levels, also are eliminated. See sucrose and dextrose.

Refiner's syrup: The residual liquid product obtained in the processing of refined sugar. It is used by food processors, but is described as having "such a salty taste and such a peculiar flavor as to be practically inedible."

Remelts: A term applied to sugars obtained by reboiling sugar liquor.

Ribose: A naturally occurring sugar produced in every cell of the body. Ribose is found, too, in red meat, especially in veal. Ribose is the only sugar used by the body to regulate and control a vital metabolic pathway (pentose phosphate). Ribose provides and sustains energy, especially for cardiovascular health.

Rice syrups: Syrups produced from rice, barley malt, and water. Enzymes in the barley malt convert the rice starch into complex sugars without the use of acid. Such products are sold in specialty outlets.

RTI-001: A synthesized high-intensity sweetener under examination, but not available commercially.

Saccharides: Carbohydrates consisting of molecular compounds of carbon, hydrogen, and oxygen.

Saccharify: To hydrolyze into a simple soluble and fermentable sugar by means of the enzyme, amylase.

Saccharin: A synthesized nonnutritive moderately high-intensity sweetener. Its calcium or sodium salts are used. Banning actions were stayed repeatedly, and ultimately dropped. It is no longer required to have a warning label on saccharin products. Chemically, saccharin is $C_7H_3NO_3S$.

Saccharometer: A hydrometer calibrated in percent solids to determine the solids in a sugar solution.

Saccharose: A term used to describe any compound sugars, such as disaccharides or trisaccharides.

Sanding sugar: A large-crystal sugar that is used mostly by bakers and confectioners to sprinkle on top of products. The large crystals reflect light and give the products a sparkling appearance.

Saponins: Naturally occurring glucosides in plants. Some of them have sweet principles.

Serendipity berry: *See* Nigerian berry.

Simple sugars: Sugars consisting of monosaccharides. These sugars dissolve readily, and are available for ready absorption from the digestive tract into the bloodstream. They supply energy rapidly. Examples are honey, maple syrup, and fruit sugars. Large quantities of simple sugars consumed repeatedly may lead to serious health problems.

Soft sugar: Sugar that has a soft grain and is coated with a film of highly refined cane-flavored syrup. It is a byproduct of the refining process.

Sorbitol: A polyol sugar. Sorbitol was found first as sorbose in the ripe berries of the mountain ash, but it occurs naturally in many other berries, as well as in fruits, seaweeds, algae, and blackstrap molasses. It is produced commercially from glucose or corn sugar. Chemically, sorbitol is $C_6H_{14}O_6$.

Sorbose: A crystalline sugar reduced to sorbitol by fermentation that is used mainly to make ascorbic acid. Chemically, sorbose is $C_6H_{12}O_6$.

Sorghum syrup: A syrup made from sorghum grain. The plant somewhat resembles sugarcane, but contains a high proportion of invert sugars, starch, and dextrin.

Stachyose: A sweet crystalline sugar found especially in the tubers of Chinese artichoke, and by hydrolysis, yields glucose, fructose, and galactose. This sugar is a tetrasaccharide. Stachyose, present in soybeans, produces flatulence in the human intestinal tract because humans lack an enzyme to digest it.

Stevia (*Stevia rebaudiana Bertoni*): A plant containing sweet principles in its leaves. It is a high-intensity sweetener that has been used traditionally in Mesoamerica.

Sucrononate: A synthesized high-intensity sweetener, but not available in commercial production.

Sucrose: A sweet, crystallizable, colorless substance that constitutes the "sugar" of commerce. It is derived from sugarcane or beet. It is a disaccharide composed of two simple sugars: glucose and fructose. Sucrose is the standard for measuring sweetness levels of all sugars and sweeteners. (*See* Appendix C.) Sucrose is known commonly as sugar, table sugar, refined sugar, or white sugar. Chemically, sucrose is $C_{12}H_{22}O_{11}$.

Sucrose palmitate: Sugar converted from starch by cereal malt enzymes. It is used as a sugar replacer in baked goods because it supports the production of carbon dioxide for leavening more efficiently than does sucrose. Baked goods may be labeled "sugar free" when sucrose palmitate is included in the baking formula ingredients to replace sugar.

Sugar alcohol: *See* polyols.

Sugar beet extract flavor base: The concentrated residue of soluble sugar beet extractives from which sugar has been recovered. It is approved for use as a food additive, but the term is not listed on food labels.

Sugar polyols: *See* polyols.

Sugar solids: Term used to represent the total amount of sugar present in a solution. Commercial liquid sugars and blends may be purchased on a dry sugar solid basis.

Sugar syrup: A liquid solution of sucrose or other sugars or sweeteners.

Syndrome X: *See* insulin resistance syndrome.

Synthesized sweeteners: Sweeteners known also as artificial sweeteners or synthetic sweeteners.

Syrup: Concentrated clarified cane juice before it crystallizes. The word syrup is applied, too, to other liquid forms of sugars and sweeteners.

Table molasses: The liquid component that results from sugar refining.

Table sugar: *See* sucrose.

Tabletop sugar: *See* sucrose. Tabletop sugar may refer to packets of sugar available in restaurants.

Tabletop sweetener: A commercial product of a synthesized high-intensity sweetener. Examples are saccharin, aspartame, and sucralose. Tabletop sweeteners may refer to packets of them available in restaurants.

Tagatose: A synthesized sweetener made by a patented process, based on a dairy byproduct, whey. The lactose (milk sugar) in the whey is hydrolyzed to galactose (another milk sugar). Then, under alkaline conditions, the galactose is converted to tagatose, which is treated in order to concentrate and crystallize it. Tagatose is a monosaccharide.

Terpenoids: Intensely sweet substances that have not been approved as sweeteners.

Tetrasaccharides: Carbohydrates that, on complete hydrolysis, yield four monosaccharide molecules. An example is stachyose.

Thaumatin I and II: Proteins isolated from the plant, *Thaumatococcus daniellii*, known as katemfe or "miraculous fruit of the Sudan." The plant is the source of high-intensity protein-based sweeteners. It is in commercial use by food and beverage processors, but is not available in retail markets.

Total invert sugar: A sugar consisting of a mixture of glucose and fructose that is formed by splitting sucrose in a process called inversion. It is accomplished by means of acids or enzymes. The product is used by food processors to keep baked goods and confections fresh and to prevent foods from shrinkage. It is sweeter than sucrose.

Treacle: A sweetener that is produced from granulated sugar liquors, and is in liquid form. Treacle somewhat resembles molasses.

Trehalose: A disaccharide found in honey, shellfish, and mushrooms, among other foods. It is made commercially by treating cornstarch enzymatically.

Trehalulose: An ingredient patented in January 1999 that is used to inhibit the decomposition of aspartame in batter mixes for sugarless baked goods.

Trisaccharides: Trisaccharides are carbohydrates that, on complete hydrolysis, yield three monosaccharide molecules. An example is raffinose.

Turbinado sugar: A partially refined cane sugar that has been washed, dried, but not yet bleached. It is off-white, yellow, or gray in color. It is 90 percent sucrose, and if properly processed, is edible. The word *turbinado* is applied because of the turbine action of the centrifuge machine as the sugar is sprayed with water.

Waffle blend: *See* imitation maple syrup.

Waffle syrup: *See* imitation maple syrup.

Wasanbon: The name of a powdered sugar that is pulverized by hand on the island of Shikoku, in western Japan. Making this artisanal sugar is time- and labor-intensive. It is reported that wasanbon is the world's most expensive sugar.

Washed raw sugar: Sugar after treatment by affination. See affination.

Water-white: Refers to a sugar solution that is clear and colorless.

White sugar: *See* sucrose.

Wood sugar: *See* xylose.

Xylan: A polysaccharide built from right-rotating xylose units and occurring in association with cellulose.

Xylitol: A sugar polyol found as xylose in numerous food plants. Commercially, xylitol is extracted from many byproducts, such as birch bark. Chemically, xylitol is $C_5H_{10}O_5$.

Xylose: A crystalline sugar widely distributed in plant materials, especially in wood, straw, and hulls. It is not found in a free state. It is found as xylan. Chemically, xylose is $C_5H_{10}O_5$, the same structure as xylitol.

Yacón: A root vegetable with a high-sugar content of oligofructose. The vegetable is *Polymnia sonchifolia* and is known as leaf cup.

Appendix C

RELATIVE SWEETNESS OF VARIOUS SUGARS AND SWEETENERS

Sucrose is used as the standard sweetener (rated at 1.0) against which all sugars and sweeteners are measured. Different methods are used to determine the degree of sweetness. Commonly, the substance is diluted in water to a threshold sweetness perception, and then, to duplicate the sweetness, in a 5 or 10 percent sucrose solution. However, different sweetness levels may be reported using different techniques for measurements. The following are the most commonly accepted figures, with secondary figures also listed.

The relative sweetness depends on several factors: the concentration of the sweetener, temperature, pH, medium used, and when humans are used for measurements—the sweetness sensitivity of the tester. Even sucrose is not constant. Due to inversion, over time, the sweetness of sucrose may decline.

Sugars and Sweeteners Less Sweet than Sucrose (<1.0)
listed in ascending order of sweetness

Sugar or Sweetener	Range	Secondary Estimates
hydrogenated starch hydrolysates	0.23–0.50	
lactitol	0.30–0.40	
polysaccharides (as a group)	0.30–0.60	
inulin	0.30–0.65	
dulcitol	0.40	
lactose	0.40	0.15–0.32
hydrolysate of neosugar	0.40–0.60	0.40–0.70
trehalose	0.45	
isomalt	0.45–0.60	0.40–0.65
sorbitol	0.50–0.70	
galactose	0.58–0.60	

glycine	0.70	
glucose (dextrose)	0.70	0.71–0.75
mannitol	0.70	0.70–1.0
maltitol	0.70	
xylitol	0.70	
erythritol	0.71	
invert sugar	0.70–0.90	
glycerol	0.80	
tagatose	0.92	
sucrose	**1.00**	

Sugars and Sweeteners Sweeter than Sucrose (>1.0)
listed in ascending order of sweetness

Sugar or Sweetener	Range	Secondary Estimates
HFCS (42 percent)	1.00	
fructose (levulose)	1.10–1.20	1.30–1.80
HFCS (55 percent)	1.10–1.50	1.10–1.15
honey	1.30	
HFCS (90 percent)	1.60	
stevia (leaf)	10.0–30.0	
cyclamate	30.0–80.0	
abrusides	30.0–100.0	
rebaudisides	30.0–450.0	
agave nectar	42.0	
glycyrrhizin (licorice)	50.0	
terpenoids	50.0–2,000	
RTI-001	58.0	
dulcin	70.0–350	
hesperidin	100	
naringen dihydrochalcones	100	100–300
acesulfame K	130	
abruside A	150	
prurin (a DHC)	160	
aspartame	150–200	100–200

osladin	300	
stevia (extract)	300	150–4,000
lo han	200-250	300
saccharin	300–500	200–700
suosan	400	
SRI-oxime V	450	
sucralose	600	320–1,000
neohesperidin	1,000–1,800	2,000
D-tryptophan derivative	1,300	
alitame	2,000	
aspartame analog	2,000	
perillaldehyde antialdoxime	2,000	
PS 99, PS 100	2,000–2,500	
thaumatin	2,000–3,000	3,000–5,000
miraculin	2,500	
monellin	3,000	
F-4000	4,000	
neotame	7,000–13,000	
SC-45647	10,000	
suosan analog	20,000	
aspartame analog	20,000	
guanidine	170,000	

Sources: These figures are compiled from several sources, including technical information from processors and from food trade journals. Additional sources include: Crosby, G. A. and R. E. Wingard, Jr. "A Survey of Less Common Sweeteners," in *Developments in Sweeteners,* E. A. M. Hough, K. J. Parker, and A. J. Vlitos, eds. London: Applied Science, 1979; Inglett, George E., "Sweeteners: An Overall Perspective," in *Aspartame, Physiology and Biochemistry,* Lewis D. Stegink and L. J. Filer, Jr., eds. New York: Marcel Dekker, 1984; and *Food Technology,* Nov 2003.

Appendix D

SOME NATURALLY OCCURRING SUGARS IN FOODS—TOLERATED BY MOST, BUT NOT BY ALL

Sugars, naturally present in foods—for example, in fruits, berries, and vegetables such as carrots, parsnips, and beets—are usually well tolerated. But certain sugars are problematic for some individuals. Intolerances to corn sugar and to polyols have already been discussed. Lactose (milk sugar), galactose (a byproduct of lactose digestion), and fructose (fruit sugar) also are problematic for some individuals who have intolerances to them.

Lactose Intolerance

Lactose intolerance is widespread, and occurs in many of the world's populations. Indeed, it is so prevalent, and at such a high level globally, that lactose *intolerance* in healthy adults has come to be regarded as *normal*, and lactose *tolerance* as *abnormal*. A large majority of entire populations are lactose intolerant. To some degree, many people cannot digest lactose.

The enzyme, lactase, is required to break down lactose. In most individuals, this enzyme declines in early childhood after weaning, unless milk consumption continues. In individuals who are genetically predisposed, the decline of the enzyme is slower, allowing for normal lactose digestion.

For the lactose intolerant, consumption of dairy products may be followed by discomfort, including abdominal pain, bloating, flatulence, and diarrhea. Formerly, sufferers were advised to shun all dairy foods. Later studies suggested that total avoidance might not be necessary. There are degrees of lactose intolerance. For those who are completely lactose intolerant—lacking in lactase entirely—total avoidance may be necessary. However, others can tolerate lactose to some extent.

Although fermented dairy products such as cheese, buttermilk, and yogurt have been recommended for lactose-intolerant individuals, not all of these products are equally well tolerated. Some fermented milk products, such as aged cheddar or Swiss cheese, are significantly reduced in lactose because the whey, not the remaining curd, contains most of the lactose. The lactose level of other fermented dairy products, such as yogurt, cultured buttermilk, and sweet acidophilus milk might be just as high as that of whole milk. The level of their lactose contents varies according to the processing techniques. For example, if nonfat milk is added to low-fat dairy products, it raises the lactose content of the product. Nonfat milk contains lactose.

Commercial food-grade lactases (beta-galactosidase enzyme preparations from microbial organisms) are used to produce lactose-hydrolyzed milk and other reduced-lactose products, which can be used instead of plain fluid milk.

Another approach is to make plain fluid milk better tolerated by using lactose-reducing products such as Lactaid, which can be added to milk at home. Such products add somewhat to the cost of milk. Also, they are inconvenient to use. They require a twenty-four-hour incubation period to be fully effective.

Lactose digestion may be helped by the addition of beta-galactosidase to milk at mealtimes. The addition is easy, improves lactose absorption, and decreases undesirable colonic hydrogen production. When added at mealtime, milk lactose can be hydrolyzed, even if solid foods are eaten at the same time.

Lactose is added, systematically, by some poultry producers to the drinking water and feed of the birds as a preventative for Salmonella. There are no special label requirements to mention the practice. Nor, has there been any investigation to learn whether, indirectly, this practice affects lactose-intolerant individuals who eat such treated birds.

Not only is lactose being incorporated into foods, directly and indirectly in novel ways, but it may be present as an unsuspected hidden ingredient. A physician reported in the *New England Journal of Medicine* (vol 14, 1991) that six children, all known to be allergic to milk, suffered adverse reactions minutes after eating certain frozen dessert products labeled "nondairy." Testing of the foods with enzyme-linked immunosorbent assays (ELISAs) showed traces of milk protein in all the food samples labeled as nondairy.

Lactose is one of the most commonly used fillers in medications, in both prescription and over-the-counter drugs. A case was reported of an asthmatic woman who was lactose-intolerant. Within two hours after inhaling a cromyln sodium product, she developed nausea, bloating, abdominal cramps, and flatulence. After a second dose, she experienced similar symptoms. Belatedly, she read the packet insert and discovered that the medication contained 20 milligrams of lactose per capsule. This case was reported by R.D. Brandstetter in *The New England Journal of Medicine* (vol. 25, 1986).

Another lactose-intolerant patient was advised to take six capsules daily of a private brand of bromelain for severe multiple allergies and other health problems. As reported in *Capsulations* (vol. 10, 1987), the patient's symptoms only worsened. When the bromelain capsules were analyzed, they were found to consist of two-thirds sugars, of which half was lactose.

Even for individuals who are not lactose intolerant, high lactose intake, resulting from the increased uses of lactose from various sources, may be undesirable. Researchers at USDA Tufts Human Nutrition Resources Center in Boston, Massachusetts, found a relationship between high lactose intake and low levels of galactokinase (an enzyme involved in lactose metabolism) and the development of senile cataracts. A high lactose intake was associated with a two-fold increase in the risk of cataract development.

Galactose Intolerance

In recent years, lactose intolerance has become better recognized. Galactose, a byproduct of lactose digestion, also creates health problems for some individuals, but presently is poorly recognized.

Galactosemia may be far less common than lactose malabsorption, but when experienced, is far more severe. The genetic disorder of galactose metabolism occurs in two forms: classic galactosemia and galactokinase-deficiency galactosemia. Both are inherited as autosomal recessive defects.

Galactose is a major component of the main carbohydrate in milk, both from humans and cows. Normally, galactose, which is formed mainly by the digestion of lactose, is metabolized by the human, and converted to glucose. However, the galactosemic individual deficient in the enzyme galactose-1-phosphate uridyl transferase (GALT) is unable to metabolize galactose, causing galactose metabolites (galactitol and galactose-l-phosphate) to accumulate in bodily tissues. Cataracts may be the only visible sign of galactokinase deficiency, which results from the accumulation of galactitol in the lens of the eye.

Estimates vary, but galactosemia may affect one in every 20,000 live births in humans. For each pregnancy in such a family, there is a one-in-four chance that the infant will be born with this genetic disorder. Mothers of affected infants are advised to adhere to a galactose-free diet during any subsequent pregnancy as a possible means of preventing brain damage in the developing fetus, and of lessening the symptoms generally present at the infant's birth.

If the newly born galactosemic baby is not treated promptly after birth with a dairy-free diet, it will fail to thrive. Acute symptoms of galactosemia (vomiting, weight loss, irritability, or lethargy) may occur a few days after birth in an otherwise apparently healthy infant who is fed either breast milk or milk-based formula.

If the galactosemic infant is allowed to continue on a milk diet, clinical effects include liver enlargement and damage, jaundice and cirrhosis; ascites (accumulated serum fluid) in the abdominal cavity; spleen enlargement; galactosuria; proteinuria; and aminoaciduria (the presence of galactose, protein, or, amino acids in the urine). Pseudotumor cerebris may occur. (This is cerebral edema and raised intracranial pressure, but without most neurological signs.) Cataracts may be present at birth, or may develop later. Severe bacterial infection may develop, accompanied by diarrhea.

Early diagnosis and therapy may heal any liver damage incurred in the first few days of life. Usually the symptoms subside after dairy foods are replaced totally by a nondairy formula based on casein hydrolysate or soy. Nutramigen or Pregestimil (both manufactured by Mead Johnson) contain no lactose or galactose.

Because the galactosemic infant responds favorably to the same diet as the lactose malabsorber, galactosemia may be unsuspected at an early stage of growth, and wrongly attributed to lactose intolerance. These two genetic diseases differ, which may become apparent only in the next stage of growth, when additional foods are introduced into the diet. The lactose malabsorber may continue to thrive when fruits, vegetables, and cereals are added, but the galactosemic child may begin to show poor growth; mental efforts such as a shortened attention span, difficulties with spatial and mathematical relationships, retardation of IQ, speech problems; and behavioral traits such as withdrawal or apathy.

A study conducted jointly by the USDA's Agricultural Research Service (ARS) and Ross Laboratories found that many common fruits and vegetables, and possibly some grains, contain galactose. As follow-up, baby food products of three leading processors were analyzed. Various amounts of galactose were identified in twelve fruits and vegetable products intended for infant feeding. High levels were found in applesauce, banana, and squash—three foods commonly introduced into the growing infant's diet when solids are added. (These foods, acceptable for normal babies, would be undesirable for galactosemics.)

The researchers examined forty-five commonly consumed fresh fruits and vegetables. They identified high galactose levels in tomato, watermelon, papaya, and persimmon. Moderately high levels were found in banana, apple, date, kiwi, pumpkin, bell pepper, and Brussels sprouts.

Unfortunately, the foods identified as galactose-free are ones not likely to be used in baby food products: artichoke, mushroom, olive, and peanut. There is not enough information at this time as to whether or not galactose is present in cereals commonly fed to infants.

Many fat-reduced dairy products now flood the marketplace. In order to formulate such products so that they approximate the texture of their traditional counterparts, a large amount of nonfat milk may be added. This procedure increases the galactose as well as lactose levels in such products.

In the 1950s, Kurt P. Richter, professor of psychobiology at Johns Hopkins Hospital, conducted studies in which rats were fed unflavored nonfat yogurt fortified with skim milk. The rats developed cataracts, Richter noted that such yogurts contain more galactose than found in whole milk. On a caloric basis, the nonfat yogurt contained 22 percent to 24 percent galactose, compared with only 14.4 percent in whole milk, and 14.2 percent in whole-milk yogurt. Although Richter had conducted these studies in the 1950s, they remained unpublished until Richter wrote an article "Cataracts Produced in Rats by Yogurt" published in *Science* (vol. 198, 1980).

Subsequent to the publication of these studies, H. Shalea et al. reported in the *Archives of Opthalmology* (vol. 2, 1980) that reduced galactokinase levels related to a greatly increased incidence of bilateral prehensile ideopathic cataracts, as well as senile cataracts, in 147 adult humans. The researchers concluded that dietary restriction in such patients might retard or prevent cataract formation. By the mid-1980s, other published reports confirmed their findings.

In 1990, another study offered strong supporting evidence that galactose may play an important role in the formation of cataracts in adults. Paul F. Jacques, an epidemiologist, compared the level of galactokinase with dairy food consumption in 100 adults, forty to seventy years of age. Seventy-three had cataracts. All but two of the individuals (both with cataracts) showed normal galactokinase levels.

Jacques defined one half of the study group with the lowest enzyme levels as "low." Those in that subgroup who abstained from consuming lactose- containing foods had the same cataract incidence as those in the "high" enzyme subgroup. However, the "low" subjects who regularly consumed even a small amount of dairy foods—for example, a cup of milk daily—had four times the risk of cataract development as those in the "high" enzyme group. The study suggested that, unwittingly, individuals with slower conversion of galactose to glucose could expose their eye lenses to a lifetime of low but chronic levels of the cataract-causing sugar.

Physicians do not screen routinely for galactokinase levels. Even if they were to do so, they might interpret the levels found in the "low" group as normal by current standards.

Fructose Intolerance

Hereditary fructose intolerance is an autosomal recessive genetically-caused inability to digest fructose due to a deficiency of the enzyme (1-phosphofructoaldolase) in the liver, kidney cortex, and small intestine. Fructosemia is also known as fructose-l-phosphate aldolase deficiency, or fructosuria.

Hereditary fructose intolerance begins in humans at birth in both genders. There is a 25 percent risk of transmitting fructosemia to offspring if both parents are carriers for a recessive disorder. Fifty percent of their offspring will be carriers. Of their offspring, one out of four children will receive normal genes from both parents, and will be genetically normal.

Early recognition of fructosemia is important in order to avoid damage to the liver, kidney, and small intestine. Soon after foods containing fructose such as fruits and sweets are added to the fructosemic's diet, there may be prolonged vomiting, failure to thrive, occasional unconsciousness, jaundice, and liver enlargement. There may be a tendency to bleed due to a deficiency of clotting factors. Glucose and phosphate blood levels will decrease. Fructose levels in the blood and urine will increase. Fortunately, there is no intellectual impairment.

Fructosemics need to be placed on a special fructose-free diet to prevent permanent physical damage. Usually, fructosemics develop a strong dislike for fruits and sweets.

Most people can convert fructose to glucose and burn it for energy. However, fructose-intolerant individuals cannot make this conversion. They are unable to absorb fructose into the bloodstream. Instead, the fructose remains in the bowel where bacterial fermentation produces carbon dioxide, hydrogen, methane, water, alcohol, and lactic acid. Both the alcohol and lactic acid can irritate the bowel lining. The gas, bloating, and abdominal distension, if chronic, can lead to hiatal hernia, or even a blowout of the thin weak-walled portion of the colon.

Fructose intolerance may have been a previously unrecognized factor associated with gluten intolerance (celiac disease) from gluten-containing grains, and in irritable bowel syndrome (IBS). Manifestations of fructose intolerance are surprisingly similar to those of lactose intolerance. A diet that has benefited some sufferers of ulcerative colitis and irritable bowel syndrome include an avoidance of fructose as well as three other poorly absorbed sugars: lactose, sorbitol, and mannitol. (For a discussion of sorbitol and mannitol, see Chapter 5 on sugar polyols.)

Not everyone with irritable bowel syndrome is fructose intolerant. Some may tolerate fructose; others may be intolerant only if the bowel already is inflamed or irritated from infections, drugs, lactose, sorbitol, or mannitol. Some may tolerate small amounts of fructose, but suffer serious effects if large amounts are consumed.

Even those individuals who are not fructose intolerant may develop health problems if this sugar is consumed at high levels. Fructose is found in fruits and honey. In recent years, with the increased use of corn-derived sweeteners and syrups in the form of high-fructose corn syrups (HFCS), fructose consumption has surpassed sucrose consumption, and offers additional challenges to fructose-intolerant individuals. (See Chapter 4 on HFCS.)

Although naturally occurring sugars such as lactose, galactose, and fructose in foods are well tolerated by most individuals, there are exceptions. The dietary needs must be addressed for individuals who have genetic deficiencies or lack of enzymes needed to digest these sugars. The use of such sugars by food and beverage processors compounds the problem for such individuals who need to monitor carefully the composition of their foods. Accurate and detailed label information is essential.

MAIN SOURCES

Introduction

Agri Res, June 1973

Am Heart J, May 1975

Am J Clin Nutr, Apr 1974

Burros, Marian, "Added Sugars, Less Urgency? Fine Print and the Dietary Guidelines." *NY Times,* Aug 25, 2004

Cohen, Aharon M., Testimony. Select Committee on Nutrition & Human Needs, U.S. Senate Hearings, Apr 30, 1973

Drug Ther, Oct 1976

Evaluation of the Health Aspects of Corn Sugar (Dextrose), Corn Syrup, and Invert Sugar as Food Ingredients. FASEB Rept to FDA, U.S. Dept Comm, NTIS, 1976

Evaluation of the Health Aspects of Sucrose as a Food Ingredient. FASEB Rept to FDA, U.S. Dept Comm, NTIS, 1976

Fd Drug Pkging, Feb 22, 1979

Fd Proc, Sept 1977; July 1978

"Food Consumption Prices & Expenditures." *Agr Eco Rept* 138, USDA, Sept 1979

Friend, Berta, "Changes in Nutrients in the United States Diet Caused by Alterations in Food Intake Patterns." *Agri Res,* USDA, 1974

Glinsmann, Walter H. et al., *Evaluation of Health Aspects of Sugars Contained in Carbohydrate Sweeteners.* Report of Sugars Task Force, Div of Nutr & Toxicol, CFSAN, FDA, 1986

Hess, John L. & Karen Hess, *The Taste of America.* NY, NY: Grossman, 1977

La Londe, Marc, *A New Perspective on the Health of Canadians.* Min Natl Health Welfare Canada, 1974

Med World News, Feb 12, 1971

Mottern, Nick, *Guidelines for Food Purchasing in the U.S.* Testimony. Select Committee on Nutrition & Human Needs, U.S. Senate Hearings, 1978

Nutr Abstracts Rev, Sept 1970; May 1977

Nutr Rev, Sept 1968

Nutr Today, Spring 1969

Page, Louise & Berta Friend, "Levels of Use of Sugars in the United States" in *Sugars in Nutrition.* Horace L. Sipple & Karen W. McNutt, eds. Wash, DC: Acad Press, 1974

Randolph, Theron G., "The Role of Specific Sugars" in *Clinical Ecology.* Lawrence D. Dickey, M.D., ed. Springfield, IL: Charles C. Thomas Pub, 1976

Reiser, Sheldon & Bela Szepesi, "SCOGS Report on the Health Aspects of Sucrose Consumption." Letter. *Am J Clin Nutr,* Vol 31, No 1, Jan 1978

Rest Bus, Aug 1, 1980

"Role of Sugar & Other Foods in Dental Caries. What Can Industry Do?" *Proceedings,* Conference of Research Institute, Am Dent Assoc Health Found, Oct 5–6, 1978

Sci, Nov 14, 1975; Feb 27, 1976

"The Sweet and Lowdown on Sugar." *NY Times*, Jan 23, 2004

World Rev Nutr Diet, Vol 22, 1975

Chapter 1: Refined Sweeteners

Am J Clin Nutr, Jan 1978

Am J Dis Childhood, Vol 49, 1935

Am J Hyg, Vol 34, 1941

Anderson, Jr., Oscar E., *The Health of a Nation.* Chicago, IL: Univ of Chicago Press, 1958

Ann Allergy, Vol 7, 1949; Vol 9, 1951

Arch Surg, Vol 61, 1950

Birch, G.G., L.F. Green, & C.G. Coulston, eds., *Glucose Syrups & Related Carbohydrates.* NY, NY: Elsevier, 1970

Cameron, Allan G., *Food Facts & Fallacies.* London: Faber & Faber, 1971

C&EN, Apr 11, 1977

Clydesdale, Fergus M., ed. "Nutritional & Health Aspects of Sugars." *Am J Clin Nutr*, Vol 62, No 1, suppl, July 1995

Duke, W. W., *Asthma, Hay Fever, Urticaria, and Allied Manifestations of Allergy.* St. Louis, MI: C.V. Mosby, 1926

Farb, Peter & George Armelagos, *Consuming Passions: The Anthropology of Eating.* Boston, MA: Houghton Mifflin, 1980

Health & Human Services News, Dec 30, 1980

J Exp Med, Vol 70, 1939

J Kansas Mad Soc, Vol 27, 1936

J Lab Clin Med, Vol 36, 1950

Rinkel, H. J. *Instructional Course.* Am Coll Allergists, 1944

Rorty, James & N. Philip Norman, *Food for Tomorrow.* NY, NY: Devin-Adair, 1956

Sugar & Sweetener Report, USDA. Dec 1967; Dec 1980

Tannahill, Reay, *Food in History.* NY, NY: Stein & Day, 1973

Wiley, Harvey Washington, *An Autobiography.* NY, NY: Bobbs Merrill, 1930

_____. *The History of a Crime Against a Food Law.* Self-published, 1929. Reprinted by Lee Foundation for Nutritional Research, Milwaukee, WI: 1935

World Rev Nutr Diet, Vol 22, 1975

Wurzberg, O. B., "Starch in the Food Industry" in *Handbook of Food Additives.* Thomas E. Furia, ed. Cleveland, OH: Chemical Rubber Co., 1968

Neosugar

Am J Clin Nutr, Vol 62 suppl, 1995

CRM, Nov 1985

Nutr Res Newsletter, Oct 1984; July 1986; July 1987

Oku, T. et al., *J Nutr,* Sept 1984

Tokunaga, T. et al., *J Nutr Sci Vit*, Vol 32, No 1, 1986

Chapter 2: Traditional Sweeteners

Brown Sugar

Baking Ind, Nov 1975; May 1976; July 1976; Aug 1977

Baking Prod & Manage, Nov 1977

Cancer Res, May 1965

CRM, Sept 2000; May 2001

Fd Proc, May 1975; Nov 1975; Dec 1978

Fd Prod Develop, Oct 1978

Health, Education & Welfare News. Release, U.S. Dept HHS, Sept 21, 1978

Snack Fd, Apr 1976

Grain-Based Syrups

Fact Sheets and Technical Sheets. Grain Millers, Inc., undated

Fd Engineer, Mar 1992; Mar 1994; May 1994; Sept 1994

Fd Proc, May 2004

Fd Prod Design, Oct 1992; June 1993; Dec 1996; Sept 2003

Fd Tech, June 1992; Feb 2001

Health Fd Bus, Nov 1987

Holder, William, "Sorghum Syrup, New Crop for Sugarmakers, Dairymen." *New England Farmer*, Feb 1992

Prep Fds, Mar 1994; May 1994; Aug 2000; Mar 2001; Aug 2003; Nov 2003

Wash Post, Apr 24, 1991

Whole Fds, Jan 1984

Honey

Accum, Frederick, *Death in the Pot*. London: Milner & Co., 1830

Am Agric, Apr 1965; Dec 1965

Am Bee J, July 1977

Ann Chem, Feb 1979

Anstice, Carroll & Embre de Persilis Vona, *The Health Food Dictionary*. Englewood Cliffs, NJ: Prentice-Hall, 1973

Arch Biochem Biophysics, Vol 79, 1959

Bakers' Digest, Aug 1974

Baking Ind., Oct 1976; May 1977

Beekeeping, Bull No 5. Florida Dept of Agric, Jan 1958

Biberoglu, M.D., "Mad Honey." Letter. *JAMA*, Apr 1, 1988

Bicknell, Franklin, *Chemicals in Food & in Farm Produce: Their Harmful Effects*. London: Faber & Faber, 1960

Bull of the Faculty of Med, Istanbul, Turkey, Vol 12, 1949

Calif Morb, July 7, 1978

C&EN, Jan 30, 1978; June 10, 1991; June 17, 1991

Clydesdale, Fergus & Frederick J. Francis, *Food, Nutrition, and You*. Englewood Cliffs, NJ: Prentice-Hall, 1977

CRM, May 2001

Fd Chem News, Dee 9, 1991; Apr 29, 2002; June 17, 2003

FDA Consumer, Feb 1979; Nov 1979; Feb 1980; Apr 1997; Nov–Dec 2002; May–June 2003

FDA Enforcement Rept, Dec 8, 1976; Mar 2, 1977; May 21, 1980; Oct 22, 1980

Fd Engineer, Feb 1974; Mar 1976; Jan 1980

Fd Proc, May 1974; Sept 1974; July 1975; Aug 1975; May 1976

Fd Prod Design, July 2003

Fd Prod Develop, May 1980

Fd Safety Newsletter, May 1993; Apr 1994; Nov-Dec 1997

Fd Tech, Aug 1974

Ferry, Elizabeth, "The Buzz about 'Laundered' Honey." *Coop News*, Hanover Consumer Cooperative Society (Hanover, N.H.) Nov–Dec 2003

Health Fd Retail, Feb 1980; Apr 1980

Infectious Dis, Sept 1979

J Assoc Official Anal Chem, Vol 62, 1979

Lampe, Kenneth F., "Rhododendrons, Mountain Laurel, and Mad Honey." Editorial. *JAMA*, Apr 1, 1988

Med Trib, Sept 20, 1978

Mirkin, Gabe, "Side Effects of Raw Honey." Letter. *JAMA*, Nov 20, 1991

MMWR, CDC, USPHS, Jan 20, 1978; Oct 20, 1978

NY Times, June 25, 1978

Prep Fds, Nov 2001

Proc Prep Fds, Sept 1979; Jan 1980

Publications & Patents, Eastern Regional Research Center, ARS, USDA, July-Aug 1979

Raloff, Janet, "The Color of Honey."*Sci News*, Sept 12, 1998

————. "Honey May Pose Hidden Toxic Risk." *Sci New*, May 18, 2002

Sci, Feb 4, 1977; Sept 1, 1978

Sci News, July 15, 1978

Snack Fd, Oct 1979

Toxicants Occurring Naturally in Foods. Pub 1354, NAS-NRC. Wash, DC: Acad Press, 1966

USDA press release, Oct 15, 1970

White, Jonathan W., "Natural Honey Toxicants." *Bee World*, Vol 62, No 1, 1981

Whole Fds, Dec 1979

Malt

Fd Engineer, Apr 1980; Sept 1980

Fd Proc, Sept 1978

Fd Prod Develop, Oct 1976; May 1978; Jan 1980

Snack Fd, July 1978; Oct 1979

Maple Syrup

Am Agric, Oct 1965; Feb 1966; Mar 1970

Am Dairy Rev, July 1976

Baking Ind, May 1977

Brattleboro [VT] *Daily Reformer*, Dec 6, 1975

C&EN, May 22, 1972

Consumer Bull, Sept 1962

Consumer Repts, Oct 1967; Oct 1968; May 1979

Dairy & Ice Cream Field, Sept 1979

FDA Consumer, Feb 1979; June 1980; Sept 1980

FDA Enforcement Rept, Feb 27, 1980; May 21, 1980; July 16, 1980

Fd Proc, Feb 1976; Sept 1977; Feb 1978; Jan 1979

Fd Prod Develop, July 1979

Media & Consumer, June 1975

Nearing, Helen & Scott, *The Maple Sugar Book*. NY, NY: John Day, 1950

NY Times, June 30, 1975

Plant Fd Ideas, June 1977; Dec 1977

That We May Eat. USDA Yearbook, 1975

Vermont Freeman, Aug 1973

Willitz, C.O., *Maple Syrup Producers Manual*. Agricultural Handbook 134, USDA, rev 1985

Molasses

All About Molasses. American Molasses Co., 1952

Corwin, Alsoph, *The Most Common Source of Chemical Contaminants*, paper, undated

Fd Proc, Jan 1979; May 1980

Morse, Roy E., *Food Facts from Rutgers*, July–Sept 1973

Nutritive Value of American Foods in Common Units. Agric Handbk No 450, ARS, USDA, Nov 1965

Pfeiffer, Carl C., *Mental and Elemental Nutrients*. New Canaan, CT: Keats Pub, 1975

Proc Prep Fds, Oct 1979

Schroeder, Henry A., *The Trace Elements and Man*. NY, NY: Devin-Adair, 1973

Snack Fd, Oct 1979

Raw Sugar

Consumer Repts, Sept 1977

CRM, Sept 2000; May 2001

JAMA, July 10, 1972

Mayer, Jean, Column. *Concord* [N.H.] *Monitor*, June 19, 1980; Feb 11, 1977

Morse, Roy E., *Food Facts from Rutgers*, July–Sept 1973

Rohe, Fred, *The Sugar Story*. Flier. Organic Merchants, Inc., undated

Yudkin, John, *Sweet and Dangerous*. NY, NY: Wyden, 1972

Sorghum

Agric Res, Mar 1972; Feb 2005

Christian Sci Monitor, Nov 19, 1973

FDA Consumer, Apr 1997

Lost Crops of Africa, Vol 1. "Grains." Wash, DC: Natl Acad Press, 1996

Neucere, Joseph N. et al., "Hemolytic Activity in Crude Polysaccharide Extracted from Grain Sorghum." *Toxicol*, Vol 24, No 3, 1986

Sugarcane Juice and Evaporated Sugarcane Juice

Fd Chem News, Mar 18, 1991

Fd Prod Design, May 2000

Health Fd Bus, Mar 1988; Jan 1989; June 1989; May 1991; Aug 1991; Feb 1992

Natural Fds Merchand, Apr 1988; Sept 1990; Sept 1991

Reichlen, Steven, "The Cane Before the Sugar." Wash Post, Mar 18, 1992

Chapter 3: Crystalline Fructose

Alive, Autumn 1979

Am J Clin Nutr, May 1979; Oct 1980

Ann Intern Med, Vol 79, 1972

Arch Intern Med, Vol 137, 1977

Biermann, June & Barbara Toohey, The Diabetic's Total Health Book. San Francisco, CA: Tarcher, 1980

Born, P. et al., "High Rate of Gastrointestinal Side Effects in Fructose-Consuming Patients." Diabetes Care, May–June 1987

Brennand, Charlotte P. & Sherrie L. Hardy, "Sucrose vs. Fructose." Utah Sci, Fall 1980

Burros, Marian, "The Conference in Chicago—A Case of Flack or Fact?" Wash Post, Oct 11, 1979

Bus Wk, May 12, 1980

Cannon, Minuha, Sweets Without Guilt: The Fructose Dessert Cookbook. Orem, UT: East Woods Press, 1981

Challem, Jack & Renate Lewin, "The Good and Bad of Fructose." Let's Live, Feb 1989

Contemp Nutr, July 1980; Aug 1980

Cooper, J. T. with Paul Hagan, Dr. Cooper's Fabulous Fructose Diet. NY, NY: Evans, 1979

"Crystalline Fructose Plays Role in Helping Increase Endurance." Prep Fds, Aug 1984

Diabetes Care, Dec 1972

Dietary Sugars in Health and Disease: Fructose. FASEB Report to FDA, Oct 1976

Doty, T.E. & E. Vanninen, "Crystalline Fructose: Use as a Food Ingredient Expected to Increase." Fd Tech, Vol 29, 1975

_____. Fructose: A Review of Nutritional, Medical and Metabolic Aspects. Helsinki, Finland: Finnish Sugar Co., Ltd., undated

Fd Chem News, May 24, 1993

Fd Engineer, Mar 1979; May 1980, Oct 1980

Fd Tech, Nov 1975

Forbes, Allan L, & Barbara A. Bowman, eds. "Health Effects of Dietary Fructose." Am J Clin Nutr, suppl, Nov 1993

Fructose Facts. ADA, 1980

"Fructose Fad Follies." Whole Fds, May 1979

Fruit Sugar: A Review of Nutritional, Medical and Metabolic Aspects. Helsinki, Finland: Finnish Sugar Co., Ltd., 1977

FTC News Summary, "Advertising Claims for Products with Fructose Are Subject to FTC Probe." Wash, DC, FTC, July 11, 1980

"The Great Fructose Debate" Health Fd Retail, July 1979

Hannigan, Kevin J., "Crystalline Fructose: Who's Using It and Why." Fd Engineer, Nov 1980

Health Fd Bus, Aug 1979

Health Fd Retail, Aug 1973; July 1979

Hollingsworth, Pierce & Chuck Wilson, "Fructose Sweetens Batter-Lite's Fortunes." Proc Prep Fds, Feb 1980

J of Nutr, May 1977; Sept 1988

Koivisto, Veikko A., "Fructose as a Dietary Sweetener in Diabetes Mellitus." Diabetes Care, July–Aug 1978

Landes, R.G. et al., "Fructose in Assessment of Protein-sparing Regimens." Letter. N Engl J Med, May 5, 1977

Lecos, Chris, "Fructose: Questionable Diet Aid." FDA Consumer, May 1980

Morris, Charles E., "First Crystalline-fructose Plant in U.S." Fd Engineer, Nov 1981

The Need for Special Foods and Sugar Substitutes by Individuals with Diabetes Mellitus, FASEB Report to FDA, May 1978

"New Fructose-sweetened Foods Have Special 'Diet Appeal.'" Fd Proc, Oct 1980

NY Times, May 7, 1980; Jan 4, 1981; Jan 20, 1981

Olefsky, Jerrold & Phyllis Crapo, "Fructose, Xylitol, and Sorbitol." Diabetes Care, Mar–Apr 1980

Palm, J. Daniel, *Fructose, the Empty Calorie Wonder Food*. Decatur, IL: Archer Daniels Midland Co, 1980

Proc Prep Fds, Feb 1979

"Pure Crystalline Fructose Opens Up New Formulation Possibilities." *Proc Prep Fds*, Aug 1980

Raloff, Janet, "Fructose Risk for High-fat Diners?" *Sci News*, Mar 26, 1988

Ratteree, Dee, "The Fabulous 14-Day Fructose Diet." *Family Circle*, Feb 20, 1979

Reese, K.M., "Effects of Fructose on Metabolism of Ethanol." Newscripts. *C&EN*, Dec 5, 1977

Skyler, Jay S. & Nadine E. Miller, "The Use of Sweeteners by Diabetic Patients." *Practical Cardiol*, Sept 1980

Snack Fd, Feb 1980; Sept 1980

Swanson, Joyce E. et al., "Metabolic Effects of Dietary Fructose in Healthy Subjects." *Am J Clin Nutr*, Vol 55, 1992

Chapter 4: High-Fructose Corn Syrup

Agric Outlook, Nov 1994

Agric Res, Oct 1992

Am Agricult, Feb 1976; Dec 1978

Am Dairy Rev, June 1976; June 1979

Apovian, Caroline M., "Sugar-Sweetened Soft Drinks, Obesity, and Type 2 Diabetes." *JAMA*, Vol 292, No 8, Aug 25, 2004

Baking Ind, Sept 1976; Feb 1977

Bantle, John P. et al., "Effects of Dietary Fructose on Plasma Lipids in Healthy Subjects." *Am J Clin Nutr*, Vol 72, 2000

Best, Daniel, "Is It Time to Address the Copper-Fructose Link?" *Prep Fds*, Sept 1987

Bremer, J. et al., "The Glycerophosphate Acyltransferesis and Their Function in the Metabolism of Fatty Acids." *Molecular Cell Biochem*, Vol 12, 1976

Bus Wk, Aug 14, 1978

C&EN, May 1, 1973

Critser, Greg, *Fat Land: How Americans Became the Fattest People in the World*. Boston, MA: Houghton Mifflin, 2003

Dairy Field, Oct 1979; May 1980; June 1980

Dairy Record, Apr 1979; May 1979; Dec 1979; Feb 1980; Mar 1980

FDA Consumer, Mar 1980; Nov 1986

Federal Trade Commission News Summary, July 11, 1980

Fd Chem News, Aug 26, 1996

Fd Engineer, Apr 1978; June 1978; Aug 1979; Apr 1980; May 1980; Mar 1983; Jan 1984; Aug 1993

Fd Proc, July 1975; June 1976; Aug 1976; Oct 1976; Nov 1980; Aug 2004

Fd Prod Design, Apr 2004

Fd Prod Develop, Sept 1979; Dec 1979; Feb 1980; Nov 1980

Fd Tech, Jan 1996; Oct 1996

Fd & Wine, Feb 1992

Fields, Meira, *Scientific Research News*, ARS, USDA, Carbohydrate Nutrition Laboratory, Beltsville, MD, July 1971

_____. "Effects of Fructose or Starch on Copper-67 Absorption and Excretion by the Rat." *J Nutr*, Vol 116, 1986

Forbes, June 26, 1978

Forristal, Linda Joyce, "The Murky World of High-Fructose Corn Syrup." *Wise Traditions*, Fall 2001

Holbrook, J., "Tissue Distribution and Excretion of Copper-67 Intraperitoneally Administered to Rats Fed Fructose or Starch." *J Nutr*, Vol 116, 1986

Hollenbeck, C. B. , "Dietary Fructose Effects on Lipoprotein Metabolism and Risk for Coronary Artery Disease." *Am J Clin Nutr*, Vol 58, suppl, 1993

Holsendorph, Ernest, "Sugar's New Rival: High-fructose Corn Syrup." *NY Times*, Oct 6, 1994

Jeffrey, Kermit & Thomas A. Mainwaring,

Sweeteners, Report No 557. Menlo Park, CA: Stanford Res Instit, Oct 1975

Klevay, L. M., "Coronary Heart Disease: The Zinc/Copper Hypothesis." *Am J Clin Nutr,* Vol 28, 1975

Ludwig, David et al., "Relation Between Consumption of Sugar-sweetened Drinks and Childhood Obesity: A Prospective, Observational Analysis." *Lancet,* Vol 357, Feb 17, 2001

Natl Fd Rev, Fall 1983

Nutr Action, Feb 1980

NY Times, July 26, 1974; Nov 17, 1976; Jan 29, 1980; Aug 21, 2004

Parks, Y. K. & E. A. Yetley, "Intake and Food Sources of Fructose in the U.S." *Am J Clin Nutr,* Vol 58, suppl, 1993

Penland, J. G., "Researching Nutritional Trace Elements." *Agric Res,* Oct 1992

Prep Fds, June 1986; Mar 1988; Mar 1995

Proc Prep Fds, Aug 1979; Apr 1980

Pure Facts, Oct 2004

Reiser, Sheldon, "Effect of Copper Intake on Blood Cholesterol and Its Lipoprotein Distribution in Men." *Nutr Rept Internatl,* Vol 36, 1987

Res Briefs, Jan–Mar 1991

Schulze, P. H., Matthias B. et al., "Sugar-sweetened Beverages, Weight Gain, and Incidence of Type 2 Diabetes in Young and Middle-Aged Women, " *JAMA,* Vol 292, No 8, Aug 25, 2004

Sci News, May 3; 19863 June 21, 1986

Starling, Shane, "High-Fructose Corn Syrup Divides Food and Beverage Industry." *Functional Fds Nutraceut,* Jan 2005

Stone, Staci, "High-Fructose Corn Syrup and Obesity: True Link or Coincidence?" *Today's Dietitian,* Sept 2006

Sugar and Sweeteners Outlook. ERC, USDA, Dec 1991; Sept 1992

Sugar and Sweeteners Outlook Yearbook. ERC, USDA, June 19, 1990

Vines, Gail, "Sweet But Deadly." *New Scient,* Sept 1, 2001

Wall St J, Aug 8, 1980

Wash Post, Apr 1976; Feb 21, 1980

Webb, Densie, "The Effects of High-Fructose Sweeteners."*NY Times,* Oct 19, 1994

Chapter 5: Sugar Polyols

Erythritol

Calorie Control Commentary, Fall 1998

Fd Chem News, June 2, 1997; July 7, 1997; Dec 8, 1997; Oct 22, 2001

Fd Proc, July 2001; Nov 2004; Apr 2005

Fd Prod Design, Aug 1997; Sept 1997; Nov 1997; Sept 2003; Feb 2005

Fd Tech, May 1997; Aug 1997; Sept 1997; Jan 1998

Lina, B. A. R. et al., "Chronic Toxicity and Carcinogenicity Study of Erythritol in Rats." *Regulatory Toxicol Pharmacol,* Vol 24, article No 0108, 1996

Mattila, Pauli T. et al., "Dietary Xylitol, Sorbitol and D-Mannitol But Not Erythritol Retard Bone Resorption in Rats." *J Nutr,* Vol 126, 1996

Prep Fds, Sept 1989; June 2003; Nov 2004; Jan 2005

Reduced-Calorie Sweeteners: Erythritol. Calorie Control Council, 2004

Wellness Fds, suppl to *Fd Proc,* Mar–Apr 2002; May–June 2003; Sept–Oct 2003

Hydrogenated Starch Hydrolysates

Calorie Control Commentary, Fall 1991

Earles, Jim, "Sugar-free Blues." *Wise Traditions,* Winter 2003

Fd Chem News, Mar 15, 1993; Apr 5, 1993; Sept 27, 1993

Fd Engineer, May 1986; May 1989; Aug 1990

Fd Safety Newsletter, Apr 1992

Fd Tech, Oct 1989; Sept 1992; July 1995

Hydrogenated Starch Hydrolysis. Brochure. CCC, 1994, rev 2004

Lycasin, Dental Bibliography. Roquette America, Inc., undated

Lycasin in Confections. Roquette America, Inc., undated

Lycasin: Maltitol Syrups for Candymakers. Roquette America, Inc., undated

Nabors, Lyn O'Brien, "Safety and Current Domestic as well as International Regulatory Aspects of Use of Sugar Alcohols in Foods." CCC, undated

_____. "Sweet Choices: Sugar Replacements for Foods and Beverages." *Fd Tech,* July 2002

Prep Fds, Aug 1986; Mar 1997

Isomalt

Isomalt. Brochure. CCC, 1994, rev 2004

Paige, David M. et al., "Palatinit Digestibility in Children." *Nutr Res,* Vol 12, No 1, Jan 1992

Prep Fds, Sept 2005; Oct 2005

Lactitol

Am J Clin Nutr, Vol 65, suppl, 1995

Calorie Control Commentary, Fall 1991

CRM, July 2003

Fd Chem News, Sept 13, 1993; Feb 14, 1994

Fd Engineer, Dec 1994

Fd Proc, Mar 2003

Fd Prod Design, Dec 1998

Fd Safety Newsletter, July–Aug 1996

Fd Tech, Jan 1985; Nov 1994; Nov 1998

Koutsou, G. A. et al., "Dose-Related Gastrointestinal Response to the Ingestion of Either [sic] Isomalt, Lactitol, or Maltitol in Milk Chocolate." *Europ J Clin Nutr,* Vol 50, No 1, Jan 1996

Lactitol. Brochure. CCC, 1994, rev 2003

Prep Fds, Aug 1993; Sept 1993; Aug 1995; Apr 1999; Apr 2000; Apr 2003; Nov 2003

Stagnito's New Prods Develop. July-Aug 2002; June 2003

Maltitol

Am J Clin Nutr, Vol 62, suppl, 1995

Fd Chem News, Mar 9, 1987; Nov 9, 1987; Feb 22, 1993; July 12, 1993; Sept 27, 1993; June 20, 1994; July 25, 1994

Fd Formulating, Oct 2005

Fd Prod Design, Aug 2002; Apr 2005; Aug 2005

Fd Tech, Oct 1989; July 1995; Jan 1998; July 2002; Mar 2005

Langkilde, A. M. et al., "Digestion and Absorption of Sorbitol, Maltitol and Isomalt from the Small Bowel. A Study in Ileostomy Subjects." *Europ J Clin Nutr,* Vol 48, 1994

Prep Fds. July 2002; Apr 2005

Reduced Calorie Sweeteners: Maltitol, CCC, 2005

Stagnito's New Prods Develop, July–Aug 2002; June 2003

Mannitol

Am J Clin Nutr, Vol 62, suppl, 1995

Baking Manage, Feb 2001

Contemp Nutr, July 1980; Aug 1980

Diabetes Care, July–Aug 1978

FDA Consumer, Feb 1980; Apr 1992

Fd Chem News, July 31, 1973; Nov 5, 1973; Sept 23, 1974; Aug 26, 1991; Dec 19, 1994; May 29, 1995; Mar 4, 1996

Fd Cos Toxicol, Oct 1971

Fd Engineer, July 1988

Fd Nutr Briefs, Apr 2003

Fd Tech, Jan 1995; Apr 1996

Fed Reg, June–Aug 1973

Functional Fds Nutraceut, June 2005

JAMA, July 18, 1980

Lancet, May 26, 1973

Moses, Frank M. "Colonic Perforation Due to Oral Mannitol." Letter. *JAMA,* Aug 5, 1988

N Engl J Med, July 12, 1979

Reduced-Calorie Sweetener: Mannitol. CCC, 2004

Sci Am, Dec 1975

"Sweet Versatile Mannitol." Agric Res, Oct 2005

Polyols

Ad Libra, Nov 1, 1989

Am J Clin Nutr, Vol 62, suppl, 1995

Baking Manage, Feb 2000; Aug 2000; Oct 2000; Feb 2001; June 2001

Best, Daniel, "Working with Sweeteners." Prep Fds, Jan 1992

Book of Abstracts, IFT, 1994

Brandt, Laura A., "Polyols Add Stability to Sugar-free Candies." Prep Fds, June 1999

_____. "The Whole Sugar-free Scoop." Prep Fds, Mar 2000

CRM, Oct 1994; Aug 2001

Decker, Kimberly J., "Sweet Without the Sugar." Fd Prod Design, Mar 1999

Diabetes Care, Mar-Apr 1980

Earles, Jim, "Sugar-free Blues." Wise Traditions, Winter 2003

Ellwood, Kathleen C., "Methods Available to Estimate the Energy Values of Sugar Alcohols." Am J Clin Nutr, Vol 62, suppl, 1995

Fd Chem News, Sept 2, 1991; May 4, 1992; Sept 14, 1992; July 11, 1994

Fd Formulating, July 1995; Sept 1995

Fd Proc, June 2003; Sept 2003; Jan–Feb 2004; Feb 2005; Apr 2005

Fd Prod Design, July 1999; Sept 1999; May 2003; Feb 2004

Fd Safety Newsletter, May 1992; July–Aug 1996

"Low Calorie Values May Have Consumers Seeing More Polyols Soon." CCC Commentary, Spring 1995

Questions & Answers About Polyols. Brochure. CCC, undated

Sugar Alcohols Fact Sheet. IFIC, Sept 2004

Sorbitol

Am J Clin Nutr, Mar–Apr 1960

Birkhed, G. Svensäter Ater & S. Edwardsson, "Cariological Studies of Individuals with Long-term Sorbitol Consumption." Caries Res, May–June 1990

Canner/Packer '77 Buyers Guide Baking Industry, Nov 1976

Calorie Control Commentary, Spring 1993

Consumer Affairs Newsletter, City of Syracuse, NY, Feb 1978

Contemp Nutr, July 1980; Aug 1980

Diabetes Care, July–Aug 1978; Mar-Apr 1980

Evaluation of the Health Aspects of Sorbitol as a Food Ingredient. FASEB, Dec 1972

Fd Chem News, Sept 28, 1987; Apr 29, 1991; Aug 5, 1991; Aug 17, 1992; Oct 26, 1992; Dec 6, 1993; Jan 8, 1996; Mar 11, 1996; Apr 22, 1996; Oct 4, 1999; Oct 25, 1999

Fd Cos Toxicol, Dec 1969

Fd Formulating, Apr 1995; Oct 1995; Nov-Dec 1995

Fd Proc, Jan 1977

Fd Safety Newsletter, July-Aug 1992

Fd Tech, Oct 1989; Jan 1994; Apr 1996; May 1997; Jan 1999

Food, Yearbook of Agriculture. Wash, DC, USDA, 1959

Gastroent, Vol 47, 1964

Hoekstra, J. H. et al., "Apple Juice Malabsorption: Fructose or Sorbitol." J Pediat Gastroent Nutr, Vol 84, 1983

Health Fd Retail, Mar 1973

Jain, Naresh K., "Low Sorbitol Tolerance Found Prevalent, Said to Threaten Control of Diabetes." Med World News, Aug 16, 1984

Jain, Naresh K. et al., "Sorbitol Intolerance in Adults." Am J Gastroent, Vol 80, No 9, Sept 1985

_____. "Sorbitol Intolerance in Adults: Prevalence of Pathogenesis on Two Continents." J Clin Gastroent, Vol 9, No 3, June 1987

JAMA, July 18, 1980; Jan 20, 1989

J Biol Chem, Vol 141, 1941

Jensen, Mark E., "Responses of Interproximal Plaque pH to Snack Foods and Effects of Chewing Sorbitol-containing Gum." *JADA,* Aug 1986

Kalfas, S., "Sorbitol and Dental Plaque. Aspect of Caries, Related Microbiological and Biochemical Factors." *Swed Dent J,* suppl, 63, 1989

Kneepkens, C. M. F. et al., "Apple Juice, Fructose, and Chronic Non-specific Diarrhoea." *Europ J Pediat,* Vol 148, No 6, Apr 1989

Koutsou, G. A. et al., "Dose-related Gastrointestinal Response to the Ingestion of Either [sic] Isomalt, Lactitol, or Maltitol in Milk Chocolate." *Europ J Clin Nutr,* Jan 1996

Lancet, Dec 25, 1971; May 26, 1973

Lederle, Frank A. et al., "An Effective Treatment of Constipation in the Elderly: A Randomized Double-blind Comparison of Sorbitol and Lactulose." *Am J Med,* Vol 89, No 5, 1990

Lipin, R. et al., "Outbreak of Diarrhea Linked to Dietetic Candies—N.H." *MMWR (CDC, USPHS),* Sept 7, 1984

MacKenzie, K. M. et al., "Three-generation Reproduction Study of Rats Ingesting Up to 10 Percent Sorbitol in the Diet—and a Brief Review of the Toxicological Status of Sorbitol." *Fd Chem Toxicol,* Vol 24, No 3, Mar 1986

Mishkin, S.R. et al., "Fructose and/or Sorbitol Intolerance in a Subgroup of Lactose Intolerant Patients, *Can J Gastroent,* Nov 1994

Need for Special Food and Sugar Substitutes by Individuals with Diabetes Mellitus, FASEB, May 1978

N Engl J Med, Sept 29, 1966; Feb 16, 1967

Nutr Action, Oct 1999

Nutr Res Newsletter, Oct 15, 1984

Polyols: A Global Strategic Business Report, 1998; 2004

Postgrad Med, Oct 1992

Prep Fds, Aug 1983

Roe, Francis J. C., ed. *Metabolic Aspects of Food Safety.* Cambridge, MA: Blackwell Scientific Pub, 1980

74th Report on Food Products, 1969. New Haven, CT: CT Agric Exp Sta, July 1970

Sorbitol. CCC, 1995; rev 2004

"Sorbitol Ban Advised at Inpatient Centers for Eating Disorders." *Clin Psychiat News,* June 1990

Smith, Melanie M. et al., "Carbohydrate Absorption from Fruit Juice in Young Children." *Pediat,* Vol 95, No 3, Mar 1995

Snack Fd, Dec 1974

Sugar Alcohol Fact Sheet. IFIC, Sept 2004

USDA News. News release, Nov 8, 1972

Xylitol

Agr Res, July 2000

Altern Med, May 2005

Am J Clin Nutr, Mar 1976; vol 62, suppl, 1995

Br Med J, Nov 8, 1996

Calorie Control Commentary, Spring 1994; Fall 1996

C&EN, Mar 14, 1977; Mar 21, 1977; Sept 12, 1977; Nov 6, 1978; Dec 7, 1987; Nov 7, 1988; Apr 10, 1989; Jan 16, 1995

FDA Consumer, Jan-Feb 1999

Fd Chem News, Oct 25, 1971; Oct 26, 1987; Nov 2, 1987; Jan 4, 1988; Jan 18, 1988, Oct 28, 1991; Jan 18, 1993; Jan 25, 1993; Mar 22, 1993; Mar 29, 1993; Jan 23, 1994

Fd Label Nutr News, July 5, 2000

Fd Proc, Apr 1976; Apr 2005

Fd Prod Develop, Feb 1979

Fd Tech, Oct 1989; Aug 1990; Mar 1993; Dec 1993; May 1994

Functional Fds Nutraceut, June 2005

Gare, Fran, *The Sweet Miracle of Xylitol.* North Bergen, NJ: Basic Health Pub, 2003

Health Fd Retail, July 1980

J Nutr, Mar 1977

Lancet, Dec 25, 1971

Let's Live, Aug 1977

Linke, Harald A. B., "Sugar Alcohols and Dental Health." *World Rev Nutr Diet*, Vol 47, 1986

Mäkinen, Kauko K. & Arje Scheinin, "Xylitol and Dental Caries." *Ann Rev Nutr*, Vol 2, 1982

Nutr Notes, Fall 1983

Nutr Res News, Mar 1988; Feb 1991

NY Times, Nov 16, 1977; Apr 24, 1978

Pediat, Vol 102, 1998

Sci, Feb 10, 1978

Sci/Med News Leads, No 5, Univ of Wash, Nov 15, 1979

Sci News, Dec 10, 1977; Apr 3, 1988; Oct 22, 1988; Oct 31, 1998

Xylitol. CCC 1988, rev 2004

Chapter 6: Licorice

Acharya, S. K. et al., "A Preliminary Open Trial on Interferon Stimulator Derived from *Glycyrrhiza Glabra* in the Treatment of Subacute Hepatic Failure." *Indian J Med Res*, Vol 98, 1993

Alloza, José-Luis, "Discolourization of Skin and Serum after Sweet Ingestion." Correspondence. *Lancet*, June 5, 1993

Altman, Lawrence K., "A Medical Mystery and How Physicians Solved It." *NY Times*, Dec 29, 1987

Ammoniated Glycyrrhizin. Technical bulletin. Camden, NJ: MacAndrews & Forbes Co., undated

Armanini, D. et al., "Reduction of Serum Testosterone in Men by Licorice." *N Engl J Med*, Vol 34, 1999

Baking Ind, May 1976

Bergner, Paul, "Licorice and AIDS." *Townsend Letter for Doctors & Patients*, Nov 1990

_____. "Licorice as a Liver Herb," *Townsend Letter for Doctors & Patients*, Dec 1994

Blachley, M. D., Jon D. & James P. Knochel, "Tobacco Chewer's Hypokalemia: Licorice Revisited." *N Engl J Med*, Apr 10, 1980

Bradbury, R. B. & D. E. White, "Estrogens and Related Substances in Plants." *Vit Hormones*, Vol 12, 1954

Bus Wk, Dec 7, 1987

"Cautions on Folk Remedies; Licorice Root." *Remedy*, Jan 2, 1993

Chamberlain, Thomas, "Licorice Poisoning: Pseudoaldosteronism and Heart Failure." Letter. *JAMA*, Aug 24, 1970

Chemicals Used in Food Processing. Pub 1274, Wash, DC: NAS-NRC, 3rd print, 1967

Choate, Mary Saucier, "Licorice: Strong Medicine or Simply Candy?" *Co-op News*, Hanover Consumer Cooperative Society (Hanover, N.H.) Sept 2003

"Comment, Time Extended on Glycyrrhizin Rule." *Fd Prod Develop*, Aug 1979

Conn, Jerome W. et al., "Licorice Linked to Blood Pressure." Letter. *JAMA*, Aug 26, 1968

Cook, Marvin K., "Ammoniated Glycyrrhizin: A Useful Natural Sweetener and Flavour Potentiator." *Flavour Ind*, Dec 1970

_____. *New Mafco-MagnaSweet Products for Food, Drugs and Cosmetics.* Technical bulletin. Camden, NJ: MacAndrews & Forbes Co., undated

Cruz, D. N. & Mark A. Perazella, "Hypertension and Hypokalemia: Unusual Syndrome." *Conn Med*, Feb 1997

Dalton, Louise, "Licorice." *C&EN*, Aug 12, 2002

Das, S. K. et al., "Deglycyrrhizinated Liquorice in Apthous Ulcers." *J Assoc Physicians India*, Vol 37, 1989

Drug Ther, Oct 1978

Edwards, Christopher R. W., "Lessons from Licorice." Editorial. *N Engl J Med*, Oct 24, 1991

Evaluation of the Health Aspects of Licorice, Glycyrrhiza and Ammoniated Glycyrrhizin as Food Ingredients. FASEB Report to FDA, 1974

Farese, Jr., Robert et al., "Licorice-induced hypermineralocorticoidism." Brief Report. *N Engl J Med*, Oct 24, 1991

Fd Chem News, Dec 11, 1995

Fd Engineer, May 1973; Nov 1973; Oct 1981; Dec 1985; May 1986; Apr 1989; June 1989; Aug 1989; Jan 1990; Apr 1990; Aug 1990; Nov 1991; May 1992; Apr 1993

Fd Nutr News, May–June 1985

Fd Proc, May 1977; Nov 1977; July 1982; Nov 1982

Fd Prod Develop, July 1979; Aug 1979

Fd Tech, Apr 1989; Oct 1989

Fed Reg, May 22, 1985

Hannigan, Kevin J., "Sugar Substitutes." *Fd Engineer,* Mar 1979

Gaby, Alan R., "Deglycyrrhizinated Licorice Treatment of Peptic Ulcer." Editorial. *Townsend Letter for Doctors & Patients,* July 1988

Good Housekeeping, Nov 1976

"GRAS Proposal for Licorice." *Canner/Packer,* Sept 1977

"GRAS Status Changed for Glycyrrhizin." *Fd Prod Develop,* July 1979

Gray, Kay Bard, "Licorice High." Letter. *Good Housekeeping,* Apr 1992

Health Fd Bus, Feb 1989

Heinkens, J. et al., "Liquorice-induced Hypertension—A New Understanding of an Old Disease: Case Report and Brief Review." *Netherlands J Med,* Vol 47, Nov 1995

JAMA, Vol 205, 1968; Aug 24, 1970

J Pharm Pharmacol, Vol 55, 2003

Josephs, R.A, et al., "Liquorice Consumption and Salivary Testosterone Concentrations." *Lancet,* Vol 358, 2001

Kaplan, Norman M., "Spitting Out the Problem." *Cortlandt Forum,* Feb 1993

Kobayashi, M. et al., "Inhibition of Burn-associated Suppressor Cell Generation by Glycyrrhizin through the Induction of Contrasuppressor T Cells." *Immunol Cell Biol,* Vol 71, 1993

Lai, Florence et al., "Licorice." Letter. *N Engl J Med,* Aug 21, 1980

"Licorice as a Culprit." Science Watch, *NY Times,* Apr 15, 1980

"Licorice-Induced Pseudoaldosternism." *JAMA,* Vol 205, 1968

"Licorice May Aid Battle against Dental Cavities." *C&EN,* Feb 6, 2006

Marderosian, Ara H. Der, "Sugar Substitutes." *Drug Ther,* Oct 1978

MD, June 1979

Moore, Ann O. & Dorothy E. Powers, *Food-Medication Interactions.* Phoenix, AZ: FMI Pub, 5th ed. Mar 1986

N Engl J Med, Vol 241, 1999

NY Times, Oct 26, 1969; Nov 20, 2001

Pennisi, E., "Enzyme Structure Points to New Drugs." *Sci News,* July 27, 1991

Penn Med, Vol 74, 1971

Picca, Stephen M., Letter. *N Engl J Med,* May 31, 1979

Prep Fds, Aug 1986; Aug 1990; Nov 1990; Aug 1995; May 1996; Aug 1997; May 2000; Aug 2003

Proc Prep Fds, Aug 1978; Feb 1979; Aug 1986; Aug 1990; Nov 1990; Aug 1995; Aug 1997; Aug 2003

Robinson, Harold J. et al., "Licorice-induced Abnormalities of Myocardium." *Modern Med,* Dec 27, 1971

Tawata, M. et al., "Anti-platelet Action of Isoliquiritgenin: An Aldose Reductase Inhibitor in Licorice." *Europ J Pharmacol,* Vol 2, 1992

Toxicants Occurring Naturally in Foods. Pub 1354, Wash, DC: NAS-NRC, July 1971

Chapter 7: Stevia

Am Perfume Essential Oil Rev, Vol 66, 1955

Bonvie, Linda, Bill Bonvie & Linda Gates, *The Stevia Story: A Tale of Incredible Sweetness and Intrigue.* Atlanta, GA: Body Ecology, 1997

Bus Wk, May 25, 1987

Calorie Control Commentary, Fall 1999; Summer–Fall 2000

Carter, James P., *Racketeering in Medicine, the*

Suppression of Alternatives. Charlottesville, VA: Hampton Roads Pub, 1992

Drake, Laurie, "So Sweet, So Natural, So L.A." *NY Times*, Mar 7, 2001

Elmore, Vicki, "Speaking Out on the Stevia Debate." *Healthy Natural J*, Apr 1999

Fd Chem News, May 27, 1991; Aug 12, 1991; Oct 28, 1991; Oct 25, 1993; Nov 15, 1993; Mar 7, 1994; Sept 7, 1998

Fd Prod Design, Oct 2001

Fd Safety Notebook, Feb 1993

Ferri, L. A. et al., "Investigation of the Anti-hypertensive Effect of oral Crude Stevioside in Patients with Mild Essential Hypertension." *Phytother Res*, Vol 20, No 9, 2006

Fillipic, Martha, "Stevia Might Not Be a Sweet Deal." Press release. Wooster, OH: Ohio State Univ, June 10, 1999

Foster, Steven, "Stevia Soured by FDA Ban" *Health Fd Bus*, Oct 1992

Gustafson, Karen, "Stevia." *Natural Health*, Feb 1990

Health Fd Bus, Feb 1990

Keville, Kathi, "The Herb Report: Stevia." *Am Herb Assoc Quarterly Newsletter*, Spring 1994

Kirkland, James & Tanya Kirkland, *Low-Carb Cooking with Stevia: The Naturally Sweet & Calorie-Free Herb*. Midlothian, TX: Crystal Health Pub, 2000

Lanar, James R., Compliance Officer, FDA, Letter. *Townsend Letter for Doctors & Patients*, Jan 1999

Lucier, James P., "How Sweet It Is." *Insight*, Aug 17, 1998

Martini, Betty, Letter. *Townsend Letter for Doctors & Patients*, Jan 1999

McKeith, Gillian, *Living Foods for Health*. Laguna Beach, CA: Basic Health Pub, 2004

Miguel, Olivido, "A New Oral Hypoglycemate." *Med Rev Paraguay*, Vol 8, No 5&6, July–Dec 1966

Natural Fds Merchand, Mar 1992; Nov 1992; May 1994

O'Neil, John, "Stevia: A Sweetener That's Not a Sweetener." *NY Times*, Mar 5, 1999

Prep Fds, July 1990; Mar 1997; Nov 2001; Apr 2002

Pure Facts, July-Aug 1998

Richard, David, *Stevia Rebaudiana: Nature's Sweet Secret*. Ridgefield, CT: Vital Health Pub, 3rd ed, 1999

Roma, Zoltan P., *Health Naturally*, Aug-Sept 1996

Sahelian, Ray & Donna Gates, *The Stevia Cookbook: Cooking with Nature's Calorie-free Sweetener*. NY, NY: Avery, 1999

Sell, Shawn, "A Sweet Alternative: Raising Stevia Instead of Cane." *USA Today*, June 22, 2001

Shock, Clinton C., "Rebaudi's Stevia: Natural Noncaloric Sweeteners."' *Cal Agric*, Sept–Oct 1982

Siegel-Maier, Karyn, "A Book-burning in Texas." *Better Nutr*, Dec 1998

Stagnito's New Prods Magazine, Oct 2001; Jan 2003

Starling, Shana, "Study Raises Hope for Stevia." *Functional Fds Nutraceut*, Mar 2005

Sugar & Sweetener, Dec 1991

Thomas, Uwanna D., "An Herb to Know." *The Herb Companion*, Dec 1991–Jan 1992

Townsend Letter for Doctors & Patients, Nov 1997; Nov 1998

Webb, Densie, "Alternative Sweetness?" *Great Life*, Apr 1998

Chapter 8: Thaumatin

Batt, Carl A. "Applying Biotechnology to Dairy Processing." Ithaca, NY: Cornell Univ NY's *Fd Life* Sc Quarterly, Vol 17, No 3, 1987

C&EN, Mar 27, 1972; Mar 11, 1985

CRM, June 1996

Fd Chem News, Nov 2, 1987

Fd Engineer, Mar 1984

Fd Tech, Apr 1987; Oct 1989; Jan 1996; Feb 1997

MD, June 1979

NY Times, Apr 9, 1977

Prep Fds, Aug 1986; Mar 1987; Mar 1997; Aug 1997; Jan 2001; Jan 2005; Apr 2005; Oct 2005

Prep Fds New Prods Annual, 1987

Pszczola, Donald E., "Sweet Beginings to a New Year." *Fd Tech*, Jan 1999

Sci News, Mar 23, 1985; May 10, 1997

Sweeteners: Issues & Uncertainties. Academic Forum, NAS. Wash, DC: Acad Press, 1975

Talin: Naturally Makes the Flavour Complete. Technical data sheets. Blauvelt, NY: RFI Ingredients, 1996

"Thaumatin: the Sweetest Substance Known to Man Has a Wide Range of Food Applications." Staff report. *Fd Tech*, Jan 1996

Van der Wel, H. & K. Loeve, "Isolation and Characterization of Thaumatin I and II, the Sweet-Tasting Proteins from *Thaumatoccus daniellii*." *Europ J Biochem*, Vol 31, 1972; Vol 35, 1973

Van der Wel, H., "Katemfe" in *Symposium: Sweeteners*. George E. Inglett, ed. Westport, CT: Avi, 1974

Witty, Michael & John D. Higgenbotham, eds. *Thaumatin*. Boca Raton, FL: CRC Press, 1994

Chapter 9: Dihydrochalcones

C&EN, Aug 25, 1975

Earles, Jim, "Sugar-free Blues." *Wise Traditions*, Winter 2003

Fd Chem News, Apr 29, 1991; Nov 11, 1991

Fd Proc, May 1977, May 1982, June 1982

Fd Proc: Foods of Tomorrow, Summer 1970

Fd Prod Develop, Jan 1982

Health Bull, Dec 20, 1969

J Agric Fd Chem, Vol 16, 1968

MD, June 1979

NY Times, Mar 16, 1977

Proc Prep Fds, Feb 1979

Sci News, July 16, 1977

USDA Daily Summary. Press release. Mar 18, 1977

USDA Service. Press release. May 1977

Chapter 10: Plant-Derived Sweeteners

Brazzein

Fd Chem News, Apr 27, 1998; Sept 13, 1999

Fd Prod Design, July 1998; Nov 1999; May 2000

Prep Fds, Sept 1998

Sci News, May 8, 1993; June 20, 1998

Hernandulcin

C&EN, Jan 28, 1985

Compadre, Cesar M. et al., "Hernandulcin: An Intensely Sweet Compound Discovered by Review of Ancient Literature." *Sci*, Jan 25, 1985

Sci 85, Apr 1985

Sci News, Jan 26, 1985

Lo Han

Fd Chem News, Jan 31, 2000

Fd Prod Design, Sept 2003

Lee, C. H., "Intense Sweetener from Lo Han Kuo." *Experientia*, Vol 31, No 5, 1975

Peilin, Guo & Dallas Clouatre, "Lo Han: A Natural Sweetener Comes of Age." *Whole Fds*, June 2003

Prep Fds, Sept 1999; Aug 2001

Stagnito's New Prods Magazine, Nov–Dec 2002

Swingle, W. T. J., (Untitled article). *Arnold Arboritum*, Vol 22, 1941

Xiang yang, Q. et al., "Effects of a *Siraita grosvenori*: Extract Containing Mogrosides on the Cellular Immune System of Type 1 Diabetes Mellitus Mice." *Mol Nutr Food Res*, Vol 50, No 8, 2006

Miracle Berry

Am Dairy Rev, Jan 1975

Chemistry, Nov 1971

Daniell, W.F., *Pharma J,* Vol 11, 1852

Drug Ther, Oct 1978

Fd Chem News, Oct 1, 1973

Health, Education & Welfare News. Press release. U.S. Dept HEW, May 23, 1977

J Agric Fd Chem, Vol 13, 1965

"Miracle Fruit Petition Denied." *Fed Reg,* May 24, 1977

NY Times, June 10, 1971; Nov 22, 1976

Press release. Ketchum, MacLeod & Grove, Inc., Nov 15, 1972

Sci, Sept 20, 1968

Osladin

Jizba, J. et al., "Polypodosaponin: A New Type of Saponin from *Polypodium vulgare L.*" *Chem Ber,* Vol 104, 1971

_____. "The Structure of Osladin: The Sweet Principle of the Rhizomes of *Polypodium vulgare L.*" *Tetrahedron Letter,* Vol 18, 1971

Sweeteners: Issues & Uncertainties. Academic Forum, NAS. Wash, DC: Acad Press, 1975

Rosary Pea

De-Vine-ly Sweet. Press release, ACS, Aug 21, 1995

Fd Engineer, Mar 1991

Fd Prod Design, May 1993

Natural Fds Merchand, July 1993

"Natural, Heat-Stable Sweetener Unveiled at ACS Meeting." *Fd Chem News,* Sept 4, 1995

Prep Fds, June 1993

Rouhi, A. Maureen, "Researchers Unlocking Potential of Diverse, Widely Distributed Saponins." *C&EN,* Sept 11, 1995

Serendipity Berry

Bus Wk, Mar 23, 1972

C&EN, Mar 2, 1972; Aug 25, 1975

Harborne, B., C. F. Van Sumere & J.G. Vaughn, eds., *The Chemistry & Biochemistry of Plant Proteins.* London: Acad Press, 1975

Inglett, George E., "Sweeteners: New Challenges and Concepts." *Symposium: Sweeteners.* Westport, CT: Avi, 1974

Inglett, George E. & J. F. Findlay, "Serendipity Berry: Source of a New Macromolecular Sweetener." Abstract paper 75A, Chicago, IL: 154th ACS meeting, 1967

JAMA, Apr 10, 1972

J Fd Sci, Vol 34, 1969

MD, June 1979

Morris, J. A. & R. H. Cagan, *Biochem Biophys,* Acta, 261, 1972

NY Times, Apr 9, 1977

Sweet Leaf Tea Plant

De-Vine-ly Sweet. Press release. ACS, Aug 21, 1995

Sweet Cicely and Hydrangea

Inglett, George E., "Sweeteners: New Challenges and Concepts" in *Symposium: Sweeteners.* Westport, CT: Avi, 1974

Sweet Shoot

Kiple, Kenneth F. & Kriemhild Coneè Ornelas, eds. *The Cambridge World History of Food.* Vol II., Cambridge, UK: Cambridge Univ Press, 2000

Yacón

Functional Fds Nutraceut, June 2005

Kiple, Kenneth F. & Kriemhild Coneè Ornelas, eds. *The Cambridge World History of Food.* Vol II, Cambridge, UK: Cambridge Univ Press, 2000

Lost Crops of the Incas. Vol 1. Grains. Wash, DC: Natl Acad Press, 1996

Chapter 11: Cyclamate

Ahmed, Farid & David B. Thomas, "Assessment of the Carcinogenicity of the Nonnutritive Sweetener Cyclamate." *Critical Rev Toxicol*, Vol 22, No 2, 1992

Am Med News, June 21, 1985

Arch Environ Health, July 1971

Barron's, Nov 17, 1969

Boffey, Philip, *The Brain Bank of America: An Inquiry into the Politics of Science.* NY, NY: McGraw-Hill, 1975

Bus Wk, Mar 22, 1969; Oct 18, 1969; Mar 25, 1972; Nov 26, 1973

Capital Times (Madison, WI) Oct 7, 1965

Calorie Control Commentary, Fall 1984

C&EN, Sept 27, 1971; Nov 26, 1973; Sept 16, 1974; Oct 21, 1974; Nov 18, 1974; Mar 24, 1975; Mar 31, 1975; Apr 7, 1975; Jan 21, 1976; Oct 9, 1978; Sept 17, 1979; Feb 18, 1980; Sept 22, 1980; Aug 6, 1984; June 17, 1985; May 22, 1989; Nov 1, 1999

Chem Abs, Vol 81, 1974

Chem Wk, July 11, 1973

Conn Med, Aug 1965

Consumer Repts, Oct 1964; May 1969; Jan 1970

Cyclamates. Hearings, Comm on the Judiciary, U.S. House of Repres, June 10, 1970; Sept 29–30, 1971; Oct 6, 1971

Dairy Fds, June 1980

Environ, Sept 1973

Evaluation of Cyclamate for Carcinogenicity. NAS-NRC. Wash, DC: Acad Press, 1985

Evening News (Newark, NJ), Sept 10, 1970

Fact, Nov–Dec, 1966

FDA Consumer, June 1976; Feb 1985

Fd Chem News, Nov 24, 1969; Aug 2, 1980; Oct 21, 1985; Feb 23, 1987; Nov 2, 1987; Dec 21, 1987; Mar 18, 1991; Nov 28, 1994; Jan 22, 1999; Aug 30, 1999

Fd Engineer, Oct 1980; Dec 1982; Feb 1985; July 1985; May 1985

Fd Proc, Nov 1976; Nov 1980

Fd Prod Design, Nov 1978; June 1979; Oct 1979; July 1992; Oct 1999

Fd Safety Notebook, Mar–Apr 1991; Oct–Nov 1992

Fd Tech, Jan 1999; Mar 2000

Health Bull, Nov 30, 1968; Oct 25, 1969

Health, Education & Welfare News. News release. Dept HHS Sept 4, 1980

Hunter, Beatrice Trum, *Food Additives & Federal Policy: The Mirage of Safety.* NY, NY: Charles Scribner's Sons, 1975

Internatl Med News, Jan 15, 1976

JAMA, Sept 4, 1967

J Am Diet Assoc, June 1965

Lancet, Dec 13, 1969

Med Letter, Sept 11, 1964

Med Trib, July 6, 1970; Aug 31, 1970; Sept 26, 1973; Dec 5, 1973; Sept 5, 1984

Med World News, Feb 13, 1970; Mar 15, 1974; Oct 11, 1974; Aug 30, 1984

Nature, Mar 25, 1967; Jan 4, 1969; May 7, 1971

New Yorker, Feb 4, 1974

Non-nutritive Sweeteners, Summary & Conclusions. Food Protection Comm, NAS-NRC. Wash, DC: Acad Press, Nov 1968

Nutr Res Newsletter, Aug 1988

NY Times, May 20, 1965; Oct 19, 1969; Nov 23, 1969; Aug 15, 1970; Sept 30, 1971; May 2, 1972; Sept 11, 1974; Nov 14, 1974; Mar 24, 1975; Dec 30, 1976; Dec 1, 1982; Aug 21, 1984; May 9, 1989; Sept 6, 1989

Policy Statement on Artificial Sweeteners. Fd & Nutr Brd, NAS-NRC, adopted Nov 1954, pub 1955, rev 1962, Wash, DC: Acad Press, 1962

Prep Fds, Aug 1984; Sept 1984; Feb 1985; July 1989; Oct 1990

Proceedings. FASEB, Dec 1969

Regulations of Cyclamate Sweeteners. Hearings. Comm Govt Oper, U.S. House of Repres, Oct 8, 1970; Oct 10, 1970

The Safety of Artificial Sweeteners. FDA Fact Sheet. Apr 3, 1969

The Safety of Artificial Sweeteners for Use in Foods. Pub No 386, Fd & Nutr Brd, NAS-NRC. Wash, DC: Acad Press, Aug 1955

Sci, Aug 26, 1967; Sept 12, 1969; Nov 1, 1974; June 28, 1985

Sci News, Aug 26, 1967; June 15, 1985

Star Ledger (Newark, NJ), Dec 11, 1975

Sugar and Sweeteners Outlook, Mar 1986; Dec 1991

Sweeteners: Issues & Uncertainties. Academy Forum, Mar 26–27, 1975. NAS-NRC. Wash, DC: Acad Press, 1975

U.S. News & World Rept, Nov 3, 1969

Verrett, Jacqueline & Jean Carper, *Eating May Be Hazardous to Your Health, The Case Against Food Additives.* NY, NY: Simon & Schuster, 1974

Walker, A. M. et al., "An Independent Analysis of the NCI Study on Non-Nutritive Sweeteners & Bladder Cancer." *Am J Public Health,* Apr 1982

Wall St J, Aug 7, 1970; Mar 10, 1972; July 25, 1972; July 2, 1973; Jan 14, 1976; July 13, 1976; Aug 26, 1999

Wash Post, Nov 17, 1960; July 8, 1987

Whole Fds, Jan 1985

Chapter 12: Saccharin

AMA Reports Saccharin Safe, Should Remain Available. Press release. CCC, Nov 7, 1985

Am Dairy Rev, Feb 1975

Am J Clin Nutr, Vol 7, 1959

Am Med News, Mar 16, 1984; Apr 10, 1985

Anderson, Oscar E., *Health of a Nation, Harvey W. Wiley's Fight for Pure Food.* Chicago, IL: Univ of Chicago Press, 1958

Arch Environ Health, July 1971

The Banning of Saccharin, 1977. Hearings, Subcomm Health Sci Res, Comm. Human Resources, U.S. Senate, June 7, 1988

Blundell, J. E. & A. J. Hill, "Paradoxical Effects of an Intense Sweetener on Appetite." *Lancet I,* No 8489, May 10, 1986

Br J Cancer, Vol 11, 1957

Br Med J, Vol 1, 1897

Bus Wk, Feb 19, 1972

Calorie Control Commentary, Spring 1988; Spring 1993; Fall 1996; Fall 1997; Fall 1998; Spring–Summer 1999; Fall 1999; Summer–Fall 2000

Cancer Res, June 15, 1998

Cancer Testing Technology & Saccharin, OTA, U.S. Congress, Oct 1977

Capital Times, (Madison, WI), Mar 21, 1977

C&EN, July 19, 1971; Apr 6, 1976; Apr 11, 1977; May 23, 1977; June 13, 1977; June 27, 1977; July 18, 1977; Sept 26, 1977; Nov 13, 1978; May 21, 1979; May 28, 1979; July 2, 1979; Jan 7, 1980; Mar 17, 1980; Apr 27, 1981; July 6, 1981; July 28, 1997; Nov 10, 1997; May 22, 2000

Chappell, Clifford I., "Saccharin Revisited." *Western J Med,* Vol 160, No 6, June 1994

Chem Wk, Feb 16, 1972; Mar 25, 1972; Apr 1, 1972

Chicago Trib, May 4, 1979

Cohen, Addad N. et al., "In Utero Exposure to Saccharin: A Threat?" *Cancer Letters,* Vol 32, No 2, Aug 1985

Comprehensive Report Documents Saccharin's Safety. Press release. CCC, July 25, 1985

Consumer Repts, July 1977

Dairy & Ice Cream Field, July 1979

Elwin, Leon B. & Samuel M. Cohen, "The Health Risks of Saccharin Revisited." *Critical Rev Toxicol,* Vol 20, No 5, 1990

Epidemiology. Brochure. CCC, May 1983

Epstein, Samuel S., *The Politics of Cancer.* San Francisco, CA: Sierra Club, 1978

Family Health, Oct 1969

FDA Consumer, Mar 1980; Dec 1980–Jan 1981; Feb 1981; Sept 1981; Feb 1985; July 1990; Dec 1990, Mar–Apr 1999

Fd Chem News, Dec 21, 1987: Jan 18, 1988; Feb 22, 1988; Apr 13, 1992; June 15, 1992; July 20, 1992; Feb 28, 1994; Mar 14, 1994; Mar 21,

1994; Apr 11, 1994; Apr 25, 1994; May 21, 1994; Apr 17, 1995; Apr 24, 1995; June 19, 1995; Oct 10, 1995; Dec 4, 1995; Feb 3, 1997; June 2, 1997; July 7, 1997; July 21, 1997; Oct 27, 1997; Nov 3, 1997; Nov 10, 1997; Feb 16, 1998; June 29, 1998; Dec 21, 1998; July 19, 1999; May 22, 2000; Jan 15, 2001

Fd Chem Toxicol, Vol 23, No 4–5, Apr–May 1985

Fd Engineer, June 1983; Sept 1984; Oct 1984

Fd Manage, Oct 1980; Dec 1982

Fd Proc, Aug 1977; Nov 1977; Apr 1983

Fd Prod Design, July 1992; Dec 1997; Apr 1999; June 2000; Feb 2001

Fd Safety Notebook, Apr 1998

Fd Tech, Oct 1989; Feb 2001; July 2002

Food & Drug Administration Talk Paper. June 20, 1977 Francesco, Negro, et al., "Hepatotoxicity of Saccharin." Letter. *N Engl J Med,* Vol 331, No 2, July 14, 1994

Frankel, Howard H., "Saccharin Revisited." *Western J Med,* Vol 160, No 6, June 1994

Good Housekeeping, Nov 1913

Health, Education & Welfare News. News release. Dept HEW, Jan 28, 1972; May 21, 1973; Jan 9, 1975; Mar 9, 1977; Apr 14, 1977; Nov 28, 1977; Jan 25, 1978; May 22, 1979; Dec 20, 1979

Hyperactive Helpline, No 183, Third Quarter, 1997

JAMA, Nov 8, 1985

J Am Diet Assoc, Vol 32, 1956

J Am Pharmaceut Assoc, Aug 1947

Lawrie, C.A., "Different Dietary Patterns in Relation to Age & the Consequences for Intake of Food Chemicals." *Fd Add Contam,* Vol 15, No 1, suppl, Jan 1998

Market Watch, Mar 1986

Med Trib, Feb 23, 1972; Nov 21, 1973

Natenberg, Maurice, *The Legacy of Dr. Wiley.* Chicago, IL: Regent House, 1957

Nature, June 8, 1973

Need to Resolve Safety Questions on Saccharin. Rept Comptroller General U.S., Aug 16, 1976

N Engl J Med, Mar 6, 1980

Newswk, Mar 21, 1977; Mar 30, 1977

Nutr Res Newsletter, June 1986

NY State J Med, Dec 1, 1955

NY Times, Oct 23, 1969; Mar 20, 1970; July 23, 1970; June 23, 1971; Nov 5, 1973; Oct 20, 1976; Mar 11, 1977; Mar 12, 1977; Mar 13, 1977; Mar 20, 1977; Mar 22, 1977; Apr 5, 1977; May 19, 1977; June 19, 1977; Oct 6, 1977; Nov 7, 1978; Mar 3, 1979; Mar 5, 1979; May 10, 1979; Dec 21, 1979; Aug 21, 1984; Nov 8, 1985; Sept 5, 1998; Dec 19, 1998; May 16, 2000

Prep Fds, Oct 1982; Mar 1983; June 1983; July 1983; Oct 1983; Sept 1984; Nov 1984; Jan 1985; Apr 1985; June 1985; July 1985; Sept 1985; Aug 1986; May 1987; Aug 2000

"The Price of Sweetness." *Tech Rev,* Jan 1990

Proceedings of the Society for Experimental Biology & Medicine, Vol 66, 1947

Progress Report to FDA from NCI Concerning the National Bladder Cancer Study. Wash, DC: NCI, Dec 1979

Proposed Saccharin Ban. Oversight Hearings, Health & Environ, Comm on Interstate Foreign Comm U.S. House of Repres, Mar 21–22, 1977

Rest Bus, Mar 15, 1981

Rest & Instit, Feb 6, 1985; Mar 6, 1985; May 29, 1985

Rest Hosp, Aug 1990

Rogers, Peter J. & John E. Blundell, "Uncoupling Sweet Taste and Calories: Effects of Saccharin on Hunger and Food Intake in Human Subjects," *Ann NY Acad Sci,* 1989

Saccharin. Brochure. CCC, Sept 1983

"Saccharin: An Update." Editorial. *Am Family Physician,* Dec 1983

"Saccharin Consumption Increases Food Consumption in Rats." *Nutr Rev,* Vol 48, No 3, Mar 1990

Saccharin: Technical Assessments of Risks & Benefits. Rept No 1. Comm for Study on Saccharin & Fd Safety Policy. NAS-NRC. Wash, DC: Acad Press, Nov 1978

Safety of Saccharin & Sodium Saccharin in the Human Diet. Subcomm on Non-nutritive Sweeteners, Comm on Fd Protection, Fd & Nutr Brd, NAS-NRC. Wash, DC: Acad Press, 1974

Sci, June 5, 1970; Feb 16, 1973; Sept 22, 1978; Mar 14, 1980; Apr 11, 1980; Oct 31, 1997

Shell, Ellen Ruppell, "Nutrition: Sweetness & Health." *Atlantic Monthly,* Aug 1985

Snack Fd, Feb 1975; June 1977; June 1979

Star Ledger (Newark, NJ), Jan 7, 1977

Stellman, S. D. & L. Garfinkel, "Artificial Sweetener Use and One-Year Weight Gain Change Among Women." *Preventive Med,* Vol 15, No 2, Mar 1986

Wall St J, Mar 17, 1970; Mar 18, 1970; Sept 18, 1970; June 23, 1971; July 23, 1973; June 20, 1977

Wash Post, July 23, 1970; May 3, 1977

Wiley, Harvey Washington, *The History of a Criime Against the Food Law.* Self-published, 1929. Reprinted Milwaukee, WI: Lee Foundation for Nutritional Research, 1955

Chapter 13: Aspartame

Allman, William F., "Aspartame: Some Bitter with the Sweet?" *Sci,* July–Aug 1984

Am Med News, July 22–29, 1983; Jan 27, 1984; Feb 3, 1984; Apr 13, 1984; June 22, 1984; Nov 23–30, 1984; Feb 15, 1985; May 10, 1985; Dec 13, 1985; Mar 14, 1986; May 9, 1986; Dec 12, 1986; June 17, 1988

Anderson, G. H. et al., "Aspartame: Effect on Lunch-Time Food Intake, Appetite and Hedonic Response in Children." *Appetite,* Vol 13, No 2, Oct 1989

"Arizona Refuses to Ban Drinks with Aspartame." *Am Med News,* Mar 23–30, 1984

Aspartame. Brochure. Atlanta, GA: CCC, Sept 1984

Aspartame Ads Mislead Consumers, Association Says. Press release. Rowland Co, Inc, Public Relations, in behalf of Sugar Assoc, Aug 14, 1984

"Aspartame Critic Faces SEC Probe in Stock Deal." *Am Med News,* Mar 9, 1984

"Aspartame Critics Persist, Recommend Avoidance during Pregnancy." *Med World News Psychiatry* edition, Feb 29, 1984

"Aspartame: Review of Safety Issues." Council on Scientific Affairs, *JAMA,* Vol 254, No 3, July 19, 1985

Barus, J. & A. Bal, "Emerging Facts about Aspartame." *J Diab Assoc of India,* Vol 35, No 4, 1994

Beardsley, Tim, "Sweet Talk." Science & the Citizen. *Sci Am,* Vol 257, No 1, July 1987

Better Homes & Gardens. Advertisement. May 1988

Blackburn, George L. et al., "The Effects of Aspartame as Part of a Multi-Disciplinary Weight-Control Program on Short- and Long-term Control of Body Weight." *Am J Clin Nutr,* Vol 65, 1997

Bleiberg, Robert M., "Low Blow at Nutra-Sweet, Food Faddists Again Are Threatening Consumer Freedom of Choice." Editorial. *Barron's,* Feb 6, 1984

Blumenthal, Harvey J. & Dwight A. Vance, "Chewing Gum Headaches." *Headache,* Vol 37, No 10, Nov–Dec 1997

Blundell, J. E., "Effects of Aspartame on Appetite and Food Intake" in *Dietary Phenylalanine & Brain Function.* R.J. Wurtman & E. Ritter-Walker, eds. Boston, MA: Birkhauser, 1988

Blundell, J. E. & A. J. Hill, "Paradoxical Effects of an Intense Sweetener (Aspartame) on Appetite." Correspondence. *Lancet 1* (8489), May 10, 1986

Blundell, J. E., et al., "Uncoupling Sweetness and Calories: Methodological Aspects of Laboratory Studies on Appetite Control." *Appetite* II, suppl 1988

Boffey, Philip M. "Diet Sweetener Risk Is Being Reassessed After New Research." *NY Times,* Aug 21, 1984

Bommersbach, Jana, "The Case Against NutraSweet: How Did It Ever Pass through the FDA?" *Valley Advocate* (Springfield, MA), Mar 28, 1984

Booth, D. A., "Evaluation of the Usefulness of Low-Calorie Sweets in Weight Control" in *Developments in Sweeteners*, Vol 3, T.H Grenby et al. London: Elsivier-Applied Science, 1987

Bradstock, M. K. et al., "Evaluation of Reactions to Food Additives: The Aspartame Experience." *Am J Clin Nutr*, Vol 43, No 3, Mar 1986

Brala, P. M. & R. L. Hagen, "Effects of Sweetness Perception & Caloric Value of a Preload on Short-term Intake." *Physiol Behav*, Vol 30, 1983

Briley, John, "FDA Unfazed by Evidence that Refrigerated Aspartame Breaks Down to Formaldehyde and DKP." *Fd Chem News*, May 5, 1997

Brody, Ira, "Aspartame & Seizures." Letter. *C&EN*, Oct 26, 1987

Brody, Jane E., "Judging Safety of Aspartame in Soft Drinks." *NY Times*, July 13, 1983

_____. "Sweetener Worries Some Scientists." *NY Times*, Feb 5, 1985

Brunner, R. L. et al., "Aspartame: Assessment of Developmental Psychotoxicity of a New Artificial Sweetener." *Neurobehav Toxicol*, Vol 1, 1979

Burros, Marian, "Approval Postponed." *NY Times*, June 22, 1983

_____. "Searching for Truth In Ads & Labels." *NY Times*. Mar 24, 1984

_____. "A Sweetener's Effects: New Questions Raised." *NY Times*. July 3, 1985

Busch, Linda, "Adverse Reaction Report under Review, FDA Rejects Aspartame Hearing Request." *Am Med News*, Mar 2, 1984

_____. "FDA to Step Up Food Reaction Monitoring Program." *Am, Med News*, Nov 22–29, 1985

Bus Wk, Aug 10, 1974; Sept 29, 1980; July 18, 1983; Aug 29, 1983; Sept 5, 1983; Jan 30, 1984

Butchko, H. H. & H. Harriett, "Aspartame

Clinical Update." Letter. *Conn Med*, Vol 54, No 4, Apr 1990

Buzzanell, Peter & Fred Gray, "Have High-Intensity Sweeteners Reached Their Peak?" *Fd Rev*, USDA, Sept–Dec 1993

Bylinsky, G., "The Battle for America's Sweet Tooth." *Fortune*, July 1982

Caballero, B. et al., "Plasma Amino Acid Levels After Single-Dose Aspartame Consumption in Phenylketonuria, Mild Hyperphenylalanine & Heterozygous State for Phenylketonuria. *J Pediat*, Vol 109, No 4, Oct 1986

Calorie Control Commentary, Spring 1984; Fall 1996; Fall 1997; Spring–Summer 1999; Fall 1999

Camfield, P. R. et al., "Aspartame Exacerbates EEG Spike-wave Discharge in Children with Generalized Absence of Epilepsy: A Double-blind Controlled Study." *Neurol*, Vol 42, 1992

Cantry, David J. & Mabel M. Chan, "Effects on Consumption of Caloric vs Noncaloric Sweet Drinks on Indices of Hunger and Food Consumption in Normal Adults." *Am J Clin Nutr*, Vol 53, 1991

C&EN, May 1, 1973; Aug 5, 1974; Dec 8, 1975; June 18, 1979; Aug 13, 1979; Feb 18, 1980; Apr 21, 1980; Oct 6, 1980; Oct 4, 1982; Jan 17, 1983; June 13, 1983; July 11, 1983; Aug 8, 1983; Aug 15, 1983; Aug 22, 1983; Sept 5, 1983; Jan 2, 1984; Jan 30, 1984; July 16, 1984; Aug 27, 1984; Feb 4, 1985; Apr 1, 1985; Dec 16, 1985; Mar 17, 1986; Sept 8, 1986; Dec 1, 1986; Jan 26, 1987; July 27, 1987; Feb 3, 1992; Nov 30, 1992; July 12, 1999; Feb 14, 2000

Chem Wk, Aug 7, 1974; Oct 2, 1974

Chicago Trib, Feb 17, 1984

"Claims about Aspartame Disputed." *Brattleboro* (VT) *Daily Reformer*, Aug 15, 1984

Cohen, Rich, "The Plot Against Sugar." *Vanity Fair*, Dec 2005

Connolly, John S., "Potential Hazards of Aspartame." Letter. *C&EN*, Sept 7, 1987

Crapo, Phyllis, "A Survey of Sweeteners." *Clin Diabet* Nov–Dec, 1983

Coulombe, R. A. & R. P. Sharma, "Neurobiochemical Alterations Induced by the Artificial Sweetener Aspartame." *Toxicol Appl Pharmacol*, Vol 83, No 1, 1986

Cruthers, Donna, "Light Desserts Heavy in Appeal." *Dairy Fds*, Dec 1988

Dairy Fds. Advertisement. June 1990

Davoli, E. et al., "Serum Methanol Concentrations in Rats and in Men after a Single Dose of Aspartame." *Fd Chem Toxicol*, Vol 24, 1986

De Bon, Umberto & Donald McLachlan, "Controlled Induction of Paired Helical Filaments of the Alzheimer Type in Cultured Neurons, by Glutamate & Aspartate." *J Neurol Sci*, Vol 68, 1985

Diomede, L. et al., "Interspecies and Interstrain Studies on the Increased Susceptibility to Metrazol Induced Convulsions in Animals Given Aspartame." *Fd Chem Toxicol*, Vol 29, No 2. Feb 1991

Dow-Edwards, D. L. et al., "Impaired Performance on Odor-Aversion Testing Following Prenatal Aspartame Exposure in the Guinea Pig." *Neurotox Teratol*, Vol 11, No 4, July–Aug 1989

Drake, Miles E., "Panic Attacks and Excessive Aspartame Ingestion." Correspondence. *Lancet* 11 (8507) Sept 13, 1986

Drewnowski, Adam et al., "Comparing the Effect of Aspartame and Sucrose on Motivational Ratings, Taste Preferences, and Energy Intake." *Am J Clin Nutr*, Vol 59, 1994

During, N. J. et al., "An In Vivo Study of Dopamine Release in Iron Striatum. The Effects of Phenylalanine" in *Proceedings of the First Internatl Meeting on Dietary Phenylalanine & Brain Function*. R.J. Wurtman & E. Ritter-Walker, eds. Wash DC, May 8–10, 1987. Boston, MA: Burkhauser, 1988

Edmeady, John, "Aspartame & Headache." Editorial. *Headache*, Feb 1988

Elsas, L. J., "Aspartame and Migraine." Letter. *N Engl J Med*, Vol 318, No 18, May 5, 1988

Elsas, L. J. & J. F. Trotter, "Changes in Physiological Concentrations of Blood Phenylalanine Produced Changes in Sensitive Parameters of Human Brain Function" in *Proceedings of the First Internatl Meeting on Dietary Phenylalanine & Brain Function*. R.J. Wurtman & E. Ritter-Walker, eds. Wash DC, May 8–10, 1987. Boston, MA: Burkhauser, 1988

Eshel, Y. & I. Sarova-Pincus, "Aspartame and Seizures." *Neurol*, Vol 43, No 10, Oct 1993

"Estimated Consumption of Aspartame and Saccharin." Chart. ERS, USDA, *Sugar and Sweeteners Outlook*, Dec 1991

European Ramazzini Found, "Study Linking Aspartame to Cancer." *Environ Health Perspect*, Mar 2006

"Evaluation of Consumer Complaints Related to Aspartame Use." CDC, MMWR. Nov 2, 1984

Everything You Need to Know about Aspartame. Flier, Wash, DC: IFIC Found, Sept 1997

Fact Sheet on Aspartame. Wash DC: Aspartame Resource Center, Community Nutr Inst, Apr 25, 1984

Farber, Steven A., "The Price of Sweeteners." *Tech Rev*, Jan 1990

FDA Consumer, Feb 1976; Feb 1985; Dec 1985; Jan 1986; Feb 1987; Apr 1987; July–Aug 1987; Nov 1987; Feb 1989; April 1989; Sept 1989; Mar 1990; Oct 1991; Sept 1996; Nov–Dec 1997; July–Aug 1998

Fd Chem News Nov 5, 1973; Feb 14, 1983; Mar 14, 1983; July 4, 1983; Aug 15, 1983; Aug 22, 1983; Sept 12, 1983; Oct 3, 1983; Oct 24, 1983; Oct 31, 1983; Dec 26, 1983; Jan 23, 1984; Apr 2, 1984; July 2, 1984; Sept 10, 1984; Apr 8, 1985; Apr 15, 1985; Aug 26, 1985; July 28, 1986; Aug 4, 1986; Oct 13, 1986; Nov 24, 1986; Dec 1, 1986; Dec 22, 1986; Aug 24, 1987; Aug 31, 1987; Sept 7, 1987; Sept 28, 1987; Oct 5, 1987; Oct 19, 1987; Oct 26, 1987; Nov 2, 1987; Nov 9, 1987; Nov 23, 1987; Dec 14, 1987; Jan 4, 1988; Jan 18, 1988; Jan 25, 1988; Feb 8, 1988; Feb 15, 1988; Feb 22, 1988; Feb 29, 1988; May 16, 1988; Apr 25, 1989; May 22, 1989; Dec 10, 1990; Feb 4, 1991; Aug 26, 1991 Dec 16, 1991; Feb 3, 1992; Mar 30, 1992; June 22, 1992; Oct 26, 1992; Nov 2, 1992; Nov 16, 1992; Dec 7, 1992; Mar 15, 1993; May 24, 1993; Aug 2, 1993; Sept

20, 1993; Jan 3, 1994; Dec 12, 1994; Jan 23, 1995; June 12, 1995; Oct 16, 1995; Dec 4, 1995; July 22, 1996; Aug 26, 1996; Oct 7, 1996; Nov 11, 1996; Nov 25, 1996; Dec 12, 1996; Mar 10, 1997; July 28, 1997; Mar 15, 1999; Aug 9, 1999

Fd Engineer, Nov 1980; Jan 1982; May 1982; June 1982; July 1982; Nov 1982; Jan 1983; May 1983; Aug 1983; Sept 1983; Nov 1983; Jan 1984; Feb 1984; Apr 1984; Aug 1984; Sept 1984; Oct 1984; Oct 1985; Nov 1985; Oct 1989; Jan 1990; June 1990; Aug 1990; Oct 1990; Jan 1991; Feb 1991; June 1991; July 1991; Apr 1992; May 1992; Feb 1993; Aug 1993

Fd Formulating, Jan 1995

Fd Proc, Sept 1974; Oct 1974; May 1975; Aug 1975; July 1982; May 1983; July 1983; Aug 1983, Sept 1983; Dec 1984

Fd Prod Design, June 1992; July 1992; Apr 1993; Aug 1993; Aug 1994; Feb 1997; Apr 2000; July 2001; Jan 2005

Fd Prod Develop, Dec 1974; Feb 1975; July 1979; Oct 1979; Nov 1979; Nov 1980

Fd Tech, July 1989; Mar 1992; Apr 1993; June 1993; Nov 1993; May 1994, Jan 1995; May 1996; Aug 1996; Jan 1997; July 2002

Ferguson, J. M., "Interaction of Aspartame and Carbohydrates in an Eating Disordered Patient." Letter. *Am J Psychiat,* Vol 142, No 2, Feb 1985

Fernstrom, J. D. & R. J. Wurtman, "Brain Serotonin Content: Increase Following Ingestion of Carbohydrate Diet." *Sci,* Vol 174, 1971

_____. "Brain Serotonin Content: Physiological Regulation by Plasma Neutral Amino Acids." *Sci,* Vol 178, 1972

Fernstrom, J. D. & D. T. Faller, "Neutral Amino Acids in the Brain: Changes in Response to Food Ingestion. *Am J Neurochem,* Vol 30, 1978

Fernstrom, J. D. et al., "Acute Effects of Aspartame on Large Neutral Amino Acids and Monoamine in Rat Brain." *Life Sci,* Vol 32, 1983

Fernstrom, J. D., "Effect of Aspartame Ingestion on Large Neutral Amino Acids and

Monoamine Neurotransmitters in the Central Nervous System" in *Dietary Phenylalanine and Brain Function,* R. J. Wurtman & E. Ritter-Walker, eds. Boston, MA: Birkhauser, 1988

Filer, Jr., L. J. et al., "Effect of Aspartame Loading on Plasma and Erythrocyte-free Amino Acid Concentrations in One-Year-Old Infants." *J Nutr,* Vol 113, 1983

Findlay, Steven, "Aspartame: The News Is Not So Sweet." *USA Today* Feb 1, 1984

Foltin, R. W, et al., "Compensation for Caloric Dilution in Humans Given Unrestricted Access to Food in a Residential Laboratory. *Appetite,* Vol 10, 1988

Freidhoff, R. et al., "Sucrose Solution vs No-calorie Sweetener vs Water in Weight Gain. *J Am Diet Assoc,* Vol 59, 1971

Friedman, Marty, "New Product Surge Wows Dairy Industry." *Dairy Fds,* Mar 1990

Functional Fds Nutraceut, Nov 2004

GAO, "Six Former HHS Employees' Involvement in Aspartame Approval." Briefing Rept to Hon. Howard Metzenbaum, U.S. Senate. Wash, DC: U.S.General Accounting Office, GAO/HRD-86-109 BR, July 1986

Garattini, S. et al., "Studies on the Susceptibility to Convulsions in Animals Receiving Abuse Doses of Aspartame" in *Dietary Phenylalanine and Brain Function.* R.J. Wurtman & E. Ritter-Walker Wash, DC: Washington Center for Brain Sciences & Metabolism Charitable Trust, 1987

Garriga, Margarita M. & D.D. Metcalfe, "Aspartame Intolerance." *Ann Allergy,* Vol 61, No 6, Part 11, Dec 1988

Garriga, Margarita M. et al., "A Combined Single-blind, Double-blind Placebo-controlled Study to Determine the Reproducibility of Hypersensitivity Reactions to Aspartame." *J Allergy Clin Immunol,* Vol 87, No 4, Apr 1991

Gellis, S. S., "More on Aspartame: The Artificial Sweetener." *Pediat Notes,* Vol 8, 1984

Gifford, Jr., Ray W., "Aspartame." Informational Report of the Council on Scientific Affairs. *AMA,* June 1985

Good Housekeeping. Advertisements. Apr 1993; May 1993

Graves, Florence, "How Safe Is Your Diet Soft Drink?" *Common Cause Magazine,* July–Aug 1984

Gray, Donna M., "Summary of Adverse Reactions Attributed to Aspartame." Memorandum to Health Hazard Evaluation Board, PHS, Dept HHS, May 23, 1996

Grebelny, D. & R. E. Galardy, "A Metabolite of Aspartame Inhibits Angiotensin Converting Enzyme." *Biochem Biophy Res Comm,* Vol 128, No 2, 1985

Grigg, Bill, "Common Cause Editor Questions Aspartame 'Process'" *FDA Talk Paper,* July 10, 1984

Guiso, G., et al., "Effect of Aspartame on Seizures in Various Models of Experimental Epilepsy." *Toxicol Applied Pharmacol,* Vol 96, 1988

_____ et al., "Effect of Tyrosine in the Potentiation by Aspartame and Phenylalanine of Metrazol-Induced Convulsions in Rats." *Fd Chem Toxicol,* Vol 29, No 12, Dec 1991

Gulya, A. J. et al., "Aspartame and Dizziness: Preliminary Results of a Prospective, Non-blinded, Prevalence & Attempted Cross-over Study." *Am J Otol,* Vol 13, No 5, Sept 1992

Gunby, Phil, "FDA Approves Aspartame as Soft-drink Sweetener." *JAMA,* Aug 19, 1983

Gurney, James G. et al., "Aspartame Consumption in Relation to Childhood Brain Tumor Risk: Results from a Case-Control Study." *J Natl Cancer Inst,* Vol 89, No 14, July 16, 1997

Guttler, F. & H. Lou, "Aspartame May Imperil Dietary Control of Phenylketonuria." *Lancet 1,* 1985

Haney, Daniel G., "Researcher Suggests Sweetener Linked to Seizures." *State Times* (Baton Rouge, LA) Nov 13, 1985

Hattan, D. G. et al., "Role of the Food and Drug Administration in Regulation of Neuroeffective Food Additives" in *Nutrition & the Brain,* R.J. Wurtman & J.J. Wurtman, eds. Vol 6. NY, NY: Raven Press, 1983

Hegenbart, Scott, "Formulating 'Lite' Bakery Products with Sweeteners." *Prep Fds,* July 1990

Henkel, John, "Sugar Substitutes, Americans Opt for Sweetness and Lite." *FDA Consumer,* Nov–Dec 1999

Herbert, W., "Mind-altering Sweetener? Bittersweet Victory for Sugar Substitute." *Sci News,* Aug 27, 1983

Heybach, J. P. & C. Ross, "Aspartame Consumption in a Representative Sample of Canadians." *Rev Assoc Can Diet,* Vol 50, 1989

Hileman, Bette, "Smoldering Aspartame Controversy Reignites." *C&EN,* Nov 25, 1996

Hines, William, "Why Critics Are Sour on New Sweetener." *Chicago Sun-Times,* Jan 25, 1984

_____ "Sweetener's Foes See It Off Shelves in Two Years." *Chicago Sun-Times,* Feb 16, 1984

Holder, M. D. & R. Yirmiya, "Behavioral Assessment of the Toxicity of Aspartame." *Pharmacol Biochem Behav,* Vol 32, 1989

Hollie, Pamela G., "Aspartame Builds a Market." *NY Times,* Sept 3, 1983

_____. "Pepsi's Diet Soft Drink Switched to NutraSweet." *NY Times,* Nov 2, 1984

Hollingsworth, Pierce, "NutraSweet After the Patent." *Fd Tech,* Feb 1993

Ingersoll, Bruce, "SEC Probe of Searle Options Raise Questions on Ethics, Inside Trades." *Wall St J,* Feb 27, 1984

Ishii, H., "Incidence of Brain Tumors in Rats Fed Aspartame." *Toxicol Letters,* Vol 7, 1981

JAMA. Advertisements. Apr 15, 1983; May 4, 1984; Feb 2, 1985; Apr 25, 1986

Janssen, F. J. C. M. & C. A. van der Heijden, "Aspartame: Review of Recent Experimental and Observational Data." *Toxicol,* Vol 50, 1988

Johns, Donald R. "Migraine Provoked by Aspartame." Letter. *N Engl J Med,* Vol 315, No 7, Aug 14, 1986

_____. "Aspartame and Headache" in

Dietary Phenylalanine and Brain Function, R.J. Wurtman & E. Ritter-Walker, eds., Boston, MA: Birkhauser, 1988

Kanarek, R. B. & R. Marks-Kaufman, "Factors Influencing the Effects of Nutritive and Non-nutritive Sweeteners on Energy Intake and Body Weight in Rats." *Appetite*, Vol 11, suppl, 1988

Kanders, B. S. et al., "An Evaluation of the Effect of Aspartame on Weight Loss." *Appetite*, Vol 11, suppl, 1988

Kiefer, Francine, "Soft-drink Makers Sweet on NutraSweet." *Transcript-Telegram* (Holyoke, MA) Aug 31, 1982

Kiritsky, P. J. & T. J. Maher, "Acute Effects of Aspartame on Systolic Blood Pressure in Spontaneously Hypertensive Rats." *J Neural Transmission*, Vol 66, No 2, 1986

Koehler, Shirley M., "A New Dietary Caution for Migraine Sufferers." *Directions in Appl Nutr*, Vol 1, 1986

Koehler, Shirley M. & Alan Glaros, "The Effect of Aspartame on Migraine Headache." *Headache*, Vol 28, Feb 1988

Koontz, Katy, "The 10 Commonist Dieting Downfalls." *McCall*, May 1987

Kruesi, Markus J. P. et al., "Effects of Sugar and Aspartame on Aggression and Activity in Children." *Am J Psychiat*, Vol 144, No 11, Nov 1987

Kulczycki, Jr., Anthony, "Aspartame-induced Urticaria." *Ann Intern Med*, Vol 104, No 2, 1986

_____. "Aspartame Allergy." *Allergy Observer*, June 1987

_____. "Aspartame-induced Hives." Letter. *J Allergy Clin Immunol*, Vol 95, No 2, Feb 1995

Kuntz, Lynn A. "Killer Food! News at 10:00!" *Fd Prod Design*, Jan 1997

Ladies' Home J. Advertisement. Nov 1990

Lapierre, Katherine A. et al., "The Neuropsychiatric Effects of Aspartame in Normal Volunteers." *J Clin Pharmacol*, Vol 30, No 5, May 1990

Lawrence, Glen & Dongmei Yuan, "Aspartame, in the Presence of Ascorbic Acid and a Transition Metal Catalyst, Can Produce Benzaldehyde via a Free Radical Attack." *J Agric Fd Chem*, Nov 1996

Lecos, Chris, "The Sweet and Sour History of Saccharin, Cyclamate, Aspartame." *FDA Consumer*, Sept 1981

Lesser, U. et al., "Relationship between Funding Sources and Conclusions among Nutrition-Related Scientific Articles." *PLoS Med*, Vol 4, No 1, 2007

Lipton, Richard B. et al., "Aspartame and Headache." Letter. *N Engl J Med*, Vol 318, No 18, May 5, 1988

_____. "Aspartame as a Dietary Trigger of Headache." *Headache*, Vol 29, No 2, Feb 1989

A Look Beyond the Taste. Brochure. Skokie, IL: NutraSweet, 1985

Low-Calorie Sweeteners: Aspartame, Saccharin, Cyclamates. Pamphlet. Summit, NJ; ACSH, July 1984

MacNeil, Karen, "Diet Soft Drinks: Too Good to Be True?" *NY Times*, Feb 4, 1987

Mahalik, M. P. & R. F. Gautieri, "Reflex Responsiveness of CF-I Mouse Neonates Following Maternal Aspartame Exposure." Research Communications. *Psychol Psychiat Behav*, Vol 9, No 4, 1984

Maher, Timothy J., "Natural Food Constituents and Food Additive: The Pharmacologic Connection." *J Allergy Clin Immunol*, Vol 79, No 3, Mar 1987

Maher, Timothy J. & F. J. Kiritsky, "Aspartame Administration Decreases the Entry of Alpha-Methyldopa into the Brain of Rats" in *Dietary Phenylalanine & Brain Function*, R.J. Wurtman & E. Ritter-Walker, eds. Boston, MA: Birkhauser, 1988

Maher, Timothy J. & Richard J. Wurtman, "Possible Neurological Effects of Aspartame, a Widely Used Food Additive." *Environ Health Perspect*, No 75, 1987

Market Watch, July-Aug 1988

Matalon, Reuben, et al., "Aspartame Consumption in Normal Individuals and Carriers for Phenylketonuria (PKU)" in *Proceedings of the First Internatl Meeting on Dietary Phenylalanine & Brain Function,* R.J. Wurtman & E. Ritter-Walker, eds. Wash, DC: May 8-10, 1987. Boston, MA: Birkhauser, 1988

Mattes, R. D. et al., "Daily Caloric Intake of Normal-Weight Adults: Response to Changes in Dietary Energy Density of a Luncheon Meal." *Am J Clin Nutr,* Vol 48, 1988

Mayer, Caroline E., "Time is Short for Nutra Sweet as the Patent on Aspartame Expires, the Competition Crystallizes." *Wash Post,* June 10, 1992

McCann, M. B. et al., "Non-caloric Sweeteners and Weight Reduction." *J Am Diet Assoc,* Vol 32, 1956

McCarthy, Michael J., "Pepsi Dates Diet Drink for Freshness in Risky Test to Gain Marketing Edge." *Wall St J,* Sept 7, 1993

McCauliffe, Daniel P. & Kevin Poitras, "Aspartame-Induced Lobular Panniculitis." Brief communications. *J Am Acad Dermatol,* Vol 24, No 2, Part 1, Feb 1991

McCormick, Richard D., "Synthetic Sweeteners —though Choice Limited by Regulatory Actions, the Need Remains." *Prep Fds,* June 1983

_____. "Demand for Low-Cal Foods Invites New Sweetener Options." *Prep Fd,* Aug 1986

Med Trib, Feb 1, 1984

Med World News, June 7, 1974; July 26, 1984; *Psychiatry ed.* Jan 1985

Miller, Bryan, "Food Trends: What Americans Are Buying." *NY Times,* Jan 5, 1983

Moller, S. E., "Effect of Aspartame and Protein Administered in Phenylalanine—Equivalent Doses on Plasma Neutral Amino Acids Aspartate, Insulin, and Glucose in Man." *Pharmacol Toxicol,* Vol 68, No 5, 1991

Monte, Woodrow C., "Aspartame: Methanol and the Public Health."*J Appl Nutr,* Vol 36, No 1, Spring 1984

"Monsanto to Acquire Searle for $2.7 Billion." *C&EN,* July 22, 1985

Morris, Charles, "Aspartame Cleared for Soft Drinks." *Fd Engineer,* Aug 1983

_____. "New Options for Soft Drinks: Aspartame." *Fd Engineer,* Sept 1, 1983

Moser, Robert H., "Aspartame and Memory Loss." 'Questions & Answers,' *JAMA,* Vol 272, No 19, Nov 16, 1994

Newswk, July 27, 1981; Nov 25, 1985; Advertisement for NutraSweet. May 9, 1988

Nolan, Anita L., "Aspartame: Too Good to Be True?" *Fd Engineer,* Mar 1984

Novick, N.L., "Aspartame-induced Granulomatous Panniculitis." *Ann Intern Med,* Vol 102, No 2, 1985

Neurotoxicity: Identifying & Controlling Poisons of the Nervous System. OTA Assessment, Congress of U.S. Wash DC:U.S. Govt Pr Off, Apr 1, 1990

NY Times, July 26, 1974; Nov 17, 1976; Apr 9, 1977; Feb 18, 1984; Mar 25, 1984; Aug 17.1984; Apr 8, 1986

NY Times, "Science Watch," Apr 23, 1986; Nov 26, 1986; Aug 16, 1987; Oct 8, 1989

NutraSweet—Health and Safety Concerns. U.S. Senate Hearings, Comm on Labor & Human Resources, Nov 3, 1987

Olney, John W., "Glutamate-Induced Neuronal Necrosis in the Infant Mouse Hypothalamus: An Electron Microscope Study." *J Neuropath Exp Neurol,* Vol 30, No 1, Jan 1971

_____. "Aspartame as a Sweetener." *N Engl J Med,* Vol 292, No 23, 1975

_____. "Another View of Aspartame" in *Sweeteners: Issues & Uncertainties.* Academy Forum, Mar 1975. Wash, DC: National Acad Press, 1975

_____. "Brain Damage in Mice from Voluntary Ingestion of Glutamate and Aspartate." *Neurobehav Toxicol Teratol,* Vol 2, 1980

_____. "Excitatoxic Food Additives—Functional Teratological Aspects in Progress in Brain Research" in *Biochemical Basis of Func-*

tional Neuroteratology: Permanent Effects of Chemicals on the Developing Brain, Vol 73, G.J. Boer, chief ed., NY: Elsevier, 1988

Olney, John W. et al., "Increasing Brain Tumor Rates: Is There a Link to Aspartame?" *J Neuropath Exp Neurol,* Vol 55, No 11, Nov 1996

Olney, John W. & Oi-Lan Ho, "Brain Damage in Infant Mice Following Oral Intake of Glutamate, Aspartate, or Cysteine." *Nature,* Vol 227, Aug 8, 1970

Oppermann, J. A. et al., "Metabolism of Aspartame in Monkey." *J Nutr,* Vol 103, 1973

O'Sullivan, Dermot, "New Sweeteners Gain Ground in Europe." *C&EN,* Jan 24, 1983

"Over 7, 000 Aspartame Complaints Since '81, FDA Says; Controversy Remains." *Nutr Wk,* Community Nutr Inst, Vol 25, No 20, May 26, 1995

Pan-Hou, H. et al., "Effect of Aspartame on N-Methyl-D-Aspartate Sensitive L-(3H) Glutamate Binding Site in Rat Brain Synaptic Membranes. *Brain Res,* No 1–2, 1990

Pardridge, William M., "Regulation of Amino Acid Availability to the Brain" in *Nutrition and the Brain,* Vol, I, R.J. Wurtman & J.J. Wurtman, eds. NY, NY: Raven Press, 1977

_____. "How Safe Are NutraSweet Products?" *Valley Advocate* (Springfield, MA), Mar 28, 1984

_____. "Potential Effects of the Dipeptide Sweetener Aspartame on the Brain." In *Nutrition and the Brain,* Vol 111, R.J. Wurtman & J.J. Wurtman, eds. NY, NY: Raven Press, 1986

_____. "The Safety of Aspartame." Letter. *JAMA,* Vol 256, No 19, Nov 21, 1986

_____. Testimony, Proceedings and Debates of the 99th Congress, First Session. *Congressional Record,* May 7, 1985

Pinto, J. M. & T. J. Maher, "Administration of Aspartame Potentiates Pentylenetetrazole & Fluorothyl-Induced Seizures in Mice." *Neuropharmacol,* Vol 27, No 1, 1988

Pivonka, Elizabeth E. A. & Katharine K. Grunewald, "Aspartame or Sugar-Sweetened Beverages: Effects on Mood in Young Women." *J Am Diet Assoc,* Vol 90, No 2, Feb 1990

Pkging Digest, Jan 1997

Porikos, K. P. & T. B.Van Itallie, "Efficacy of Low-Calorie Sweeteners in Reducing Food Intake: Studies with Aspartame" in *Aspartame: Physiology and Biochemistry,* L.D. Stegink & L.J. Filer, eds. NY, NY: Marcel Dekker, 1984

Porikos, K. P. & H. S. Koopmans, "The Effect of Non-nutritive Sweeteners on Body Weight in Rats." *Appetite,* Vol 2, No 11 suppl, 1985

Potenza, Daniel D. & Rif S. El-Mallackh, "Aspartame: Clinical Update." *Conn Med,* Vol 53, No 7, July 1989

Prep Fds, Mar 1979; Buyers' Guide 1983; Feb 1983; Apr 1983; May 1983; Aug 1983; Oct 1983; Nov 1983; Mar 1984; Apr 1984; May 1984; Sept 1984; Oct 1984; Nov 1984; Sept 1985; Nov 1985; Mar 1986; May 1986; June 1986; Buyers' Guide 1987; Feb 1987; Mar 1987; May 1987; June 1987; Aug 1987; Jan 1988; Aug 1988; Oct 1988; Nov 1988; May 1989; Oct 1989; July 1990; Aug 1990; Oct 1990; Jan 1991; May 1991; Mar 1992; May 1992; Sept 1992; May 1993; Jun 1993; Aug 1993; Feb 1995; Mar 1995; May 1996; Aug 1996; Mar 1997; Aug 1997; Sept 1998; May 2005

Progressive Grocer, June 1974

Przybyla, Ann, "Aspartame to Appear as an Ingredient in New Prepared Foods, "*Prep Fds,* Aug 1982

_____. "Dietary Revolution Creates a Demand for Variety of Low-Calorie Sweeteners." *Prep Fds,* Sept 1985

Raloff, Janet, "A Sweet Taste of Success to Drink In." *Sci News,* Apr 27, 1985

Randal, Judith, "'The Most-Tested Additive: Lingering Question." *Wash Post,* Apr 15, 1984

Reed, B. B. et al., "Orofacial Sensitivity Reactions and the Role of Dietary Components. Case Reports." *Austral Dent J,* Vol 38, No 4, Aug 1993

Reference Guide to Aspartame Scientific Research. Skokie, IL: G.D.Searle, 1984

Reisch, Marc, "Monsanto Plans to Split in Two." *C&EN*, Dec 16, 1996

Remington, Dennis W., "Neurological & Metabolic Effects of Artificial Sweeteners." Paper. *Am Acad Environ Med*, annual meeting. Wichita, KS: AAEM. 1988

Remington, Dennis W. & Barbara W. Higa, *The Bitter Truth About Artificial Sweeteners.* Provo, UT: Vitality House Internatl, 1987

Rest Hosp, Mar 1983; Apr 1983; Dec 1986; Jan 1987; Nov 1987; Oct 1988; Sept 1989

Rest & Instit, July 1982; Feb 1984; Feb 29, 1984; June 6, 1984; May 1, 1985; June 10, 1988

Robbins, Paula & Laurence Raymond, "Aspartame and Symptoms in Carpel Tunnel Syndrome." *J Environ Occup Med*, Vol 41, No 1, 1999

Roberts, H. J., "Complications Associated with Aspartame (NutraSweet) in Diabetics." *Clin Res*, Vol 3, 1988

_____. "Neurological, Psychiatric, and Behavioral Reactions to Aspartame in 505 Aspartame Reactors" in *Dietary Phenylalanine & Brain Function*. R.J. Wurtman & E. Ritter-Walker, eds. Boston, MA: Birkhauser, 1988

_____. "Aspartame and Brain Cancer." Correspondence. *Lancet*, Vol 349, No 362, Feb 1, 1997

_____. "Aspartame as a Cause of Allergic Reactions, including Anaphylaxis." *Arch Intern Med*, Vol 156, No 9, Sept 1996

_____. *Aspartame Disease: An Ignored Epidemic*. West Palm Beach, FL: Sunshine Sentinel Press, 2001

_____. *Aspartame (NutraSweet) Is It Safe?* Philadelphia, PA: The Charles Press, 1990

_____. "Aspartame, Tryptophan, and other Amino Acids as Potentially Hazardous Experiments." *Southern Med J*, Vol 83, No 9, Sept 1990

_____. "Does Aspartame (NutraSweet) Cause Human Brain Cancer?" *Clin Res*, Vol 38, 1990

_____. "Reactions Attributed to Aspartame-Containing Products: 551 Cases." *J Appl Nutr*, Vol 40, No 2, 1988

Rodin, Judith, "Comparative Effects of Fructose, Aspartame, Glucose and Water Preloads on Calorie and Micronutrient Intake." *Am J Clin Nutr*, Vol 51, No, 3, Mar 1990

Rogers, P. J. et al., "Uncoupling Sweet Taste and Calories. Comparison of the Effects of Glucose and Three Intense Sweeteners on Hunger and Food Intake." *Physiol Behav*, Vol, 43, l988

Rogers, Ron, "Monsanto Exits Food Ingredients with Sale of NutraSweet." *C&EN*, Apr 3, 2000

Rolls, Barbara J., "Sweetness and Satiety" in *Sweetness*, J. Dobbing ed. London: Springer-Verlag, 1987

_____. "Effects of Intense Sweeteners on Hunger, Food Intake, and Body Weight: A Review." *Am J Clin Nutr*, Vol 53, 1991

Rolls, Barbara J. et al., "Hunger and Food Intake Following Consumption of Low-Calorie Foods." *Appetite*, Vol 13, No 2, Oct 1989

Ross, Walter S., "Artificial Sweeteners: Are They Safe?" Reprint. *Readers' Digest*, Dec 1985

Rovner, Sandy, "A Craving for Sweets." *Wash Post Health*, May 26, 1987

Saravis, Susan et al., "Aspartame: Effects on Learning, Behavior and Mood." *Pediat*, Vol 86, No 1, July 1990

Sardesai, V. M. et al., "Effect of Aspartame in Diabetic Rats" in *Dietary Phenylalanine & Brain Function*. R.J. Wurtman & E. Ritter-Walker, eds. Boston, MA: Birkhauser 1988

Schiffman, Susan S. et al., "Aspartame and Susceptibility to Headache." *N Engl J Med*, Vol 317, No 19, Nov 5, 1987

Sci, Feb 22, 1980

Sci News, Aug 11, 1979; July 25, 1981; Aug 27, 1983; June 16, 1984; July 28, 1984; Apr 19, 1986; June 21, 1986

"Science Fair Study Shows Effects of Aspartame in Learning." *Pure Facts*, Sept 1998

Scott, Carlee R., "NutraSweet Says Sweetener

Cleared for Expanded Use." *Wall St J*, June 8, 1988

"Searle: Rallying a Drug Company with an Injection of New Vitality." *Bus Wk*, Feb 8, 1982

Seligmann, Jean & Mary Hager, "Good News for Sweet Teeth." *Newswk*, May 11, 1992

Shell, Ellen Ruppel, "Nutrition: Sweetness and Health." Reports and comments. *The Atlantic*, Aug 1985

Shephard, S.E. et al., "Mutagenic Activity of Peptides and the Artificial Sweetener Aspartame after Nitrosation." *Fd Chem Toxicol*, Vol 31, No 5, May 1993

Sloan, A. Elizabeth, "Boomers." *Fd Engineer*, Nov 1985

Smith, R. Jeffrey, "Aspartame Approved, Despite Risks." *New Scient*, Aug 28, 1981

Sonnewald, U. et al., "Effects of Aspartame on 45CA Influx and LDH Leakage from Nerve Cells in Culture." Research Council of Norway, *Neuroreport*, Vol 6, No 2, 1995

Spiers, Paul A. et al., "Aspartame and Human Behavior: Cognitive and Behavioral Observations" in *Dietary Phenylalanine & Brain Function*. R.J.Wurtman & E. Ritter-Walker, eds. Boston, MA: Birkhauser, 1988

_____. "Aspartame: Neuropsychologic and Neurophysiologic Evaluation of Acute and Chronic Effects." *Am J Clin Nutr*, Vol 68, 1998

Squires, Sally, "Sweeteners Face Scrutiny Over Safety." *Wash Post Health*, Apr 24, 1985

Stegink, Lewis D. et al., "Effect of Aspartame- and Aspartate-loading upon Plasma and Erythrocyte Free Amino Acid Levels in Normal Adult Volunteers." *J Nutr*, Vol 107, 1977

_____. "Effect of an Abuse Dose of Aspartame upon Plasma and Erythrocyte Levels of Amino Acids in Phenylketonuric Heterozygotes and Normal Adults." *J Nutr*, Vol 110, 1980

_____. "Blood Methanol Concentrations in Normal Adult Subjects Administered Abuse Doses of Aspartame." *J Toxicol Environ Health*, Vol 7, 1981

_____. "Blood Methanol Concentrations in One-Year-Old Infants Administered Graded Doses of Aspartame." *J Nutr*, Vol 113, 1983

_____. "Plasma Amino Acid Concentrations in Normal Adults Fed Meals with Added Monosodium L-glutamate and Aspartame." *J Nutr*, Vol 113, 1983

_____. "Repeated Ingestion of Aspartame-sweetened Beverages: Effect on Plasma Amino Acid Concentration in Normal Adults." *Metabol*, Vol 37, No 3, Mar 1988

_____. "Effect of Repeated Ingestion of Aspartame-sweetened Beverages on Plasma Amino Acid, Blood Methanol, and Blood Formate Concentrations in Normal Adults." *Metabol*, Vol 38, No 4, Apr 1989

_____. "Effect of Sucrose on the Metabolic Disposition of Aspartame." *Am J Clin Nutr*, Vol 52, No 2, Aug 1990

_____. "Repeated Ingestion of Aspartame-sweetened Beverages; Further Observations in Individual Heterozygous for Phenylketonuria." *Metabol*, Vol 39, No 10, Oct 1990

Steinmetzer, R. V. et al., "Aspartame and Headache." Letter. *N Eng J Med*, Vol 318, No 8, May 5, 1988

Stellman, Steven D. & Lawrence Garfinkel, "Artificial Sweetener Use and One-Year Weight Change Among Women." *Preventive Med*, Vol 15, 1986

Stern, Judith S., "Your Diet: Sweet Talk."*Vogue*, July 1987

Stokes, A.F. et al., "Effects of Alcohol and Chronic Aspartame Ingestion upon Performance in Aviation Relevant to Cognitive Tasks." *Aviat Space Environ Med*, Vol 65, No 1, 1994

"Straight Answers about Aspartame." Nutrition Fact Sheet sponsored by CCC. *J Am Diet Assoc*, June 2003

Sweet Choices. Pamphlet. Atlanta, GA: CCC, 1985

"Sweeteners: Are Any of Them Safe? The Health Aspects of Sweeteners without Calories." *Consumer Repts*, Nov 1985

Sweet Misery: A Poisoned World (DVD) Tucson, AR: Sound & Fury Productions, 2004

Thomas-Dobersen, Deborah, "Calculation of Aspartame Intake in Children." *J Am Diet Assoc,* June 1989

Tollefson, L. & Robert J. Barnard, "An Analysis of FDA's Passive Surveillance Reports of Seizures Associated with Consumption of Aspartame." *J Am Diet Assoc,* Vol 92, No 2, 1992

Tordoff, Michael G., "How Do Nonnutritive Sweeteners Increase Food Intake?" *Appetite,* Vol 11 suppl. 1988

_____. "Sweeteners and Appetite" in *Sweeteners: Health Effects.* G.M. Williams, ed. Princeton, NJ: Princeton Scientific, 1988

Tordoff, Michael G. & Annette M. Alleva, "Oral Stimulation with Aspartame Increases Hunger." *Physiol Behav,* Vol 47, Mar 1990

_____. "Effect of Drinking Soda Sweetened with Aspartame or High Fructose Corn Syrup on Food Intake and Body Weight." *Am J Clin Nutr,* Vol 51, No 6, June 1990

Trocho, C. et al., "Formaldehyde Derived from Dietary Aspartame Binds to Tissue Components in vivo." *Life Sci,* Vol 63, No 5, May 1998

Uribe, Misael, "Potential Toxicity of a New Sugar Substitute in Patients with Liver Disease." Letter. *N Engl J Med,* Vol 306, No 3, Jan 21, 1982

Urquhart, John, "Monsanto's NutraSweet Ordered to Drop 'Anti-Competition' Practices in Canada." *Wall St J,* Oct 5, 1991

"Use of Noncaloric Sweeteners." Position statement. *Diabetes Care,* Vol 10, No 4, July–Aug 1987; Vol 13, suppl 1, Jan 1990

Van Den Eeden, S. K. et al., "Aspartame Ingestion and Headaches: Randomized Crossover Trial." *Neurol,* Vol 44, No 10, Oct 1994

Vettel, Phil, "The Latest on Artificial Sweeteners: How Sweet It Isn't." *Chicago-Sun Times.* May 27, 1984

Wall St J, Dec 5, 1975; Apr 9, 1976

Walton, Ralph G., "Seizure and Mania after High Intake of Aspartame." Case report. *Psychosomatics,* Vol 27, No 3, Mar 1986

_____. "The Possible Role of Aspartame in Seizure Induction" in *Proceedings of the First Internatl Conference on Phenylalanine and the Brain.* R.J.Wurtman & E. Ritter-Walker, eds. Cambridge, Center for Brain Science and Metabolism Charitable Trust, 1987

_____. "Survey of Aspartame Studies: Correlation of Outcome and Funding Sources." www.dorway.com (date accessed) March 1, 2007

Walton, Ralph G. et al., "Adverse Reactions to Aspartame: Double-blind Challenge in Patients from a Vulnerable Population." *Biol Psych,* Vol 34, No 1–2, 1993

Ward, Stephen, "NutraSweet Blues" *Vt Vanguard Press,* Feb 12–19, 1984

Wash Post, Apr 8, 1976; Nov 20, 1985

Watts, R. S., "Aspartame Headaches and Beta Blockers." *Headache,* Vol 31, No 3, 1991

Wayne, Leslie, "Searle's Push into Sweeteners." *NY Times,* Oct 24, 1982

Whole Fds, Sept 1983; Feb 1984

Wolraich, Mark L. et al., "Effects of Diets High in Sucrose or Aspartame on the Behavior and Cognitive Performance in Children." *N Engl J Med,* Vol 330, No 5, Feb 3, 1994

Wurtman, Richard J., "Aspartame Effects on Brain Serotonin." *Am J Clin Nutr,* Vol 45, No 4, Apr 1987

_____. "Aspartame's Possible Effect on Seizure Susceptiblity." Correspondence. *Lancet II,* (8463) Nov 9, 1985

_____. "Effects of Aspartame and Glucose on Rat Brain Amino Acids and Serotonin." *N Engl J Med,* Vol 309, No 7, 1983

_____. "Neurochemical Changes Following High-Dose Aspartame with Dietary Carbohydrate." Letter. *N Engl J Med,* Vol 309, No 7, 1983

_____. Testimony. Proceedings and Debate of the 99th Congress, 1st Session. *Congressional Record,* May 7, 1985

Wurtman, Richard J. & J. D. Fernstrom, "Control of Brain Monoamine Synthesis by Diet and Plasma Amino Acids." *Am J Clin Nutr*, Vol 28, 1975

Wurtman, Richard J. & Timothy J. Maher, "Calculation of the Aspartame Dose for Rodents that Produces Neurochemical Effects Comparable to Those Occurring in People" in *Dietary Phenylalanine & Brain Function*. R.J. Wurtman & E. Ritter-Walker, eds. Boston, MA: Berkhauser, 1988

Yellowlees, H., "Aspartame," *Br Med J*, Vol 287, 1983

Yokogoshi, Hidehiko et al., "Effects of Aspartame and Glucose Administration on Brain and Plasma Levels of Large Neutral Amino Acids and Brain 5-Hydroxyindoles." *Am J Clin Nutr*, Vol 40, July 1984

Yokogoshi, Hidehiko & Richard J. Wurtman, "Acute Effects of Oral or Parenteral Aspartame on Catecholamine Metabolism in Various Regions of Rat Brain." *J Nutr*, Vol 116, 1986

Ziesenitz, S. C. & G. Siebert, "Nonnutritive Sweeteners as Inhibitors of Acid Formation by Oral Microorganisms." *Caries Res*, Vol 20, No 6, Nov–Dec 1986

Zinman, David, "Experts Still Troubled by Aspartame, Safety of NutraSweet for Children, Pregnant Women Disputed." *Wash Post Health*, July 3, 1995

Chapter 14: Neotame

C&EN, Jan 5, 1998; July 12, 1999; July 19, 2002

Earles, Jim, "Sugar-free Blues." *Wise Traditions*, Winter 2003

Fact Sheet Insert, "Neotame." *Stagnito's New Prod Magazine*, Aug 2003

FDA Approves New Non-Nutritive Sugar Substitute, Neotame. Talk paper. FDA press release, July 5, 2002

FDA Consumer, Sept-Oct 2002

Fd Chem News, Sept 4, 1995; Dec 29, 1997; Apr 13, 1998; June 22, 1998

Fd Prod Design, Feb 1998; Mar 1999; Sept 2002

Fd Tech, Mar 1999; Aug 2002

Gallo-Torres, Julia M., "Neotame-ing the Beast." *Prep Fds*, May 2005

Hollingsworth, Pierce, "Artificial Sweeteners Face Sweet 'n Sour Consumer Market." *Fd Tech*, July 2002

Horvath, Stephanie M., "Monsanto's NutraSweet Division Gets Approval for Artificial Sweetener Neotame." *Wall St J*, July 8, 2002

Monsanto Chemical Co., *1998 Annual Rept*

Nabors, Lyn O'Brien, "Sweet Choices: Sugar Replacements for Foods and Beverages." *Fd Tech*, July 2002

Prakash, Indra et al., "Neotame: The Next-Generation Sweetener." *Fd Tech*, July 2002

Chapter 15: Acesulfame-K

Acesulfame-K. Flier. CCC, 1989

Acesulfame Potassium. Flier. Wash, DC: IFIC Found, undated

Boston Globe (Boston, MA), Feb 15, 1989

Bus Wk, Mar 2, 1987

Calorie Control Commentary, Spring 1988; Fall 1991; Spring 1992; Spring 1993; Spring 1995; Spring 1996; Fall 1996; Fall 1998

C&EN, Aug 1, 1988; July 6, 1998,

CRM, May 1987; Oct 1988

FDA Consumer, Sept 1995; Nov–Dec 1998; Dec 1999

Fd Chem Codex, Aug 23, 1994

Fd Chem News, Oct 18, 1982; Oct 12, 1987; Jan 18, 1988; Sept 5, 1988; Aug 6, 1990; Nov 5, 1990; Dec 10, 1990; Oct 30, 1991; Nov 11, 1991; Feb 24, 1992; Mar 2, 1992; Mar 16, 1992; Mar 30, 1992; June 15, 1992; Sept 21, 1992; Nov 2, 1992; Nov 16, 1992; Dec 14, 1992; Sept 13, 1993; Nov 19, 1993; Jan 10, 1994; Dec 5, 1994; Mar 13, 1995; May 8, 1995; June 5, 1995; Mar 4, 1996; Mar 23, 1996; May 27, 1996; June 17, 1996; Aug 5, 1996; Sept 2, 1996; Nov 10, 1997; July 6, 1998; July 13, 1998; Aug 3, 1998; Aug 17, 1998

Fd Engineer, Mar 1984; Aug 1989; Feb 1990; Aug 1990; Oct 1990; Apr 1993; Dec 1994

Fd Prod Design, Sept 1983; July 1992; Nov 1994; Oct 1998; Mar 2004; July 2005

Fd Tech, Oct 1989; Jan 1991; Apr 1992; May 1992; Dec 1992; Apr 1993; Oct 1993; Nov 1994; June 1995; Jan 1996; Nov 1998; June 1999; Sept 1999; July 2002; Oct 2002; Feb 2004

Health Professionals' Opinions on Acesulfame Potassium. CCC, 2004

NY Times, July 28, 1988; Sept 5, 1989

Prep Fds, May 1984; Aug 1986; Oct 1988; Oct 1989; Apr 1990; July 1990; Aug 1990; Oct 1990; May 1991; Aug 1991; Nov 1991; June 1993; Aug 1993; Sept 1993; Apr 1994; Mar 1995; June 1995, June 1996; Aug 1998; Sept 1998; Sept 1999; May 2000; Nov 2003; Feb 2004

Mayer, D. G. & F. H. Kemper, eds. *Acesulfame-K.* NY, NY: Marcel Dekker, 1991

Stagnito's New Prods Magazine, July–Aug 2002; June 2003

Wall St J, July 28, 1988; Feb 6, 1989

Wash Post, July 8, 1987

Chapter 16: Sucralose

Burros, Marian, "Splenda's 'Sugar' Claim Unites Odd Couple of Nutrition Wars." *NY Times,* Feb 14, 2005

Bus Wk, Mar 2, 1987

Calorie Control Commentary, Fall 1991; Spring 1993; Spring 1994; Spring 1995; Spring–Summer 1999; Fall 1999; Summer–Fall 2000

C&EN, Dec 6, 2004

CRM, Oct 1990

Dairy Fds, June 1990

Earles, Jim, "Artificial Sweeteners." Letter. *Wise Traditions,* Spring 2005

_____. "Sugar-free Blues." *Wise Traditions,* Winter 2003

Everything You Need to Know About Sucralose. Brochure. Wash, DC: IFIC Found, May 1998

The Facts: The Only Low-Calories Sweetener Made from Sugar. Brochure. Berkeley Heights, NJ: McNeil Specialty Products Co., undated

FDA Approves First Low-Calorie Sweetener Made

from Sugar. Press release. McNeil Specialty Products Co./Hill & Knowlton, Apr 1, 1998

FDA Consumer, July–Aug 1998; Dec 1999

Fd Arts, Mar 2001

Fd Chem News, Apr 6, 1987; May 11, 1987; Oct 5, 1987; Nov 23, 1987; Dec 7, 1987; Feb 26, 1990; Mar 11, 1990; Aug 13, 1990; Nov 12, 1990; Mar 11, 1991; May 20, 1991; July 1, 1991; Sept 16, 1991; Oct 14, 1991; Oct 21, 1991, Nov 11, 1991; Mar 2, 1992; Apr 6, 1992; Apr 27, 1992: Sept 28, 1992; Nov 16, 1992; Nov 23, 1992; Dec 14, 1992; Dec 21, 1992; Feb 8, 1993; Oct 18, 1993; Dec 14, 1993: Aug 29, 1994; Apr 7, 1997; Aug 23, 1997; Apr 6, 1998; Apr 13, 1998; Aug 30, 1999

Fd Engineer Apr 1985; Oct 1985

Fd Formulating, Sept 1995

Fd Proc, Mar 2003; July 2003; Feb 2005

Fd Prod Design, July 1992; Nov 1993; May 1994; May 1998; Mar 2001; Sept 2000; Apr 2004; June 2005

Fd Safety Notebook, Oct–Nov 1992

Fd Tech, Apr 1989; Dec 1993; May 1998; Feb 1999; June 1999; Sept 1999; May 2000; July 2002

Filipic, Martha, "Sucralose Sweet for Calorie-Counters." News release, *Chowline.* Wooster, OH: Ohio State Univ, Oct 3, 2004

Functional Fds Nutraceut, Feb 2005

High Intensive Sweeteners from Sucrose. South Orange, NJ: Reach Associates, Inc., 1985

Hollingsworth, Pierce, "Sucralose Approval Sweetens Low-Cal Market." *Fd Tech,* May 1998

J Fd Sci, May–June 1983

LaBell, Fran, "Sucralose Sweetener Approved." *Prep Fds,* May 1998

Layman, Patricia, "UK's Dextra Laboratories Enjoy Sweet Success." *C&EN,* Oct 8, 1990

Less Sugar Can Be Sweet. Promotional brochure. McNeil Specialty Products Co., Splenda, Inc., 2003

NY Times, Sept 5, 1989; Oct 28, 1992

Prep Fds, May 1987; Oct 1989; Apr 1990; Oct 1990; Oct 1991; June 1993; Nov 1994; Mar

1997; June 1998; Apr 1999; June 1999; Sept 1999; Mar 2000; May 2000; Aug 2000; Mar 2001; Sept 2001; Mar 2002; Sept 2002; Nov 2003; June 2005

Prep Fds New Prods Annual, 1987

Prep Fds NutraSolutions, Spring 2004

Pszczola, Donald E., "Sweet Beginnings to a New Year." *Fd Tech*, Jan 1999

Schettler, Renée, "Is Splenda America's Sweetheart?" *Valley News* (upper NH-VT), Mar 16, 2005, reprinted from *Wash Post*

Singer, Beth Wolfensberger, "Go Ahead, Splurge." *Health*, Sept 1998

Stagnito's New Prods Magazine, Oct 2003

"Sucralose." *CRM*, Oct 1990

Sugars & Sweeteners, Dec 1991

Wash Post, July 8, 1987

Chapter 17: Alitame

Calorie Control Commentary, Fall 1991; Spring 1994; Spring 1995

C&EN, Sept 1, 1986

Earles, Jim, "Sugar-free Blues." *Wise Traditions*, Winter 2003

Fd Chem News, Oct 5, 1987; Jan 19, 1988; Apr 15, 1991; Mar 16, 1992; June 15, 1992; Mar 28, 1994

Fd Engineer, May 1989; Jan 1990; Mar 1991

Fd Formulating, June 1995; Jan 1996

Fd Tech, Apr 1989, Oct 1989

Hunter, Beatrice Trum, "Alitame." *CRM*, Mar 1992

Nabors, Lyn O'Brien, "Sweet Choices: Sugar Replacements for Foods & Beverages." *Fd Tech*, July 2002

Prep Fds, Aug 1988; Oct 1990; Apr 1992; Mar 1997

Chapter 18: Trehalose, Tagatose, and Agave Nectar

Agave and Maguey

Fd as Med, Fall 2005

Fd Tech, June 1999

LaBell, Fran, "Ancient Agave Yields Modern Sweetener." *Prep Fds*, June 1999

Maguey Fact Sheet. Springville, CA: Botanical Products, Inc., 1992

Prep Fds, July 2000; Aug 2000

Prep Fds suppl, "NutraSolutions," July 2003

Shugr

Fd Prod, Apr 2005

Pure Facts, Apr 2005

Tagatose

CRM, June 2002

Earles, Jim, "Sugar-free Blues." *Wise Traditions*, Winter 2003

Fd Chem News, Sept 8, 1997; Aug 9, 1999; Sept 13, 1999; Nov 19, 2001

Fd Prod Design, June 2002; Mar 2003; Sept 2003

Fd Tech, Jan 2003; June 2003; Nov 2003

Functional Fds Nutraceut, Mar 2005

Hollingsworth, Pierce, "Artificial Sweeteners Face Sweet 'n Sour Consumer Market." *Fd Tech*, July 2002

Katz, Frances, "A New Generation of Sweeteners." *Fd Proc*, May 2004 Prep Fds, *Apr 1992; Aug 1996; May 2001; June 2001; Jan 2003; Nov 2003; Jan 2005*

Pszczola, Donald E., "*Sweet Beginnings to a New Year.*" Fd Tech, *Jan 1999*

Stagnito's New Prods Magazine, *Mar 2003*

Trehalose

CRM, Sept 2001

Earles, Jim, "Sugar-free Blues." *Wise Traditions*, Winter 2003

Fd Chem News, July 2, 2001

Fd Prod Design, Aug 2002

Fd Tech, May 1999; June 2003

Katz, Frances, "A New Generation of Sweeteners." *Fd Proc*, May 2004

Prep Fds, Nov 2003

Stagnito's New Prods Magazine, July–Aug 2002

Chapter 19: Designing New Sweeteners

Bilger, Burkhard, "The Search for Sweet: Building a Better Sugar Substitute." *NY Times*, May 22, 2006

Dairy Fds, Oct 1995

Fd Chem News, Mar 11, 1991; Dec 4, 1995

Kevin, Kitty, "Naturally Sweet, New Research Uncovers a Family of Sweet Natural Compounds." *Fds of Tomorrow*, Oct 1995

Prep Fds, Feb 1992

Symposium, Div Agr Fd Chem & Div Computers Chem. ACS, national meeting, Boston, MA, 1990

Acetosulfam

Fd Proc, May 1977

Proc Prep Fds, Feb 1979

Glycine and Kynurenine

Chemistry and the Food System. NAS-NRC. Wash, DC: Acad Press, 1980

Conference on Foods, Nutrition and Dental Health. Am Dent Assoc Health Found, Oct 1978

Fd Proc, Nov 1982; July 1983

Packard, Jr., Vernal S., *Processed Foods and the Consumer*. Minneapolis, MN: Univ of MN Press, 1976

Sci News, May 30, 1970

Leashed Polymers

Bus Wk, May 14, 1979

C&EN, Aug 25, 1975

Fd Engineer, Sept 1978

Fd Proc, Jan 1978

Fd Prod Develop, Oct 1978

Newswk, Apr 4, 1977

Left-rotating Sugars

Sweet Solutions. NOVA television program, Natl Sci Found, 1979

PS 99 and PS100

Prep Fds, Nov 1988

RTI-001

C&EN, May 13, 1985

Fd Inst Rept, May 25, 1985

Improved Artificial Sweetener. Press release. ACS, Apr 30, 1985

Prep Fds, Sept 1985

Seltzman, Herbert H. et al., *Peptide Sweeteners*. Presentation. 189th annual meeting, ACS, Apr 1985

SRI

C&EN, Aug 25, 1975

Newswk, Apr 4, 1977

Sweetness Modifier

Ritter, Steve, "Flavor Enhancers and Taste Modulators." *C&EN*, Aug 29, 2005

Warner, Melanie, "Better Disguises Through Chemistry." *NY Times*, Apr 6, 2005

Chapter 20: Sugars and the Glycemic Index

Atkinson, Mark, "Infant Diets and Type I Diabetes." *JAMA*, Vol 290, No 13, Oct 1, 2003

Brand-Miller, Jennie C. et al., "Low-Glycemic Food Improves Long-term Glycemic Control in NIDDM." *Diabetes Care*, Vol 14, 1991

_____. "Importance of glycemic index in diabetes." *Am J Clin Nutr*, Vol 59, suppl, 1994

_____. *The Glucose Revolution: The Authoritative Guide to the Glycemic Index*. NY, NY: Marlowe & Co, 1999

_____. "Glycemic Index and Obesity." *Am J Clin Nutr*, Vol 67, suppl, 2002

Davy, R.D. et al., "The Effect of Fiber-rich Carbohydrates on Features of Syndrome X." *J Am Diet Assoc*, Vol 103, No 1, 2003

Deis, Ronald C., "Down on Low-Carb." *Fd Prod Design*, Feb 2005

_____. "Measuring Glycemic Index." *Fd Prod Design*, Nov 2005

Esquivel, Teresa, "Clarifying Glycemic Terminology." *Fd Prod Design*, Nov 2006

Fernandes, Glen et al., "Glycemic Index of Potatoes Commonly Consumed in North America." Current research. *J Am Diet Assoc*, Vol 105, No 4, Apr 2005

Fd Proc, Apr 2005

Fd Prod Design, Feb 2001; Dec 2003

Fd Tech, July 2003

Filipic, Martha, "Glycemic Factor Gets Complex in Real Life." News release. *Chowline*, Wooster, OH: Univ of Ohio, May 20, 2001

_____. "Some Carbs are Better than Others." News release. *Chowline*. Wooster, OH: Univ of Ohio, Feb 22, 2004

_____. "Glycemic Index Still Controversial Topic." News release. *Chowline*. Wooster, OH: Univ of Ohio, Feb 29, 2004

_____. "Don't Be Fooled by '0' Carbs, Cholesterol." News release. *Chowline*. Wooster, OH: Univ of Ohio, Mar 21, 2004

"Formulating Glycemic Strategies." *Fd Prod Design*, suppl, July 2006

Glycemic Index: Summary of Current Status and Future Prospects. CCC, 2004

"Glycemic Index: What Is It and How Can Polyols Help?" *Fd Prod Design*, Feb 2004

Goodnough, Abby, "New Doctor, New Diet, But Still No Cookies." *NY Times*, Oct 7, 2003

Halpern, Marc, "Sugar Snap Low-Glycemic Diets Lie Ahead on the Low-Carb Horizon." *Fd Creation*, 2003

Hoover-Plow, Jane et al., "The Glycemic Response to Meals with Six Different Fruits in Insulin-Dependent Diabetics Using a Home Blood-Glucose Monitoring System." *Am J Clin Nutr*, Vol 45, 1987

Internatl Clin Nutr Rev, July 1986

Jenkins, D. J., "Glycemic Index: An Overview of Implications in Health and Disease." *Am J Clin Nutr*, suppl, 2000

_____. "Low-Glycemic Index Carbohydrate Foods in the Management of Hyperlipidemia." *Am J Clin Nutr*, Vol 42, 1985

_____. "Low-Glycemic Index Starchy Foods in the Diabetic Diet." *Am J Clin Nutr*, Vol 48, 1988

_____. "Metabolic Effects of a Low-Glycemic Index Diet." *Am J Clin Nutr*, Vol 46, 1987

Jenkins, D. J. et al., "Glycemic Index of Foods: A Physiological Basis for Carbohydrate Exchange." *Am J Clin Nutr*, Vol 34, 1981

Katz, Frances, "Diabetes Under Control." *Fd Proc Wellness Fds* suppl, Apr 2005

Leeds, A. R., "Glycemic Index and Heart Disease." *Am J Clin Nutr*, suppl, 2002

Liu, Simin et al., "A Prospective Study of Dietary Glycemic Load, Carbohydrate Intake, and Risk of Coronary Heart Disease in U.S. Women." *Am J Clin Nutr*, Vol 71, 2000

"Low-Carb Slump Gives Way to Slow-Carb Revolution." *Functional Fds Nutraceut*, Feb 2005

Ludwig, David S., "Dietary Glycemic Index and Obesity." *J Nutr*, Vol 130, 2000

_____. "The Glycemic Index at 20 Years." *Am J Clin Nutr*, suppl, 2002

_____. "The Glycemic Index: Physiological Mechanisms Relating to Obesity, Diabetes, and Cardiovascular Diseases." *JAMA*, Vol 287, No 18, May 8, 2002

Ludwig, David S. et al., "High-glycemic Index foods, Overeating, and Obesity." *Pediat*, Vol 103, 1999

"Net Carb Claims." *Fd Prod Design*, Feb 2004

Norris, Jill M. et al., "Timing of Initial Cereal Exposure in Infancy and Risk of Islet Autoimmunity." *JAMA*, Vol 290, No 13, Oct 1, 2003

Nutr Today, Mar–Apr 1984; July–Aug 1984

Pereira, Mark A. et al., "Effects of a Low-Glycemic Load Diet on Resting Energy

Expenditure and Heart Disease Risk Factors During Weight Loss." *JAMA*, Vol 292, 2004

_____. "Low-Glycemic Load Diet and Resting Energy Expenditure." Letter. *JAMA*, Vol 283, No 10, Mar 9, 2005

Pi-Sunyer, P. X., "Glycemic Index and Disease." *Am J Clin Nutr*, suppl, 2002

Shelke, Kantha, "Must Have Healthful Ingredients." *Fd Proc*, Sept 2005

Starling, Shana, "GI Labelling Continues to Grow—and Confuse." *Functional Fds Nutraceut*, Apr 2005

"U.S. Moves beyond Low Carb." *Functional Fds Nutraceut*, June 2005

Willett, Walter C. et al., "Glycemic Index, Glycemic Load, and Risk of Type I Diabetes." *Am J Clin Nutr*, suppl, 2002

Wolever, T. M. et al., "The Use of the Glycemic Index in Predicting the Blood Glucose Response in Mixed Meals." *Am J Clin Nutr*, Vol 43, 1986

_____. "Second-Meal Effects: Low-Glycemic Index Foods Eaten at Dinner Improve Subsequent Breakfast Glycemic Response." *Am J Clin Nutr*, Vol 8, 1989

_____. "The Glycemic Index: Variation between Subjects and Predictive Differences." *J Am Coll Nutr*, Vol 8, 1989

_____. "The Glycemic Index: Methodology and Clinical Implications." *Am J Clin Nutr*, Vol 54, 1991

_____. "Beneficial Effect of Low-Glycemic Index Diet in Overweight NIDDM Subjects." *Diabetes Care*, Vol 15, 1992

Woolf, Sarah L., "The Glycemic Index Concept." *Fd Prod Design*, Sept 2005

Ziegler, Annette G. et al., "Early Infant Feeding and Risk of Developing Type I Diabetes-Associated Autobodies." *JAMA*, Vol 290, No 13, Oct 1, 2003

Chapter 21: Sugar Consumption Statistics

Hunter, Beatrice Trum, "Confusing Consumers about Sugar Intake." *CRM*, Jan 1995

Mooney, Chris, *The Republican War on Sciences*. NY, NY: Basic Books, 2005

Nestle, Marion, *Food Politics: How the Food Industry Influences Nutrition and Health*. Berkeley, CA: Univ of Calif Press, 2002

Sugar and Sweeteners Outlook Yearbook. ERS, USDA, 1980; 1999; 2004

Wells, Malaike Geuka, "Sugar's Sweet Surprise." *Fd Prod Design*, Feb 2001

Woolf, Sarah L., "Sugar Seeks New Label Requirements." *Food Prod Design*, Oct 2005

Chapter 22: Avoiding the Sweetener Trap

Brownell, Kelly D. & Kathleen Battle Horgen, *Food Fight: The Inside Story of the Food Industry, America's Obesity Crisis, & What We Can Do About It*. NY, NY: McGraw-Hill, 2004

Choi, S. B. et al., "Effect of Cola Intake on Insulin Resistance in Moderate Fat-Fed Weaning Male Rats." *J Nutr Biochem*, Vol 13, 2002

"'Compelling Evidence' Links Child Advertising to Obesity." *Fd Proc*, Jan 2006

Food Marketing to Children and Youth; Threat or Opportunity? IOM, NAS, Wash, DC.: Natl Acad Press, Dec 6, 2005

Fusaro, Dave, editor-in-chief, "Misplaced Blame and Ignorance." *Fd Proc*, Jan 2006

Hampton, Tracy, "Biomedical Journals Probe Peer Review." Medical News & Perspectives. *JAMA*, Vol 294, No 18, Nov 9, 2005

Kleinfield, N. R., "Diabetes and Its Awful Toll Quietly Emerges as a Crisis." (Part 1 of series), *NY Times*, Jan 9, 2006

_____. "Living at an Epicenter of Diabetes, Defiance & Dispair." (Part 2 of series), *NY Times*, Jan 10, 2006

Kolata, Gina, "Obese Children: A Growing Problem." *Sci*, Vol 232, 1986

Mayer, Caroline E., "Lawyers Ready Suit Over Soda, Case Being Built Linking Obesity to Sale in Schools." *Wash Post*, Dec 2, 2005

Mitka, Mike, "Experts Target Heart Disease from Birth," *JAMA*, Nov 23–30, 2005

Mooney, Chris, *The Republican War on Science.* NY: NY: Basic Books, 2005

A Review of Low-Calorie Sweetener Benefits. Atlanta, GA: CCC, 1988

Santora, Marc, "East Meets West, Adding Pounds & Peril." (Part 4 of series), *NY Times,* Jan 12, 2006

Schulze, M. B. et al., "Sugar-sweetened Beverages, Weight Gain, and Incidence of Type 2 Diabetes in Young and Middle-aged Women." *JAMA,* Vol 292, 2004

Siener, K. et al., "Soft Drink Logos on Baby Bottles: Do They Influence What Is Fed to Children?" *J of Dent Child,* Vol 64, 1997

Toops, Diane, News & Trends ed., "I'm Lovin' It; So Should You." *Fd Proc,* Jan 2006

Urbina, Ian, "In the Treatment of Diabetes, Success Often Does Not Pay." (Part 3 of series) *NY Times,* Jan 11, 2006

Winkelmayer, Wolfgang C. et al., "Habitual Caffeine Intake and the Risk of Hypertension in Women." *JAMA,* Vol 294, No 18, Nov 9, 2005

Appendix D: Some Naturally Occurring Sugar in Foods

Fructose Intolerance

Gibbons, D. L., *The Self-Help Way to Treat Colitis and Other Irritable Bowel Conditions.* New Canaan, CT: Keats Pub, 1992

Hunter, Beatrice Trum, "Some Problematic Food Sugars." *Environ Med,* Vol 9, No 3, 1993

Galactose Intolerance

Cramer, D. W., "Galactose Consumption and Metabolism in Relation to the Risk of Ovarian Cancer." *Lancet,* No 8654, 1989

Donnell, George N., ed., *Galactosemia: New Frontiers in Research.* NIH Pub No 93-3436. Wash, DC: Natl Instit Child Health, Feb 1993

Galactosemia. Fact sheet. Center Grove, NJ: Am Liver Found, 1992

Gropper, S. S., et al., *The Galactose Content of Selected Fruits and Vegetables in Baby Foods: Implications for Infants on Galactose-Restricted Diets.* Auburn, AL: Auburn Univ, 1992

Gross, K. C. & F. B. Acosta, "Fruits and Vegetables Are a Source of Galactose: Implications in Planning the Diets of Patients with Galactosemia." *J Inher Metabol Dis,* Vol 14, 1991

Professional Guide to Diseases. Springhouse Pub Staff. Springhouse, PA: Springhouse Pub, 3rd ed, 1989

Richter, C. P., "Cataracts Produced in Rats by Yogurt," *Sci,* Vol 198, 1980

Skalke, H. et al., "Prehensile Cataract Formation and Decreased Activity of Galactosemic Enzymes." *Arch Opthal,* Vol 2, 1980

Lactose Intolerance

Brandstetter, R. D., "Lactose Intolerance Associated with Intal Capsules." *N Engl J Med,* Vol 25, 1986

Bronson-Adatto, Corinne, ed., *Lactose Intolerance. The Food Sensitivity Series.* Chicago, IL: ADA, 1985

Carper, Steve, *Milk Is Not for Every Body; Living with Lactose Intolerance.* NY, NY: Facts on File, Inc., 1995

Gern, J. E. et al., "Allergic Reactions to Milk-Contaminated 'Nondairy' Products." *N Engl J, Med,* Vol 14, 1991

"Hidden Lactose: Are Your Patients Safe from It?" *Capsulations,* Vol 10, 1987

Hunter, Beatrice Trum, "Lactose Intolerance."' *CRM,* Mar 1986

"Hydrolyzed Lactose Concentrate Sweeteners in Soft Drinks." *Fd Engineer,* Aug 1991

Jacques, P., "Lactose Intake and Senile Cataract." *J Am Cell Nutr,* Vol 7, 1988

Prep Fds, May 1991

Zukin, Jane, *Raising Your Child Without Milk.* Rocklin, CA: Prima Pub, 1996

INDEX

ABOUT THE AUTHOR

Beatrice Trum Hunter has written nearly thirty books on food issues, including *Consumer Beware: Your Food & What's Been Done to It* (Simon & Schuster, 1971), *The Mirage of Safety: Food Additives and Public Policy* (Charles Scribner's Sons, 1975), *The Sugar Trap & How to Avoid It* (Houghton Mifflin, 1982), *Food & Your Health* (Basic Health, 2003) and *A Whole Foods Primer* (Basic Health, 2007). As food editor for more than twenty years at *Consumers' Research Magazine,* her monthly columns and feature articles brought cutting-edge issues before general recognition.

Hunter has received many awards and recognitions for her work. The International Academy of Preventive Medicine made her an hononary fellow. Other honorary memberships include: the American Academy of Environmental Medicine, the Price-Pottenger Nutrition Foundation, the Weston A. Price Foundation, and Nutrition for Optimal Health Association. She received the prestigious Jonathan Forman Award for outstanding contributions to the field of environmental medicine, was honored by the International College of Applied Nutrition, and was recipient of the President's Award for the National Nutritional Foods Association.